UNBALANCED

Mental Health Policy in Ontario, 1930–1989

For Eileen

UNBALANCED

Mental Health Policy in Ontario, 1930–1989

Harvey G. Simmons
York University

WT

WALL & THOMPSON
Toronto

Thompson Educational Publishing, Inc.
11 Briarcroft Road, Toronto, Ontario, Canada M6S 1H3

Wall & Emerson, Inc.
Six O'Connor Drive, Toronto, Ontario, Canada M4K 2Kl

The publication of this volume has been made possible by a grant from Associated Medical Services Incorporated and the Hannah Institute for the History of Medicine in Toronto.

Canadian Cataloguing in Publication Data
Simmons, Harvey G. (Harvey Gerald), 1935-
Unbalanced: mental health policy in Ontario, 1930–1988

Bibliography: p.
Includes index.
ISBN 0–921332–16–5

1. Mental health policy - Ontario - History.
2. Mental health services - Ontario - Evaluation.
3. Mental health facilities - Ontario.
I. Title.

RA790.7.C3S55 1989   362.2'09713   C89-093469-X
ISBN 0–921332–16–5

Cover photograph: This photograph was taken in the 1920s at the Hamilton Psychiatric Hospital as part of a campaign to recruit nurses for the hospital. Patients were placed on a canvas lining and then covered with water kept between 78° and 80° Fahrenheit. Patients remained in the bath for around two hours, although at some institutions they might be submerged for up to twelve hours. For less benign treatments, see Chapters 1 and 12. *Photograph courtesy of the Hamilton Psychiatric Hospital Museum.*

Printed in Canada.
1 2 3 4 5   94 93 92 91 90

Table of Contents

Preface vii

Introduction ix

PART 1: 1930–1960

1. Insanity in the 1930s 3
2. Postwar Plans 35
3. Mental Health Clinics and Public Health 47
4. The Psychiatric Unit System 65

PART II: 1960–1970

5. The 1960s—An Era of Change 87
6. The Dymond Era 103
7. The System Under Scrutiny 125

PART III: 1970–1985

8. Internal Politics in the Ministry of Health 141
9. Deinstitutionalization in a Vacuum 157
10. Policy Under Attack 181
11. End of an Era 197
12. Lobotomy and the Decline of Psychiatric Authority 209
13. The Politics of Mental Health Law 225

PART IV: CONCLUSIONS

14. Conclusion 241

Postscript 263

Interviews 270
Ministers of Health 271
Index 273

List of Tables

Table 1.1:	Fourteen Diagnostic Categories	5
Table 1.2:	Percent of Mentally Ill Due to Organic Factors	5
Table 1.3:	Percent of Patients Discharged Whose Diagnosis Was Mental Illness Without Organic Cause	6
Table 1.4:	Occupations of Mentally Ill People in Provincial Asylums, 1851–1904	7
Table 4.1:	Psychiatric Units	76
Table 6.1:	Residential Units in Ontario Hospitals	113
Table 9.1:	Number of Patients in Hospital and Residential Units	158
Table 9.2:	Rate of Mentally Ill in Psychiatric Hospitals	159
Table 10.1:	Mental Health Expenditures	182
Table 14.1:	Mental Health Expenditures as a Percentage of MOH Expenditure	242

Preface

I began research on mental health policy in 1983 after finishing a book on mental retardation policy. Once again, I made extensive use of the Archives of Ontario. The archivists at the AO were extremely helpful, especially Barbara Craig who knows the health area like the back of her hand. The Scott and Administrative Studies libraries at York University have good collections of documents, periodicals and monographs relating to mental health policy and I made extensive use of them. I firmly believe that one cannot understand how policy is made without speaking to people who formulate, authorize and implement policy. I interviewed a wide spectrum of people: ex-patients, nurses, attendants, psychiatrists, politicians and bureaucrats. Every interview illuminated one or another aspect of policy and put flesh on the bare bones of scholarly theories. Everyone I interviewed spoke frankly and freely and all contributed immensely to this book. Only three people I contacted absolutely refused, despite repeated requests, to be interviewed: an NDP member of the legislative assembly, a civil servant who played a crucial role in shaping mental health policy during the 1960s, and a psychiatrist. I have listed those interviewed at the end of the book, although a few people wished to remain anonymous.

It took five years to do the research for, and to write this book. During two of those years I was able to devote full-time to research and writing thanks to a sabbatical year and a research grant from the York Faculty of Arts. I have always found York University extremely generous in providing time and funds to support scholarly research. Partial support during sabbatical year was provided by a grant from the Social Science and Humanities Research Council, while the Faculty of Arts provided minor research grants to help defray the costs of photocopying and other expenses.

There are a number of people in Toronto who know mental health policy well, but few as well as Cyril Greenland and Dr. J. D. Griffin. For years they have struggled to interest scholars and researchers in the history and evolution of mental health policy in Canada, and they have selflessly devoted their time to developing and opening to the public the archives at the Queen Street Mental Health Centre. They deserve our thanks.

The lively talks and discussions at the Luna Circle, a study group on the history of mental health in Canada, kept my interest in the project alive and often led me to rethink strongly held ideas.

I would like to thank Associated Medical Services and the Hannah Institute for the History of Medicine for their generosity in providing publication assistance for this book.

Finally, all opinions expressed are my own and nothing said here should be interpreted as expressing the views of those who were interviewed for this book.

Introduction

The 1986/87 edition of *Regional Allocation of Estimated Expenditures on Mental Health Services by Ministry of Health* tells the story of mental health policy in Ontario in a nutshell. In 1986/87 the ten provincial psychiatric hospitals consumed 35.2 percent of mental health expenditures, 22.5 percent went to the more than 60 psychiatric units located in the provincial general hospitals, and a mere 4.9 percent was devoted to community mental health. Ontario Health Insurance Plan (OHIP) payments and homes for special care consumed an additional 31 percent. In Ontario's unbalanced tripod of services, community mental health is the weak leg.

Focusing on government policy-making from the 1930s, this account explains how Ontario's lopsided mental health system developed out of a policy-making process that was firmly grounded in "ad hocery," or the art of muddling through.

In 1930 responsibility for mental health was transferred from the office of the Provincial Secretary to the Department of Health. The 1930s ushered in a period of change and, for many psychiatrists, of optimism. Institutional psychiatrists agreed that mental illness was a disease similar to physical illness and should be treated by techniques similar to those used in general medicine. With the inception of new, radical therapies flooding in from Europe, psychiatrists glimpsed the possibility of permanently curing patients of mental illness and reducing the population of the psychiatric hospitals. Throughout Ontario's psychiatric hospitals, doctors subjected thousands of patients to insulin coma therapy, metrazol shock treatment, electroshock therapy, or lobotomy. Psychiatrists grasped and used any treatment which gave the public the impression that psychiatry was as scientific and deserving of the same status, salary and working conditions, as physical medicine.[1] In their eagerness to apply the new therapies, they overlooked the fact that these treatments were painful, physically or mentally injurious, and in the end, mostly ineffective. It was in the 1930s, then, in their cavalier use of radical treatments that psychiatrists embarked on the road that would lead directly to the antipsychiatry critique of the 1960s.

Beginning in the 1960s mental health laws gradually restricted the ability of psychiatrists to commit and compulsorily treat people in Ontario's psychiatric hospitals. Today patient advocates are stationed in each of Ontario's ten psychiatric hospitals, lawyers specializing in mental health law are busily engaged in courtroom challenges of mental health law, and a myriad of patients' rights and mental health pressure groups jealously guard the rights of mentally ill people in their encounters with the Mental Health Act.

The radical decline in psychiatric authority is only one facet of the revolution in mental health policy that began in the 1960s. The inception of new drugs in the 1950s made it easier to control the gross behavioural symptoms of major mental illnesses such as schizophrenia. Shortly afterward, because of the drugs or, depending on which critics one reads, because of economic, humanitarian or other reasons, governments drastically began to reduce the patient populations of the large psychiatric institutions. Some ex-mental patients were simply transferred from psychiatric hospitals to privately run homes for special care or to nursing homes. Others found accommodation in downtown boarding homes or hostels. The lucky ones returned to their families—the unlucky ones slept rough in the streets.

In the 1930s some mental health authorities realized that hospital treatment was only a partial answer to the problem of mental illness and that some kind of community or aftercare system had to be established for the less seriously mentally ill and for ex-patients. In 1935, one of the most original thinkers in the history of mental health policy in Ontario, deputy minister of health Dr. B. T. McGhie, noted that the "serious problem" caused by the increasing number of mentally ill and mentally retarded people seeking places in the Ontario Hospital system,

> could be met only partly by increasing bed accommodation in existing hospitals. The possibility of caring for patients outside the hospital proper was greatly extended by the adoption of the policy of placing carefully selected patients in approved "boarding homes" where their supervision could be carried on by the outpatient staff of the hospital, but where their maintenance was much less expensive. The re-establishment of improved or recovered patients from mental hospitals has been made increasingly difficult by general economic conditions.[2]

In 1944, Dr. McGhie proposed to a committee of the House of Commons in Ottawa a radical and comprehensive plan for a community-based system of mental health care. But McGhie's plan was never adopted, nor were any of the myriad of plans, proposals and recommendations for community mental health care that followed. Instead, in the 1950s, with the enthusiastic support of the psychiatric community, including the physicians who staffed the Department of Health, from the Minister on down, the province began to open psychiatric units in general hospitals. By the 1960s the psychiatric unit system had developed into the second major leg of Ontario's unbalanced tripod of mental health services.

In 1930, apart from the Minister of Health, the top ranks of the Department of Health were staffed by the deputy minister of health, the deputy minister of hospitals, a chief director of hospital services, a part-time senior assistant physician for the Ontario Hospitals and the inspector of hospitals and charitable institutions. All, including the Minister of Health, were medical doctors. By the 1980s the number of medical doctors at the top of the civil service hierarchy had been sharply reduced and replaced by civil servants with business or management training.[3] At the same time, the post of medical superintendent at the provincial psychiatric hospitals had given way to a system of divided responsibility, with a professional administrator looking after the business affairs of the institution and a psychiatrist in charge of medical matters.

Over the years, the level of funding increased enormously. In 1988, total provincial expenditures on all aspects of mental health was close to $1 billion, compared to $3.5 million expended on mental health and mental retardation policy in 1930.

Successive Mental Health Acts have narrowed the grounds for involuntary commitment to mental hospitals and vastly extended the legal basis on which patients in mental hospitals can refuse treatment or commitment. Whereas in the 1930s, the only institutions providing inpatient care were the crowded, underfunded and understaffed mental hospitals, by the 1980s there were over sixty psychiatric units in general hospitals. By the 1960s they had begun to admit more people than the provincial psychiatric hospitals. Whereas in the 1930s the tiny approved homes program was the only residential alternative in the community for mentally ill people, by the 1980s housing and aftercare services were much more extensive. The number of psychiatrists in public service had increased from 1936, when 69 physicians looked after 10,903 patients in the Ontario Hospitals, to 1988, when 140 psychiatrists were employed to care for 4,000 patients. But 50 positions were vacant, a shortfall of 26 percent.[4]

Finally, there had been an enormous change in the paradigm of mental health. Whereas until the 1950s it was assumed that mental illness required treatment by psychiatrists in a hospital setting, by the 1960s the antipsychiatry movement had begun to question the very nature of mental illness, and, in Thomas Szasz's famous phrase, to talk about the "myth of mental illness." In addition, self-help pressure groups composed of former psychiatric patients, or, as some called themselves, "ex-inmates" or "ex-prisoners" sprang up in Vancouver, Toronto and Montreal, and began to criticize government and psychiatrists alike for their authoritarian treatment of mentally ill people and their unwillingness to provide community mental health care services.

Yet, as we approach the 1990s, more than half a century after McGhie's proposed reform, Ontario's mental health system is still plagued by the problem of underfunded and understaffed psychiatric hospitals and an inadequate community care program.

What explains the low priority of mental health policy in government and its egregious failures? Briefly summarized, the major explanations are as follows:

1. The phenomenological explanation argues that mentally ill people have to be seen as part of a larger category of deviants including mentally retarded people, the physically disabled and others whose appearance or behaviour marks them off as substantially different from the majority of people.[5] According to Alexander Leighton:

> One could argue that all diseases seen as chronic and life threatening or incurable make people uneasy, and I would accept this general uneasiness as a com-

> ponent in the emotions inspired by madness... But I think that the response to insanity has additional dimensions of intensity and irrationality. There is something particular in these disorders that evokes in human beings existential apprehension that is akin to the fear of the dead and of ghosts, demons, trolls and other apparitions.[6]

Whereas after years of publicity and campaigning, mental retardation pressure groups succeeded in getting the public to abandon terms like "idiot," "imbecile," and "moron," and to think of mentally retarded people in positive ways, despite years of effort by mental health groups, many people still think of mentally ill people as bizarre, offensive or dangerous. These ideas about mental illness have political consequences. Time and again in the course of this study, mental health bureaucrats, politicians and psychiatrists emphasized that lack of public sympathy for mentally ill people translated into weak support for mental health policy.

2. Some scholars argue that mental health policy cannot be viewed in isolation from other social welfare policies. In Western capitalist societies, so this argument goes, social policies are not intended to help the unemployed, the poor and the disadvantaged, but rather to maintain social control over them. Consequently social welfare and mental health policies are underfunded and poorly administered. Worst off are the chronically mentally ill, who combine low socioeconomic status with the stigma of mental illness. Although they consume a disproportionately large percentage of mental health expenditures, they are the most disadvantaged in terms of funding and programs.[7] Thus, community mental health programs or the large psychiatric hospitals serving mainly poor, unemployed or seriously mentally ill people suffer in comparison with psychiatric units serving a more middle class, less seriously incapacitated population.

3. A sociological explanation of mental health policy concentrates on the psychiatric profession and on the claims of the psychiatric discipline. Since the 1960s the antipsychiatrist attack has borne fruit. Psychiatrists no longer have the prestige, legal power or professional standing they had during the immediate postwar period. Women, gays and blacks attacked psychiatrists for trying to delegitimize and reduce to mental illnesses what these groups claimed were alternative life-styles or political choices. In the process, alternative therapies emerged to challenge psychiatry's monopoly over the treatment of mental illness. Moreover, most psychiatrists avoid working at comparatively low-paying jobs in psychiatric hospitals, or in community programs, preferring to work in general hospitals, or if interested in research, in medical schools. Even the assumption that the cutting edge of research in psychiatry lies in the chemistry of the brain draws psychiatrists away from the psychiatric hospitals and community care, and further devalues work in those areas. All this helps account for the low priority of mental health policy in government.

4. Finally, political reasons are given for the state of mental health policy. For example, one cannot understand how the American mental health system was reshaped without knowing something about pressure groups, the congressional system and the power of the Presidency in the United States. Nor can one understand the nature of the mental health system in Ontario without knowing something about how the political process works in the Ontario bureaucracy.

Although the phenomenology of deviance, the political economy of advanced capitalism, and the sociology of the psychiatric profession all bear on the question, the focus of this book is on how political factors influenced the evolution of mental health policy in Ontario.

Any explanation of the evolution of policy must take a variety of political forces into account. Government, pressure groups, psychiatrists, the media, opposition parties, and the public all influenced policy. Mental health policy also unfolded against a background of changing ideas on the nature and treatment of mental illness, an evolving legal structure and competing political ideologies. In the end, however, it was government that formulated, adopted and implemented policy. Thus, it is to government that one must turn for an explanation of the current unbalanced state of mental health services in Ontario. By government I mean the Cabinet, the various Ministers of Health, those civil servants, or as I call them, "mental health bureaucrats" in the Ministry of Health responsible for mental health policy, and the opposition political parties.

There is a good reason for focusing on this narrow circle of decision-makers. Until the 1950s, political scientists devoted an inordinate amount of attention to the "input" side of politics, that is, to those political forces that made policy demands on government. A plethora of studies looked at voting behaviour, elections, pressure groups, political parties, legislatures and legislators. But few people asked how government actually made policy. Government appeared to be a mysterious "black box" in which policy demands were somehow converted into "outputs"—actual policies. However, by the 1970s there was an enormous increase in the number of works that examined government's role in policy-making. This book is part of that literature.

In Ontario, mental health policy derived from a process of "incremental politics." This has been defined by David Braybrooke and Charles Lindblom as "decision-making through small or incremental moves on particular problems rather than through a comprehensive reform program."[8] In incremental politics, decision-makers look at alternatives which differ only marginally from existing policies, no one claims to have the right solution to the problem and the best solution is the one which gets the most support. Policies are intended to resolve existing problems or difficulties, not to conform to some long-term, coherent, overall plan for the future.[9]

Incremental politics has always been the order of the day in Ontario. Yet, decision-making did not have to follow the incremental model. Almost every five years from 1930 to 1985, a report, analysis or critique of Ontario's mental health system appeared, recommending major changes and reforms. Without exception, each recommended a major extension of community mental health services. The major reports are listed below.

Except for the 1988 Graham Report (which the government supports but has not yet implemented), not once did the government do more than adopt a few recommendations or tinker with the system. This is not to say that the mental health system did not change, but changes always resulted from the accretion of short-term, minor alterations intended to deal with immediate and pressing policy problems. For example, the psychiatric units were established initially to serve as examination and observation centres for the courts, and then to reduce the intake of the provincial psychiatric hospitals and to attract federal cost-sharing funds. Inspired by a small circle of mental health bureaucrats, the psychiatric unit system was endorsed by the various Ministers of Health and implemented with little public discussion or debate. It was not informed by any coherent vision of the future of mental health services in Ontario, nor was it based on the kind of fact-gathering exercise that usually accompanies major policy initiatives. Nor was this an exception, for, from 1930 to 1985, mental health policy developed in response to specific problems. Like Topsy, it seems to have just "growed." But mental health policy did not evolve in a purely contingent fashion. The evolution of mental health policy in Ontario was influenced by specific political forces and structures. The task of this book is to describe these forces and structures, to show how incremental decision-making dominated mental health politics in Ontario for more than half a century and to explain why Ontario's mental health system evolved into the unbalanced tripod we have today.

The book is divided into three parts and a postscript.

Part I: 1930–1960.

In 1930, all matters relating to health were removed from the Department of the Provincial Secretary and transferred to the newly-created Department of Health. The provincial psychiatric hospitals began to use a variety of heroic methods to treat the insane. A discussion of the various treatment therapies during this period illustrates how patients were treated, provides a background to the decline in psychiatric authority, and helps explain the growing disrepute of the provincial psychiatric hospitals. Dr. B. T. McGhie's reform proposals of 1943 and 1944 are described and the establishment of the mental health clinic program is discussed.

Part II: 1960–1970.

In 1955 the National Scientific Planning Council of the Canadian Mental Health Association appointed a committee to look into the state of psychiatry and mental health services in Canada. After years of discussion and hearings, its report *More for the Mind* was published in 1963. *More for the Mind* confirmed the trend toward establishing psychiatric units as an alternative to the large mental hospital, while insisting on the primacy of the psychiatrist in all phases of mental health policy. Under Minister of Health Dr. Matthew B. Dymond, the Department of Health slowed and finally stopped constructing large mental hospitals. But chronic and elderly patients in the provincial psychiatric hospitals became pawns in a game intended to obtain federal cost-shared funds, and were shunted aside into special residential units in the hospitals. When this failed to attract federal funds, they were transferred to the Homes for Special Care Program, which then became an object of severe criticism.

Part III: 1970–1985.

During this period thousands of ex-mental patients were deinstitutionalized into an unprepared, sometimes hostile and completely underserviced community. The result was a series of dramatic incidents and crises, especially at the Queen Street Mental Health Centre and in the Parkdale area of Toronto. Yet, the Ministry of Health seemed unable to formulate a coherent, long-term response, and fell back on a series of short-term measures directed at resolving immediate problems. Thus, in 1985, when the Progressive Conservative government left office after 42 years in power, mental health policy seemed to be as diffuse, confused and unbalanced as ever.

Postscript: 1985–1989

Immediately upon assuming power in 1985, the Liberals promised major changes in mental health policy, including increased funding for community care. The radical proposals of the 1988 Graham Report are summarized and discussed.

Notes

[1] In the course of his presidential address to the Canadian Psychiatric Association on June 18, 1963, Dr. C. A. Roberts, stated: "We believe that we and our patients should be accepted as are other doctors and patients…we want the same social recognition, the same rewards in kind and we want similar equality for our patients as compared to other patients." C. A. Roberts, "Psychiatry at the Crossroads," *Canadian Psychiatric Association Journal*, 10 (1965): 449. Andrew Scull argues that psychiatric explanations for, and treatment of mental illness were heavily influenced by the psychiatrist's search for the same prestige and rewards as medical doctors. See Andrew Scull, *Museums of Madness* (New York: Penguin Books, 1982) 164–171.

[2] Ontario, *Sessional Papers*, "Annual Report of the Hospitals Division, Department of Health, for the year ending 31 October 1934 upon Hospitals for Mentally Ill, Subnormal and Epileptics," Volume 67, Pt. IV, No. 15.

[3] However, the two most recent deputy ministers of health, Dr. A. Dyer and Dr. M. Barkin were respectively a Ph.D. in pharmacy and a medical doctor.

[4] For statistics on number of psychiatrists employed, see G. F. Heseltine, *Towards a Blueprint for Change: A Mental Health and Policy Perspective: Discussion Paper* (Ontario: Ministry of Health, December 1983) 196. For recent statistics see *The Globe and Mail* 8 March 1988.

[5] Two classics in the field are Edwin M. Lemert, *Human Deviance, Social Problems and*

Social Control (New Jersey: Prentice-Hall, 1972) and Howard Becker, *Outsiders* (New York: Free Press, 1963).

6 Alexander Leighton, *Caring for Mentally Ill People* (London: Cambridge University Press, 1982) 8.

7 S. J. J. Freeman states that although the chronic mentally ill comprise only 20 percent of the mentally ill population, they "consume over 40 percent of mental health funding." See "The Chronic Patient Rediscovered: Ten Propositions," *Canada's Mental Health*, 31 (1983): 15–16. For a marxist approach to the question see Andrew Scull, *Decarceration* (New Jersey: Prentice-Hall, 1977).

8 David Braybrooke and Charles Lindblom, *A Strategy of Decision* (New York: Free Press, 1963) 71.

9 See James E. Anderson, *Public Policy-Making* (New York: Praeger Publishers, 1975) 12–14.

PART I: 1930–1960

1

Insanity in the 1930s

> I noticed the cruelty at Buffalo when I was interning. There was a black girl who had a baby who couldn't think of a name for it, and she heard a beautiful word she thought would make a good name; the word was "placenta," and the staff encouraged her on this. But I blew the whistle on it and the staff said: "What, are you crazy, imagine this kid will go around called 'Placenta,' Ha." There was this funny duality of very sacrificing, caring people, and there was also the frustration that people were so sick and miserable and the families were so horrible and you couldn't do anything, you couldn't do a goddam thing. Either you developed a callus around your heart, or you said you can't take it anymore and went to do research. So the mental hospitals ended up with funny authoritarian people who couldn't make it elsewhere.
>
> A Toronto psychiatrist

Setting the Scene

In the 1930s, the mental health system in Ontario centered almost exclusively around the twelve mental hospitals that had sprung up over the previous one hundred years. They ranged in size from the enormous 1,550 patient institution at Whitby to the comparatively small 235 patient institution at Woodstock. Of the twelve, seven had been constructed in the nineteenth century, the oldest among them being the Toronto asylum which was first opened in 1846. However, in a system notable for administrative stagnation and institutional inertia, the 1930s did bring some changes. In 1931 the provincial health service was transferred from the office of the Provincial Secretary—where it had competed with prisons, charities and other public institutions for funds and for administrative attention—to the Department of Health. The appointment of Dr. B. T. McGhie as director of hospital services brought to the office a dynamic and innovative administrator. McGhie immediately began establishing a network of mental health clinics associated with the mental hospitals, an approved home network to provide residences for patients who could live outside the hospital, and a probation system whereby patients were released from hospital in the custody of friends or relatives. The 1930s also saw the inception of radical new therapies for mental illness in the form of insulin coma therapy, metrazol, fever therapy for syphilis, and electroshock treatment.

Despite these innovations, the provincial mental hospitals were in dreadful shape. They were overcrowded, the rate of admissions continued to grow inexorably, and they had become catch-all institutions housing not only mentally ill people but those whose mental illness was caused by serious organic diseases such as cerebral arteriosclerosis, epilepsy and mental retardation.[1] Because the province lacked specific facilities for their treatment, the psychiatric hospitals also housed large numbers of alcoholics and elderly people.

Patients

From 1930 to 1940 the patient population in Ontario's psychiatric hospitals rose from 8,453 (excluding those in the Ontario Hospital, Orillia, the provincial institution for mentally retarded people) to 10,384. The numbers continued to rise over the next two decades. During this time the provincial statistician distinguished between those patients whose insanity stemmed from organic causes such as syphilis, mental deficiency, epilepsy, cerebral arteriosclerosis, and alcoholism and those whose insanity stemmed from non-organic causes. In the latter category fell those patients who had been labelled as insane, but for whose insanity one could find no apparent organic or neurological cause. Although most jurisdictions ultimately established separate institutions for people suffering from mental illness caused by organic problems, the lack of financial resources in the 1930s led to the institutionalization of people whose primary problem was not mental illness but an underlying organic disease. For example, in 1940, there were 14,314 people listed on the books of all Ontario hospitals, including Orillia. Of this total, 2,884 suffered from "mental deficiency without psychosis." Since, in 1940, Orillia housed 2,073 patients, 811 mentally retarded people who might have been in Orillia were housed in mental hospitals. In addition, there were 599 patients diagnosed as suffering from "psychoses with mental deficiency." How many of these could have been placed in Orillia if there had been more room is hard to say, but clearly if the province had established larger, separate institutions for mentally retarded people, the numbers of patients in the mental hospitals would have been reduced. In 1940 as well, official statistics record the presence of 562 patients suffering from "epilepsy without psychosis." Although the province had set aside the Woodstock hospital mainly for epileptics, in the official statistics they were counted among the mentally ill. Three hundred and sixty-four patients were diagnosed under the heading "senile psychoses," and 337 under "psychoses with cerebral arteriosclerosis." Here too, it is likely that if the province had provided suitable accommodation for the elderly, numbers in the two latter categories would have been substantially reduced.

Although 40 percent of the institutionalized population suffered from mental illness caused by identifiable organic diseases, some scholars have argued that many of those labelled as mentally ill suffered from nothing more than a tendency to depart from accepted political or social norms and that the historical function of the mental hospitals was to impose social control over these deviants. Writing about the origins of the asylum system in Ontario in the nineteenth century, Thomas E. Brown states that "the move to segregate the insane in their

Table 1.1
Fourteen Diagnostic Categories

1.	Dementia Praecox
2.	Manic-depressive Psychoses
3.	Psychoses with Mental Deficiency
4.	Senile Psychoses
5.	Epileptic Psychoses
6.	Mental Deficiency without Psychosis
7.	G.P.I. and Cerebral Syphilis
8.	Psychoses with Cerebral Ateriosclerosis
9.	Involutional Psychoses
10.	Paranoia and Paranoid Conditions
11.	Alcoholic Psychoses
12.	Alcoholism without Psychosis
13.	Epilepsy without Psychosis
14.	All Other

Table 1.2
Percent of Mentally Ill Due to Organic Factors (Diagnostic categories 3–8, 11–14)

Year	*Percent*
1934	41.1
1935	41.1
1936	42.3
1937	42.4
1938	43.0
1939	43.0
1940	43.0
1941	42.8
1942	43.2
1943	43.5
1944	44.0
1945	44.2
1946	44.1
1947	45.6

[Source: *Annual Reports*, Department of Health, 1934–1947]

Table 1.3
Percent of Patients Discharged Whose Diagnosis Was Mental Illness Without Organic Cause

Year	*Percent*
1934	61.2
1935	56.8
1936	44.8
1937	67.6
1938	72.5
1939	60.0
1940	60.4
1941	64.5
1942	62.1
1943	63.5
1944	63.6
1945	67.3
1946	69.1
1947	67.1

[Source: *Annual Reports,* Department of Health, 1934–1947]

own special institution was not an isolated political act but part of a much larger design to identify, classify and contain deviancy and dependency in general."[2]

From 1934 the annual report for Ontario mental hospitals distributed patients among fourteen diagnostic categories, as shown in Table 1.1. A quick glance at this listing will show that except for diagnoses 1, 2, 9, and 10, all other forms of mental illness were caused by organic factors such as epilepsy, mental deficiency and senility, or by alcoholism.

Except, perhaps, for alcoholism, it would be difficult to argue that those suffering from mental illnesses caused by organic factors were institutionalized as a means of social control. Table 1.2 shows that from 1934 to 1947 a large percentage of those institutionalized in the Ontario mental hospitals would, because of the nature of their illness, have been institutionalized under any political or economic system.

It is hardly likely that those diagnosed as suffering from mental deficiency, cerebral arteriosclerosis, alcoholism or epilepsy would have escaped institutionalization no matter under what economic or political system they lived. Moreover, statistics also show that the vast majority of those discharged suffered from mental illness without any apparent organic cause. Put another way, those people whose mental illness was occasioned by alcoholism, epilepsy, mental deficiency or senility were less likely to be discharged than those whose mental illness stemmed from non-organic or non-neurological causes. This difference argues

Table 1.4
Occupations of Mentally Ill People in Provincial Asylums, 1851–1904

Occupation	*Number*	*Percent*
Housekeepers	5,094	18.4
Labourers	4,522	16.3
Farmers	4,232	15.2
Domestic Servants (all kinds)	3,671	14.8
Unknown or other employment	2,917	10.5
No occupation	1,393	5.0
Wives	650	2.3

[Source: Ontario Sessional Papers, volume 37, Pt. 9, Department of Health, *Thirty Seventh Annual Report*, 1905, Table 12. Out of 164 different occupations listed in the 1904 report only the most important categories are listed, comprising 82.5 percent of the total number of patients.]

either in favour of the remarkable skill of the hospital authorities in normalizing those who were previously deviant, or, more likely, in favour of the fact that many mentally ill people undergo spontaneous recoveries which then permit them to leave the mental hospital for a greater or lesser period of time.

Moreover, it is clear from first admission figures that the majority of those who became the chronic, long-stay patients in the mental hospitals suffered from neurological or organic diseases. Figures from 1933 to 1946 consistently show that those who suffered from mental illness without organic or neurological causes comprised a minority of admissions. Fewer of this group came in, and more of it went out than the group composed of those suffering from organically caused mental illness. Clearly then, the mental hospitals were caring for two apparently distinct groups: one suffering from mental illness caused by organic or neurological diseases, the other suffering from mental illness caused by non-organic factors. The first group was more likely to stay in the hospital for a longer time than the second, to make up a good percentage of the long-stay chronic population, and less likely than the second group to leave the hospital.[3] (See Table 1.3.)

In addition to using the mental hospitals for people with organic diseases, the institutions were also used for welfare purposes. This was not an innovation of the 1930s. In 1860, Dr. Joseph Workman, the superintendent of the Provincial Lunatic Asylum at Toronto (which came to be known as "999 Queen Street") observed with some acerbity: "In the present hard times, no doubt the 'authorities' regard every person, who has nothing to eat, as dangerous to be at large; and as the Asylum is known as a good boarding house, they conclude that it cannot be turned to better purpose than that of relieving themselves of the duty of supporting the poor."[4]

In 1904, the provincial statistician provided a table listing 164 different occupations (plus "unknown or other employment") and the numbers of people in those occupations who had been institutionalized in all Ontario asylums since 1851, 27,667 people in all. (See Table 1.4)

Over the following years the largest single categories consisted of housewives and people with no occupation. In 1934, for example, 20.6 percent of the patients were housewives, and 24.4 percent had no occupation. Those from the "professional" and "commercial" categories usually comprised no more than 12 percent of the total asylum population in any given year. Of course, among the "housewives" there were probably large numbers of women from middle class and professional homes, but because data was not collected on the class or occupational background of women patients, it is impossible to tell what percentage of the total they comprised.

During this time, the institutions were under the authority of the provincial government, but, in fact, were run in an authoritarian fashion by the medical superintendent. They were, according to psychologist Ray Berry who worked at the London and St. Thomas institutions in the 1950s, "like fiefdoms."

> It was the superintendent who made all the decisions. He held the conference at which patients were discussed, but in fact the superintendent would decide no matter what the hell, no matter what anybody else said, what he thought the patient was.[5]

According to Dr. S. Freeman the medical superintendent was,

> the last of the feudal lords. The medical superintendent, he was everything, he had responsibility for 2,000 or 2,400 patients and 1,000 staff, and for the fields, and the cows. He knew enough about them to know that the cow on their home farm was about to calve, and he would make a point of asking about it. Dr. Fletcher of the Whitby Hospital would do rounds every Sunday after church and he knew the name of every patient whom he addressed as a lord of the manor would have done.[6]

In these circumstances, and given the stigma from which mental patients suffered at this time, abuses were bound to occur.

The Royal Commission on the Operation of the Mental Hospital Act

In the 1930s, as had been the case for nearly 100 years, responsibility for mental health policy in Ontario lay securely in the hands of a small and exclusive body of decision-makers—all of them medical doctors. At the top was the Minister of Health assisted by the deputy minister of hospitals and the director of hospital services. Aside from two inspectors of hospitals, the department was staffed by secretaries and clerks. The mental hospitals were headed by the medical superintendents of the twelve mental hospitals, including one institution for the mentally retarded.

Since the press rarely interested itself in the mental health system, and the legislature hardly ever, policy was made by the Minister of Health, the mental health bureaucracy in the Department of Health and the medical superintendents.[7] There were occasions, as during the early part of the twentieth century, when the myth of the menace of the feeble-minded roused the press and the public and led to a widespread public debate about policy toward mentally retarded people, but the day-to-day operations of the mental hospital system were usually closed to public view and the administration of that system rarely became the focus of attention and debate.[8]

One occasion when the public got a rare glimpse of how the system actually worked occurred in the fall of 1938 with the appointment of the Royal Commission on the Operation of the Mental Health Act. The Royal Commission was appointed as a direct result of the complaint of John R. Green, a lawyer who claimed that he had been incarcerated in the London mental hospital for nearly three years despite the fact that, according to the *Toronto Star*, he was "believed by many who knew him to be perfectly sane."[9]

Green's case was headline news in 1938. Green was an acquaintance of Premier Mitchell Hepburn and he lived in St. Thomas, the Premier's constituency. Shortly after his release from the London mental hospital, he visited Premier Hepburn at his farm and told him his story. Hepburn was obviously impressed and angered because at the same time as he announced the appointment of the Royal Commission he commented:

> I have reason to believe that lots of sane people are railroaded to mental hospitals and kept there under pressure to serve the interests of those responsible for their improper detention. I can't think of anything more inhuman than to keep a person, in his right mind, cooped up—often for long periods—with others who are undoubtedly insane. That this has been going on in many instances in our own province is awful to contemplate.[10]

One of the main findings to emerge from the Commission's hearings was how poorly protected individuals were during commitment proceedings. Under the law, a person charged with any offence could be sent by a magistrate to an institution, whether a mental hospital, examination unit or institution for the mentally retarded, for observation for not more than sixty days. Whereas a person charged with a criminal offence could obtain bail, this was not the case with those committed under the Mental Hospitals Act. If, during the observation period, the superintendent found the person either mentally ill or mentally defective then that person had to be examined by two medical doctors. The legislature had intended that the two doctors should examine the patient separately so as to give him the benefit of doubt but the Royal Commission found that in every provincial mental hospital the hospital gave to the two examining doctors the history, case and clinical records of the person under observation. It was not surprising that the Commission did not find a single instance in which the two independent doctors came to a conclusion which differed from that of the hospital staff.

The Commission also heard evidence of hospital staff beating patients, accusations of murder and, after exhumation of the body of a patient whose death was purportedly due to perforation of the bowel caused by falling out of bed, testimony from a provincial coroner that the likely cause of death was "external violence."[11] The Commission was also told by the deputy minister of public works that, because of its dilapidated state, the entire London mental hospital should be abandoned.[12] After reviewing this and other evidence, the Royal Commission recommended that "psychopathic wards be established in all general hospitals" where magistrates could send people to be assessed, rather than sending them directly to mental hospitals. The evidence of at least one medical doctor would be required before the magistrate could commit to the psychiatric ward, and of two doctors for committal to a mental hospital.

In addition, the Commission questioned the superintendents about the establishment of a board or boards of review to assess regularly those patients whose detention might be unwarranted. Except for Dr. Fletcher of the Whitby institution, the superintendents unanimously supported the idea, differing mainly over the question of whether the board should be composed exclusively of psychiatrists or should have lay participation, and over the question of whether there should be one or a series of such boards.[13] The Royal Commission also made recommendations concerning treatment of alcoholics, sterilization, coroner's reports and administrative procedure at the various provincial institutions. However, except for changes in the law regarding committal proceedings and some other minor changes few of the Royal Commission's recommendations were implemented. It was not until twenty-nine years later, in 1967, that review boards were established in provincial psychiatric hospitals.

The criticisms and recommendations of the 1938 Royal Commission were neither surprising nor novel. Just a few years before, under the leadership of Dr. Clarence M. Hincks, the Canadian National Committee on Mental Hygiene (CNCMH) had criticized the overcrowding and poor conditions in Ontario's mental hospitals. At this time Hincks was the head of the CNCMH as well as of the American National Committee on Mental Hygiene. In 1936, the CNCMH received a grant of $16,000 from the Rockefeller Foundation for the establishment of a Mental Hospital Survey Committee, but it was unable to get the Ontario government to allow a Canadian Survey Committee to visit the Ontario mental hospitals and make an assessment.[14] However, the government did agree to the establishment of a two-man committee staffed by Dr. Samuel W. Hamilton, formerly medical director of the Bloomingdale hospital and Dr. G. A. Kempf, associate medical director of the U.S. Public Health Service—both were Americans.[15]

The Mental Hospital Survey Committee

The 1937 Mental Hospital Survey Committee report was highly critical of the Ontario mental hospital system. Overcrowding was rampant, the hospitals were underfunded, and, above all, there were major drawbacks to Ontario's centralized administration of the hospital system.

Hamilton and Kempf noted that the provincial authorities had a penchant for saving money by converting older buildings for use as mental hospitals. The mental hospital at Kingston had been a stable, the institution at Malden had been an army barracks, the Cobourg institution had been a college, and the immense 1,800 bed (in 1936) institution for mentally retarded people at Orillia had started life as a summer hotel.[16] Hamilton and Kempf estimated that the system was overcrowded by 30 percent: with a formal bed capacity of 9,920 beds, the 12 Ontario institutions actually had 12,914 beds.

> The patients must spend their time in turmoil, so thrown together that peace is impossible, when an able-bodied patient must spend months in bed because of the danger of combat if he is up in narrow quarters, when there is not space for eating together because beds have supplanted all other accommodations, then it must be time for radical action in the field of construction.[17]

Action was taken when Premier Hepburn gave the go-ahead for the construction of an enormous 3,600 bed hospital located in the southwestern part of the province, near the small city of St. Thomas. Because the hospital was to be built in his constituency on land owned by the Premier, the government hoped to kill two birds with one stone: to increase the number of mental health beds and to curry political favour for the Premier and his Liberal government.[18] In 1939 the St. Thomas Hospital received 1,054 patients, transferred from the provincial hospital system, but in the fall it was taken over by the Royal Canadian Air Force and the patients were transferred back again. Despite the initial projections, by the 1950s St. Thomas housed approximately 1,600 patients. Yet, by North American standards St. Thomas was not unusually large. In 1939, 24 American state hospitals had populations between 3,000 and 4,500, and three held more than 4,500 people.[19]

Once built, Ontario's mental hospitals were subjected to severe financial constraints. Every penny spent was carefully accounted for, and the authorities tried wherever possible to pass on to the public some of the cost of running the system. Although the majority of the patients in the Ontario mental hospital system were indigents, the Minister of Health admonished the superintendents to exercise the "utmost vigilance...to see that maintenance should be paid, where the people are financially able to do so."[20] In 1931 and in 1938, the Department of Health told the superintendents that wherever possible relatives should supply clothing for patients.[21] The Department also took a hard look at the farms attached to most of the institutions. Despite the general feeling that they were unprofitable, in 1935 the Minister of Health "stressed the importance of the farms as giving facility [*sic*] for occupational therapy, and commended them in that regard, although financially they may be a losing proposition."[22]

Hamilton and Kempf had criticized the Ontario mental hospitals for shoddy construction, dangerous lack of fireproofing and inadequate facilities. Cobourg they characterized as a "makeshift institution," Fort William was "a frame structure that is not very suitable for a hospital service," and one wing of the Kingston hospital should be "pulled down." At London they noted that a Royal Commission in 1930 had recommended "the abandonment of the whole institution," New Toronto was "so crowded that it functions poorly," the institution at 999 Queen Street in Toronto should, they suggested, be abandoned, and resold "to a railroad or other purchaser," and Toronto Psychiatric Hospital was "too small for its purpose and not well arranged." Despite the fact that both men were experts with wide experience in the health system, they were shocked to discover that: "A curious, amazing and distressing condition prevails in many hospitals. Bedrooms are unheated. In the bitter cold of winter there are disturbed patients who negligently discard part or all of their clothing while quartered in such rooms."[23]

Finally, in comparison with Massachusetts and New York, which they felt most nearly resembled Ontario, Hamilton and Kempf found mental health policy in Ontario to be inferior by almost every standard. Ontario's institutions were more overcrowded, there were fewer physicians per patient, and per capita expenditures were lower than in Massachusetts and New York. In terms of the ratio of nurses and attendants to patients, however, Ontario ranked slightly above the two states.[24] The reason for this was that the Depression had thrown a large number of people on the job market, and given the scarcity of jobs and the attractive prospect of secure, long-term provincial employment, people were attracted to the mental hospital system who might otherwise have obtained jobs elsewhere. Perhaps such comparisons were not completely fair since historically per capita expenditures on mental health had always been higher in Massachusetts and New York than the United States average, but the Ontario authorities often compared Ontario favourably with the major northeastern states, and so Hamilton and Kempf were merely returning the compliment.[25]

Hamilton and Kempf did not assign specific blame for these shortcomings, but it is apparent from their report that the highly centralized and politicized administrative system of the Ontario mental health system must have been a contributing factor. What struck them most forcefully was the absence of any intermediate authorities or regulatory bodies between the mental health bureaucrats in the Department of Health and the mental hospitals. Of course, this situation obtained in some parts of the United States, but Hamilton and Kempf, as representatives of the mental hygiene movement, favoured administrative arrangements which gave some autonomy to local hospital boards of trustees and to an independent board or agency which would mitigate the powers of the central authorities.

> Since 1931 this Division [the hospitals division of the Department of Health] has operated as a highly centralized service with a more or less permanent

> Deputy Minister at its head... This type of organization dispenses with any local boards. The local Member of Parliament may be interested helpfully or otherwise in the Department, but has no specific relation to it. The distribution of all personnel, medical, nursing, mechanical and other, is determined in the offices of the Department. Appointments are made by the Civil Service Commissioner on the recommendation of the Minister. No examinations, competitive or non-competitive, are held for appointment or promotion. Any institution head may recommend discharge but can of his own authority go no farther than to suspend the offender.[26]

The result was that employment staffing policies at the mental hospitals were determined by political considerations, or as Hamilton and Kempf put it delicately: "There remains...a curious political link in their relation to the appointing power."[27] It is very difficult, of course, to document the manner in which politics intruded into the appointment process at the various mental hospitals, but one may surmise that the local MPP or the Minister often played a hand in determining the allocation of positions.[28] One egregious example, albeit from 1960, can be found in correspondence between the Minister of Planning and Development and the superintendent of the Kingston Psychiatric Hospital. In a letter dated April 7, 1960, the Minister complained to the superintendent about a letter that had been sent to another MPP,

> to the effect that your personnel manager at your hospital indicated that to get employment at your institution, I had to be contacted. That statement is not in accordance with the facts. I have never asked a person their politics concerning any employment, nor do I take the position or assume authority for having the right to veto who to employ and who not to employ at your fine hospital.

About two weeks later, however, the superintendent received a letter from the Minister concerning a constituent whose father had been killed in World War I. "I am not prepared," the Minister wrote,

> having served overseas with her father, who gave his life that we might enjoy the privileges we do today in this land of ours, to have my old comrade's daughter go hungry, and that is just what the situation amounts to. I want to get her employed... It is the rarest of occasions when I ask for employment...but this is a desperate case that demands immediate action.

One week later the Minister wrote to the superintendent telling him that he "would appreciate very much indeed if you would telephone me about employment for Miss———." In the end, it seems that the superintendent found a job for the woman in the occupational therapy department or as a part-time librarian.[29]

In addition to providing a source of political patronage for local members of parliament, Hamilton and Kempf noted another nefarious feature of the centralized administrative system in Ontario—its suffocation of creativity and initiative. It is important to remember that Kempf and Hamilton spoke for the National Committee for Mental Hygiene and in doing so expressed the interests of the psychiatric profession. They did not look kindly on a system which gave primacy of place to bureaucrats—even if these bureaucrats were themselves physicians—and where the Minister of Health "is in a position to dictate about the last detail of hospital activity…but [where] he has no formal advisory organization of those who are unselfishly interested in the hospitals."[30] The problem was that the superintendents were seriously constrained by the Department of Health and were unable to develop new initiatives or make innovations that might depart from departmental guidelines. Moreover, because the superintendent did not have the power to hire or fire subordinates, there was no way he could build up around himself a "capable and loyal organization in his hospital." The result was to "subordinate genius to regularity."[31] The hospital also did not have the benefit of links with the community that might come with the establishment of a board system. "Strong hospitals in other regions often have a lay group with some powers, some responsibilities and much knowledge of the problems of the hospital."

Clearly Hamilton and Kempf were thinking of states like Massachusetts and New York where governments had established autonomous agencies to administer the mental health system and where, as well, local boards of trustees were attached to the various state mental hospitals.[32] Above all, Hamilton and Kempf advocated more autonomy for the superintendents and the medical staff attached to the hospitals, additional resources for the hospitals, an increase in the number of physicians and an improvement in the various services offered by the Department of Health.

Despite the thoroughness of their investigation and the wide-ranging nature of their recommendations, Hamilton and Kempf had practically no influence on mental health policy in Ontario. Part of the reason had to do with the lack of funds. North America was in the grip of an unprecedented depression. The conventional wisdom held that the only way toward recovery was to cut costs, balance the budget and hope that business would begin to improve. Given the fact that governments are usually very reluctant to spend money on mental health care and given the economic circumstances of the time, it is not surprising that the mental hospital system remained underfunded, overcrowded and centrally controlled. Although the Canadian National Committee on Mental Hygiene fully endorsed the Hamilton and Kempf report, it had little influence on government.

During this time, only a scandal or a dramatic death could provoke the interest of the press or of government. Most of what went on behind the locked doors of the provincial mental hospitals was hidden from public view. The public was vaguely aware that conditions in the mental hospitals were poor and that staff sometimes abused or injured patients, but most people were indifferent to the mental hospital system. Under the guidance of Dr. Hincks, the CNCMH deliberately followed a low-key policy of trying to influence government by providing it with information through personal contacts Hincks had in government and in the medical community.[33] Unlike the United States, therefore, where the internal operations of the mental hospitals were subject, in principle at least, to the scrutiny of boards of trustees or semi-independent government agencies, in Ontario the mental hospital system operated in obscurity, with mental health policy determined by a very small number of mainly medical decision-makers.

In these circumstances, the hospital staff had to cope on a day-to-day basis with enormous and increasing numbers of people suffering from a wide variety of mental and physical illnesses, often behaving in a bizarre, disruptive or violent fashion. It is no wonder that, lacking any other means, staff sometimes resorted to brute force and violence or to mechanical restraints in order to deal with difficult patients.

Radical Treatments

In the 1930s, Canadian institutional psychiatrists began to use new, radical, and intrusive therapies which had been developed in Austria, Hungary, Italy and Portugal.[34] Psychiatrists injected patients with insulin, inducing a coma which often brought the patient close to the point of death until it was relieved with an injection of glucose; they administered a camphor-based drug called metrazol which provoked spine-cracking convulsions; they indiscriminately administered forty, fifty or even hundreds of shock treatments and, in lobotomy operations they drilled holes in patients' skulls and excised portions of their brain.[35] Although radical treatments were justified in terms of medical science and expertise, archival documents show that treatments were administered haphazardly, with little understanding of how they worked and with scant regard for the wishes of the patient. The choice of treatment often was dictated by the ease with which it could be administered, the speed with which it took effect, the lack of side effects, safety and cost. Only after a good deal of random experimentation were specific illness linked to treatments. But even then, radical treatments might be administered not because they ameliorated the illness, but as a means of punishment or because they calmed the patient and made work easier for the ward and medical staff. Moreover, psychiatrists fought hard to maintain their professional image and their freedom of action. When films about psychiatrists or mental illness depicted psychiatry in a negative light, Ontario psychiatrists were able to get the offending films censored. And when questions of patients' consent to treatment threatened their authority, Ontario psychiatrists tried to narrow the grounds of consent, or to eliminate consent procedures altogether.

Insulin Coma Therapy

Insulin coma therapy was developed in Vienna in the 1930s by Dr. Manfred Sakel. After injecting a morphine addict with insulin and accidentally inducing a coma, Sakel noticed the craving for morphine disappeared. Sometime later, Sakel again accidentally brought about a deep coma in a mental patient, and again noticed the symptoms were alleviated after the patient recovered. After further experiments, Sakel told the world that insulin coma therapy was effective in treating schizophrenia and by the late 1930s it was widely used throughout North America.

However, at the provincial hospital in St. John, New Brunswick, insulin was given to patients who were thought "definitely unsuitable cases for treatment" because relatives "insisted" and, according to hospital authorities, because of "our own curiosity regarding the effect of insulin."[36] In 1939, the CNCMH reported that insulin had been used to mitigate withdrawal symptoms in the treatment of alcoholics and drug addicts at the Verdun Hospital in Quebec.[37] Insulin was first used in Ontario on May 31, 1937, at the New Toronto psychiatric hospital. According to the director of the provincial hospitals division, "the work at New Toronto was a unique experiment… at present limited to females."[38] Typically, when new treatments were introduced women were selected as the guinea pigs.[39] When Dr. C. B. Farrar reminded his fellow superintendents at a conference that "the risks in the treatment were very great and could not be minimized," the director of hospitals edited the minutes, eliding the phrase "were very great."[40] By 1939 the CNCMH was warning the Department of Health of reports from New York of a 16 percent death rate after insulin treatments.[41] However, according to Dr. N. L. Easton, superintendent of the New Toronto psychiatric hospital and director of research for Ontario's psychiatric hospitals, early results from the use of metrazol and insulin were encouraging because 80 percent of the cases treated recovered and were returned to the community.[42]

In March 1939, the deputy minister of health claimed an 84 percent success rate for insulin administered to patients with "dementia praecox."[43] During this time the Department of Health continued to publish statistics on shock therapies gathered by Dr. Easton, the major champion of insulin coma therapy in the province. However, in 1946, Dr. Fletcher, superintendent of the Whitby institution, wrote to the director of the hospitals division about Easton's claims. "Those claims were, I think, in direct contradiction to the statistics…by the Provincial Statistician and personally I think it is far from having been proven…that the results are better than if the same amount of attention was given with any other type of drug or indeed with no drug at all if it were possible to arouse the same enthusiasm…"[44] Nonetheless, insulin treatment continued until it was replaced by the more effective and safer electroshock therapy in the 1950s.[45]

Metrazol

Shortly after the inception of insulin coma therapy, another dramatic treatment arrived from Hungary. This involved metrazol, a convulsion-inducing drug first used on mental patients by the Budapest physician Ladislas von Meduna. Along with many other psychiatrists, Meduna assumed (incorrectly as it turned out) that patients with epilepsy did not have schizophrenia. He therefore concluded that there was an antagonism between epileptic convulsions and schizophrenia. As had been the case with insulin, early experiments with metrazol proved effective in ameliorating schizophrenia, and by 1938 metrazol was adopted by psychiatrists the world over.[46]

As is usually the case with new drugs, early reports indicated a large degree of success. However, the theories advanced to explain how metrazol worked were extremely simple. In early 1938, Dr. N. L. Easton wrote that "[t]he theoretical basis for the metrazol therapy lies in the assumption that a certain biochemical antagonism exists between the convulsive state and the schizophrenic process… To my way of thinking, the convulsion acts as a 'battering-ram' to the psychosis and as such should have some favourable therapeutic effect."[47] Another explanation suggested by Dr. J. E. Edlin, a Chicago psychiatrist, was that metrazol "causes convulsions and literally snaps the patient out of his psychosis."[48] The justification for the use of metrazol, insulin and, later, electroshock therapy was purely empirical: although no one knew why, the treatments seemed to work.[49]

One of the side-effects of metrazol was that just before the convulsions began, patients experienced a horrible sense of foreboding and impending doom. Dr. J. D. Griffin recalls that after observing metrazol treatment at the Cook County Hospital in Chicago in 1940:

> What I saw I shall never forget. They would line up about thirty or forty male chronic schizophrenic patients, they looked older than they were, they were all dressed in long nightshirts and they were herded like sheep into a pen of some sort. One at a time they were injected with metrazol and they went into horrible seizures that were horribly painful. They were frightened and were in excruciating pain for a few seconds or even longer, and then gradually they would recover and staggering, they would be led out. Then they would lead in another patient with all the patients listening to all this if not actually looking at it. They were partially screened from seeing the actual procedure but they could hear and they were terrified. I felt that whatever value this had, this was not the way to do it.[50]

One ex-superintendent stated that "patients would run as fast as they could in the other direction" when they saw metrazol coming.[51] Dr. N. L. Easton observed the administration of metrazol in Buffalo in 1938 and noted: "The treatment appears very drastic to one observing it for the first time. The patients themselves all hate it and make all manner of excuses to avoid taking the injections. Even after treatments have been completed the patients have nothing nice to say about it."[52] One year after metrazol treatments began, the CNCMH sent the Department of Health a "strictly confidential and not for publication" bulletin noting that some investigators in the United States had discovered compression fractures of the spine in patients who had undergone the treatment.[53] There were also some indications of a higher rate of tuberculosis among patients treated with metrazol.[54] The Department of Health moved quickly to determine whether patients in Ontario institutions suffered from these problems. Whereas investigators in New York found that 43.1 percent of 58 patients who received metrazol suffered compression fractures, a survey of 100 patients in Ontario found only one instance of injury, and the investigators were not certain that it had been caused by metrazol.[55] Thus, the Department decided to continue the metrazol treatments. However, just a few days after that decision, Dr. Easton suggested that in view of the better results obtained through insulin, the number of metrazol units be decreased and the number of insulin units be increased.[56] In its May 27,

1939 bulletin, the CNCMH noted that "[t]he general consensus at the meeting [of the American Psychiatric Association from May 8–12] was that metrazol was not living up to previous expectations. More complications, more dangers, and less favourable results than had been expected were consistently reported."[57] Despite these warnings metrazol treatment continued, and when the division of medical statistics did a survey in 1941, it found that for every patient who had received insulin, six had been given metrazol. In addition to its apparent therapeutic value, metrazol, like the other therapies, appears to have been given to make easier the work of ward staff. Dr. J. S. Stewart of the Kingston Hospital wrote to the director of the hospitals division:

> I know quite definitely that at Hamilton, Metrazol therapy was used for a number of chronic continued-treatment cases who had been in the hospital for a considerable period of time. It was not expected at the time that a recovery would be obtained, but it was hoped that following Metrazol treatment some improvement might be found in the institutional adjustments of the patients. If this same procedure occurred at other hospitals, and it is reasonable to think that perhaps it may have, the swollen numbers that received Metrazol should be taken into consideration.[58]

In 1941, the division of medical statistics undertook an examination of the results of metrazol and insulin therapy. It found that by June 30, 1941, 1,316 patients had been treated with metrazol alone, 217 with insulin alone, and 30 patients had been treated with metrazol and insulin at different times.[59] Three hospitals accounted for two-thirds of all treatments.[60] The survey found that the success rate with both insulin and metrazol treatments was much less dramatic than had been reported at their inception some three years before. Of the 217 patients treated with insulin, only 34 percent had made a full recovery, 23 percent were in "social remission," 21 percent were "improved," and 22 percent were "negative." However, if one combines the first two categories, the 57 percent who had either fully recovered or who were in social remission is a far cry from the 80–84 percent success rate that the Department of Health had claimed in 1939.

With regard to metrazol, 26 percent of the patients were described as "fully recovered," 21 percent as in "social remission," 28 percent "improved," and 25 percent as "negative."

There were striking differences in the results reported at different hospitals. For example, whereas 56 percent of the patients given metrazol at New Toronto were reported to have had "negative" results, only 16 percent of the patients at Kingston had the same results. After controlling for other variables, the division of medical statistics concluded that "the standards used to evaluate outcome are not altogether uniform from centre to centre."[61]

Despite the fact that, by November 1941, Dr. Easton had found that 23 percent of patients who had been treated with metrazol and then x-rayed had compression fractures of the spine, the use of metrazol continued. By 1943, however, the director of the hospitals division ordered that no more metrazol be purchased because electroshock machines were beginning to replace metrazol.[62]

In November 1944, the provincial statistician, L. S. Penrose, did a study of 3,866 patients who had received shock therapies during the period 1938 to 1944.[63] He discussed the report at a superintendents' conference on April 25, 1945. Penrose found that there was a significantly high correlation between the administration of metrazol and deaths from tuberculosis. According to Penrose, "the net result of the enquiry...suggests strongly that metrazol is a hazardous form of treatment from the mortality rate and that it increases the risk of tubercular disease in patients who receive it." In the cover letter he appended to the report and sent to the director of hospitals, Dr. R. C. Montgomery, Penrose also observed, "I think that it is likely there are some deaths which have not been reported."[64] On May 22, 1945, Dr. Montgomery wrote to Penrose: "In the light of the statistical evidence it appears highly advisable to discontinue the use of metrazol treatment." Two weeks later, Montgomery wrote to Penrose, "I do not see how this information can be published."[65] Although metrazol treatments were discontinued in 1945, electroshock and insulin coma therapy continued apace until the 1950s.[66]

Electroshock

Electroshock treatment entered the mental health system in the same unobtrusive way as had insulin and metrazol. The Department of Health learned of some interesting experiments that had been done elsewhere, means were acquired to administer the technique, initial results were encouraging and the press hailed the technique as a highly effective treatment for mental illness.[67] In November 1943, the *The Globe and Mail* reported that electroshock was "safe, harmless and highly beneficial in 90 percent of 250 cases treated," and noted that patients who had been in hospital for six to eighteen months were "apparently, permanently cured in three to four weeks." The reporter mentioned that electroshock was particularly valuable in cases of involutional depression in women.[68] As with the other techniques, however, there was no theoretical basis to explain why electroshock worked—except that it produced results. In a flippantly headed article, "Electric Shot in Brain Said Sure, Those Dreary Monday Blues to Cure," *The Toronto Star* observed that electroshock "was an outgrowth" of the discovery that insulin and metrazol shock "would cure some of the insane."[69] The reporter stated that: "Exactly what happens to the brain in this period is not certain," but he noted that there was widespread agreement that electroshock treatments were less dangerous than metrazol. In addition to these advantages the CNCMH noted that patients were more willing to accept electroshock than metrazol. The CNCMH noted that, in contrast to the after-effects of insulin and metrazol, there seemed to be little problem with compression fractures of the spine after electroshock. When one adds to these advantages the fact that electroshock was cheaper and much easier to administer than either metrazol or insulin, it is not surprising that from the date of its adoption in 1941 to 1945, 2,003 patients had received electroshock treatments. By 1950, that total had increased by 400 percent with 9,480 patients having received electroshock treatments, and by 1964, 24,652 treatments had been administered.[70] Unfortunately statistics on the total number of men and women receiving electroshock are not available, but at Whitby from January to December 22, 1964, women received 2,175 treatments and men 884.[71]

Although, in 1944, Penrose had found that electroshock was not effective in treating schizophrenics, the technique was used indiscriminately to treat a variety of illnesses, including schizophrenia and syphilis. The assistant director of the hospitals division of the Department of Health noted that "most every patient is getting shock therapy" at the hospital in London.[72] At the Hamilton hospital it was used on schizophrenics "[b]ecause it was the only form of 'shock' therapy available."[73] It was also used because it was less expensive than insulin. At the London hospital: "All suitable schizophrenic patients...receive the quickly acting economic electrotherapy first. The more slowly acting, expensive insulin therapy is held in reserve for suitable 'electroshock failures'..."[74]

L. S. Penrose's statistical studies continued to be a thorn in the side of the superintendents. On April 25, 1945, the director of hospitals convened a superintendents' conference to discuss Penrose's "Results of Special Therapies in the Ontario Hospitals, Coma, Convulsion and Leucotomy up to November, 1944." Penrose was not at the conference. In an analysis of 1,600 cases treated with insulin and metrazol, 182 patients treated with electroshock and 19 cases treated with prefrontal leucotomies, Penrose criticized the conventional wisdom with regard to mental patients and shock treatment therapies. He argued that the view was "fallacious" which held that early treatment of mental illness through shock therapy would produce favourable results. He found that the results of electroshock treatment were less favourable than with metrazol or insulin therapy, that "schizophrenics do not react favourably to electroshock treatment" and that in fact it might be "harmful in cases diagnosed schizophrenia." Lobotomy also had better results than other forms of treatment.[75] As regards shock treatments, Penrose concluded that "shock therapy tends to speed up recovery in cases who are heading eventually toward recovery so that these patients are discharged sooner than would otherwise be expected; there is no evidence, however, that the ultimate outcome after a five year period is in any way altered by these treatments."

Finally, Penrose criticized the notion that one of the signs of good treatment results was a high discharge rate from the hospital. Penrose pointed out that the discharge rates took no account of readmissions. Thus, the secular increase in discharge rates from Ontario mental hospitals from 1882 to 1944 meant only that "patients were being admitted, discharged and readmitted and discharged more rapidly than at any previous time in Ontario hospital history."

Despite Penrose's findings, the superintendents' conference in April 1945 recommended the continuation of shock treatments. Since Penrose found that the main value of shock treatments was in hastening the recovery of those who were on the mend anyway, the superintendents argued that shock therapy was important because by shortening the length of stay in hospital it helped to restore people, "especially wage earners...to remunerative employment... It provides a quicker turnover of hospital patients and in regard to the indigent patient is a financial saving to the government."

But the superintendents still had to deal with the fact that 42.7 percent of the shock treated cases remained in hospital five years after admission. Here the superintendents pointed out that, although they had not improved sufficiently to return to the community, they were "less destructive on the wards, and more amenable to other forms of therapy." Shock therapy also "greatly eased the nursing problem."[76] In 1946, Dr. N. L. Easton recommended to the director of the hospitals division that electroshock be used "on one of the refractory wards with the purpose of treating chronically disturbed patients...the nursing problem would be greatly alleviated and the destruction almost eliminated."[77] One observer noted that electroshock was used with the patient who "so often reacts aggressively to deprivation of his liberty."[78]

In the 1940s, the Ontario mental hospitals used fever cabinets for the treatment of syphilis. This involved placing the patient in an insulated box and raising the temperature to 105–106 degrees in order to kill the syphilis spirochete. The treatment was extremely uncomfortable and patients naturally resisted, or, as one doctor from New Toronto put it: "The biggest delaying factor is an untoward mental state of the patient." A brief dose of electroshock, it was found, helped to overcome this obstacle.[79]

So pleased with electroshock was one doctor at London that he recommended that patients return once a month for "prophylactic shock treatments." The rationale was that since "electroshock quickly dissipates manic excitement or depression...it should act in a similar way in the subclinical state." The authorities at London notified 46 patients in the community about the existence of the program and sent a social worker to encourage them to return to the hospital for monthly electroshock treatments. Nineteen responded and participated in the program with good results.[80]

However, there was increasing evidence that electroshock was not the unmitigated success it seemed to be. Despite the earlier reports from the CNCMH and other sources claiming that the danger of compression fractures and other injuries from electroshock was minimal, evidence of such injuries began to appear. In the late 1940s the Ontario authorities learned that in some cases amnesia and brain damage accompanied electroshock. Although in 1943, Dr. Easton observed that the incidence of compression fractures in electroshock was lower than in metrazol treatment, in October 1944, the director of the hospitals division noted that electroshock resulted in fractures of the spine in anywhere from five to 25 percent of the cases treated.

The authorities at the London hospital felt that the fractures were so innocuous and had so little effect on the patient that the routine x-rays taken after treatment were discontinued. After all, it was noted,

> nothing specific is done for the fractured vertebrae. During the years, post-treatment x-rays of spines have been taken by the thousand, viewed, diagnosed and filed... What benefit has this radiological procedure brought to the patient, therapist or preventive technique? Only that the patient does not know he has a compression fracture, the therapist that he has, the preventive technique remains unchanged and the fracture incidence remains more or less constant.[81]

At the mental hospital in Toronto , it was found that spinal x-rays were taken of male but not female patients since "[t]he assumption is that female patients do not have spinal compression fractures."[82] In addition to the compression fractures, there seemed to be additional problems associated with electroshock. In 1947, the Offner Electronics Company sent a letter to the director of the hospitals division noting that one of the merits of the Offner machine was that it caused less brain damage and less amnesia than competing machines. The reduced amnesia, however, was considered to be a disadvantage since patients who could remember events just before and after electroshock were reluctant to consent to the treatment.[83] According to the director of research for Ontario mental hospitals, some patients thought of suicide in order to escape further electroshock treatments.[84]

The problem of the compression fractures was dealt with in 1953 when the American Psychiatric Association published its "Standards for Electroshock Treatment." The APA noted that the most common "complication in electroshock therapy is vertebral fractures... and these cannot be prevented on occasion regardless of what techniques are used." Despite the fact that the complication was "unpredictable," the APA maintained that "vertebral fractures... generally heal without difficulty and without any special orthopedic treatment."[85] In view of this evidence, the administration of electroshock continued.

The superintendents also argued that shock treatments improved the morale of the nursing staff because they had "the feeling that they are accomplishing something. Further to raising the morale of the staff this form of therapy showing rapid results has a profound effect on relatives who actually see an active treatment unit and do not consider the term hospital a misnomer."[86] By 1949, however, the incidence of compression fractures was causing some concern to the Department of Health. A survey of 4,774 post-treatment x-rays from 1944 to 1950 showed that 616 patients, or 12.8 percent suffered fractures of one or more vertebrae, with an enormous difference in the rate between hospitals, ranging from 5.1 percent to 28 percent.[87]

These figures occasioned some surprise because, as one superintendent noted, it had been decided at a previous superintendents' conference that the "compression fractures were of academic interest only."[88] Despite the criticism, however, the mental health authorities decided to continue with the electroshock program.

Psychiatrists and Public Responsibility

Until very recently, mental hospitals were crammed with people who manifested gross behavioural abnormalities that have since completely disappeared.

Patients were often violent, abusive, or lacked control over bodily functions. This is not to justify the way in which staff dealt with difficult patients but it does explain why mental hospital staff desperately grasped at any therapeutic straw that might allow them to dispense with physical force or mechanical restraints.

There was another reason why the doctors and staff embraced new therapies. Suffering from the low esteem that clung to those who worked with mentally ill people, they were eager to improve their image. Drugs such as insulin or metrazol and techniques such as electroshock and psychosurgery gave to doctors and nurses the feeling that they were using scientific methods and working in a hospital system much like their brethren in the general hospitals.

In Britain, the growing use by psychiatrists of insulin, metrazol, electroshock and lobotomy apparently helped to convince general hospital physicians of the scientific nature of the psychiatric enterprise which they usually viewed with suspicion or even with outright hostility. According to a 1943 editorial in the *British Medical Journal*, the "tangibility" of these physical treatments,

> makes them easily acceptable to the layman, sometimes perhaps dangerously acceptable; and for the same reason they have an appeal to medical men in general who...are still apt to regard mental diseases as things apart from their concern. The actual physical treatment of mental disease...should have the effect on many people of bringing mental diseases within the same category of thought as physical ill-health.[89]

The desire for professional recognition was a powerful force impelling the mental health authorities to imitate the techniques and forms of general medicine. Given the newspaper stories about successful new treatments, and basking in the "scientific" aura that accompanied the use of new drugs and techniques, it is no wonder that the superintendents were reluctant to accept the negative conclusions of L. S. Penrose's statistical studies. To do so would have been to abandon the attempt to convince the public and the rest of the medical profession that psychiatry and the mental hospitals were as deserving of respect (and public funds) as medical doctors and general hospitals.

In the 1930s, patients were chosen for drastic therapies for a variety of reasons: for experimental purposes, out of "curiosity," to control violent or difficult patients and, of course, in the hopes of ameliorating or even curing mental illness. Treatments were also administered for public relations purposes—to convince the public that mental hospitals were "hospitals" just like general hospitals. Patients' rights hardly entered into the question. The superintendent ruled supreme within the hospital, the patients were his subjects and however kindly an individual superintendent might feel toward these subjects they were, ultimately, at his mercy and the mercy of the hospital staff. By claiming they were acting in the patients' best interests, psychiatrists could solemnly invoke intrusive and cruel treatments without anyone raising an eyebrow.[90] And the press, always vigilant in watching for abuses of the commitment power, cheered each new development, raising false hopes and pressuring psychiatrists to implement untested therapies.

Although it is important to try to understand the historical context in which actions take place and to guard against imposing current values on past practices, it is equally important to avoid a complete suspension of judgment. Certainly mental health authorities thought they were acting for the patients' benefit. In interviews, some psychiatrists defended their colleagues of the 1930s by pointing out that their actions were well within accepted practice. But those psychiatrists who administered radical therapies were not acting within a closed system. They were not merely passive social actors, unthinking reflectors of the values of their profession. It was always possible to choose whether or not to use any or all of the radical therapies, to which patients they should be applied, and whether or not consent should be obtained. Within psychiatry itself there was always some dispute about the effectiveness and the morality of administering radical therapies.[91] It is true most criticisms emanated from the United States, but Canadian psychiatrists were members, and some were officers of the American Psychiatric Association and as such they could hardly have been unaware of crosscurrents in the profession.[92] In 1938, for example, Dr. Oskar Diethelm of Cornell University read a paper at the annual meeting of the American Psychiatric Association in which he criticized psychiatrists' tendency to indiscriminate use of "somatic treatment," and he warned his colleagues that:

> In any scientific treatment which is not fully understood there is the serious danger of not being able to predict possible damage. It should be an inflexible duty to become thoroughly familiar with the drug or procedure to be employed... No one has the right to invent theories to suit his desires without having given full consideration to what has been established or found plausible.[93]

However, psychiatrists did not take kindly to criticism emanating from outside the profession. Beginning in the 1940s, criticism appeared in an unexpected quarter—the cinema. Perhaps it was inevitable that mental hospitals and psychiatrists would catch Hollywood's attention. After all, every North American was dimly aware of the existence of the "looney bin" or the "nut house," with its bizarre patients and mysterious atmosphere. And the theme of insanity ran through many nineteenth and twentieth century novels. By the 1940s, however, in a typical attempt to sentimentalize changing attitudes toward the mentally ill and at the same time to cash in on the public's morbid interest in the new shock treatments, Hollywood began to produce films with a psychiatrist playing a central—and highly ambiguous role. At least that is how Ontario psychiatrists felt in 1940 when they saw *Young Dr. Kildare's Dilemma.* Officials in the Department of Health objected to a scene portraying insulin coma therapy because, as Dr. Easton put it,

> the picture does not portray the therapy in its proper perspective, and would create a false impression as well as undue apprehension on the part of anyone considering this form of treatment... I would not recommend that this picture be shown to the public as it would leave the impression that insulin shock treatment

is very dangerous, and probably painful and hard to take, all of which experience has proved to be untrue.[94]

The deputy minister of health complained to O. J. Silverthorne, head of the provincial board of censors, and within two weeks Silverthorne replied that the offending scenes had been eliminated and the film "altered in such a way as to make it...quite acceptable to the theatre-going public."[95] In 1946, the deputy minister informed the medical director of the CNCMH that it had been common practice "for some years, for the Censor Board to request an opinion from this Department on motion pictures with a medical background."[96]

But even under existing standards there seem to have been serious violations of the law. The wholesale administration of radical treatments often occurred with scarce regard to the question of consent. In the 1940s, the law was unclear regarding the question of whether a superintendent could order that a mental patient be given treatments such as electroshock or insulin coma therapy without the consent of relatives.[97] In fact, these treatments were routinely administered without seeking consent. Dr. Stevenson of the London hospital mentioned that as regards electroshock and insulin coma therapy, "several years ago it was decided that we did not need to receive relatives' consent for these treatments." He also noted that other superintendents pressed the Department of Health to require relatives to give to the superintendent "blanket consent for any treatment which may, in our judgment, be of benefit to the patient."[98]

Consent procedures differed from one hospital to another. In 1938, Dr. T. D. Cumberland, medical superintendent of the Ontario Hospital at New Toronto referred to sending out consent forms to relatives of patients about to undergo metrazol treatment.[99] When informed that the Department of Health was not in favour, Dr. Stevenson argued: "When any patient comes to us for psychiatric treatment we should not be interfered with in giving adequate treatment by the withholding of consent by relatives."[100] In the mid–1940s, however, the question of consent was an important consideration in psychosurgery because lobotomies were surgical procedures which were supposed to be performed in a hospital. In these circumstances, the law required the written consent either of the patient or of his legally constituted representative. However, according to the provincial solicitor, the law permitted the superintendent to act as the "committee of the patient" and, as such, "could direct the course of treatment of the patient."[101] Moreover, refusal to grant consent might rebound against the patient. At a superintendents' meeting in 1948, Dr. Stokes of the Toronto Psychiatric Hospital said "it was quite plain that if a voluntary patient refuses to accept a recognized form of treatment which is recommended, his status as a voluntary patient is open to question."[102]

Today, the major therapies of the pre- and postwar period have disappeared—with the exception of electroshock. People in psychiatric hospitals are better protected than ever before against abuses of psychiatric authority. Competent patients can refuse to give their consent to psychiatric treatment, while under no circumstances can a lobotomy be performed in an Ontario psychiatric hospital.

Yet, if there is any lesson to be learned, it is that good intentions are not enough. That conditions in the mental hospitals were abominable from the 1930s to the 1950s, and that patients were extremely difficult to handle cannot be denied. But these are explanations, not justifications for the way in which patients were treated. Many psychiatrists chose to treat patients as guinea pigs, to use radical therapies for social control rather than therapeutic purposes, to ignore or seek to override the question of consent, and to censor negative information about these therapies. Unless we support the notion of historical inevitability and wish to exculpate all historical actors, including psychiatrists, from moral judgment, then we must assess moral blame on those institutional psychiatrists who abused their positions of authority in the administration of radical therapies.[103]

Notes

1 In his report for the 1939 Royal Commission on Dominion-Provincial Relations, A. E. Grauer wrote: "Overcrowding in mental institutions in Canada is of such proportions as to constitute a national disgrace." A. E. Grauer, *Public Health* (Ottawa: Royal Commission on Dominion-Provincial Relations, 1939) 42.

2 T. Brown, "The Origins of the Asylum in Upper Canada: 1830–1839," *Canadian Bulletin of Medical History* 1 (1984): 38. For a critique of this and similar views see Harvey G. Simmons, "The New Marxist Orthodoxy: a Critique," *Canadian Bulletin of Medical History* 2 (1985): 97–114.

3 According to Wendy Mitchinson: "Focusing on the socioeconomic characteristics of the insane shows clearly that the asylum was not being used as a place to hide away the deviant or the idle (as is often suggested in the social control literature) except to the extent that mental illness was defined as deviancy and led to an inability to work." "Gender and Insanity as Characteristics of the Insane: A Nineteenth Century Case," *Canadian Bulletin of Medical History* 4 (1987): 99.

4 Province of Canada, *Sessional Papers*, 1861, V. 19, no. 24.

5 Interview, Ray Berry.

6 Interview, S. Freeman.

7 Six of the first eight Ministers of Health were medical doctors. From 1930 to 1970, the five deputy ministers were medical doctors.

8 On the myth of the menace of the feeble-minded in Ontario, see Harvey G. Simmons, *From Asylum to Welfare* (Toronto: National Institute on Mental Retardation, 1982): 65–100.

9 *The Toronto Star*, 8 September 1938.

10 *The Toronto Star*, 8 September 1938.

11 *Telegram*, 3 November 1938.

12 *Globe and Mail*, 16 September 1938.

[13] Clifford R. Magone, Chairman, *Report of the Royal Commission on the Operation of the Mental Health Act 1938* (Ontario: Royal Commission on the Operation of the Mental Health Act, 1938).

[14] On the establishment of the Mental Health Survey Committee see Gerald Grob, *Mental Illness and American Society, 1875–1940*, (New Jersey: Princeton, 1983) 310.

[15] According to Dr. J. D. Griffin, McGhie explained to Hincks that the reason for not permitting a Canadian survey team to visit the Ontario hospitals was because they were "too local." The result was that despite the fact that Hincks chose the team, it was not identified as being associated with the National Committee on Mental Hygiene, even though Hamilton was the head of its New York office. Interview, J. D. Griffin.

[16] Dr. Samuel W. Hamilton and Dr. G. A. Kempf, *A Survey of the Ontario Hospitals*, (Ontario: Mental Hospital Survey Committee, Feb. 1937) 1. On the early history of the Orillia institution see Simmons, *Asylum* 18–48.

[17] Simmons, *Asylum* 8.

[18] The figure of 3,600 comes from Dr. Burdette McNeel who held a variety administrative posts in mental health in the Department of Health. Interview.

[19] Grob 315.

[20] According to Dr. James Faulkner, Minister of Health, speaking at the Conference of Superintendents, Ontario Hospital, Toronto, Feb. 9, 1935. AO, RG 10, 10–20-A–1.

[21] AO, RG 10, 10–20-A–1. May 1, 1931, and Jan 25, 1938.

[22] AO, RG 10, 10–20-A–1, February 9, 1935.

[23] Hamilton and Kempf 43 ff.

[24] Whereas institutions in Massachusetts were overcrowded by 16.4 percent and in New York by 13.5 percent, overcrowding in Ontario reached 30.3 percent. Whereas in Ontario the ratio of physicians to patients was 1 : 216, in New Hampshire it was 1 : 190, in New York 1 : 192 and in Massachusetts 1 : 196. According to standards established by the American Psychiatric Association, there should have been at least 6.7 physicians to each 1,000 patients. In Ontario, the ratio was 4.6 : 1,000, while in New Hampshire, New York, and Massachusetts the ratio was around 5.2 : 1,000. With regard to the adequacy of the nursing staff and the number of attendants, Ontario fared less badly. In Ontario the ratio of nurses and attendants for each 100 patients was 12.2 : 100, while in New Hampshire it was 14.9 : 100, in New York 11.3 : 100 and in Massachusetts 14.3. Finally, in terms of per capita maintenance expenditures, Ontario spent $316.32 per year per patient, New York spent $358.45 and Massachusetts $357.00.

[25] Grob 217.

[26] Hamilton and Kempf 3.

[27] Criticism of political interference in the hiring of medical staff had already led the government in 1935 to appoint a three-man board of examiners to vet medical appointments to the provincial hospital services. See "Psychiatry in the Ontario Provincial Service," *American Journal of Psychiatry* 91 (1935): 94–95.

[28] There was no question that the asylums were embedded in a system of political patronage in many American jurisdictions. Albert Deutsch noted that in 1934 the American Psychiatric Association revealed that "[i]n several states there was a general turnover of state hospital personnel—from superintendent down—every time one political party was supplanted by another in state power. Some superintendents had to base their appointments of subordinate officers on nominations forwarded by politicians…in 14 states, officers and employees of state hospitals were forced to contribute a portion of their salary to the reigning political party." Albert Deutsch, "Psychiatry as State Medicine," *American Journal of Psychiatry*, 100 (1944): 188.

[29] Letters from W. M. Nickle, Minister of Planning and Development to Dr. E. A. James, superintendent, Ontario Hospital, Kingston, April 7, 1960 and April 23, 1960. In author's possession.

[30] Hamilton and Kempf 11.

[31] Hamilton and Kempf 13.

[32] Grob 210.

[33] According to Dr. J. D. Griffin, former general director of the Canadian Mental Health Association: "Dr. Hincks had a policy which he carried out systematically of not making public in an exposed way any criticisms he had of the mental health services, but to go quietly to the government with his complaints or observations and try to get the government to correct the situation without there being any public blowup or publicity." Interview.

[34] Lobotomy is discussed in chapter 12.

[35] The use of drugs in mental hospitals has a long and varied history. Traditionally, drugs were intended to pacify noisy or violent patients and to make the task of nursing or control easier for the staff. In the nineteenth century, Daniel Hack Tuke noted: "Hypodermic injections of morphia, the administration of the bromides, chloral hydrate, hypocymine, physotigma, cannabis indica, amyl nitrate, conium, digitalis, ergot, pilocarpine, the application of electricity, the use of the Turkish bath and the wet pack, and other remedies too numerous to mention have had their strenuous advocates during late years." Daniel Hack Tuke, *History of the Insane* (1882; Amsterdam: E. J. Bonset, 1968) 485.

[36] Canadian Mental Health Association, Bulletin No. 16, "Recent Advances in the Treatment of Dementia Praecox, Insulin Shock at the Provincial Hospital, St. John New Brunswick," January 17, 1939.

[37] Canadian Mental Health Association, Bulletin No. 20, "Research at Verdun Hospital, Verdun Que." March 14, 1939.

[38] AO, RG 10, HS 1–2, Series 107, August 27, 1937, Central Files, Medical Staff Conferences, Superintendents' meeting.

[39] The exact reason why women were selected is unclear. In 1937 there were 6,611 men and 6,408 women in the various provincial hospitals. It might be argued that the new treatments were thought most appropriate for illnesses where women were overrepresented. But insulin coma therapy was thought particularly appropriate for schizophrenia, or dementia praecox, which was the term used in the Ontario hospital system in the 1930s. However, in 1937, 3,013 women and 3,004 men were classified

as suffering from dementia praecox, a statistically insignificant difference. According to Dr. J. D. Griffin, the reason for initially selecting women for new treatments simply may have been that they were more tractable than men. Interview, J. D. Griffin.

40 AO, RG 10, HS–1–2, Series 107, Central Files, Medical Staff Conferences, Superintendents' Meeting, August 27, 1937. Edited version of the minutes appears in same file on September 2, 1937.

41 Bulletin No. 25, June 16, 1939 from the CNCMH in file of Department of Health notes an article in the *American Journal of Psychiatry* on coma deaths from insulin.

42 *The Toronto Star*, 25 October 1938.

43 *The Toronto Star*, 23 March 1939.

44 AO, RG 10 Gen 1–9–4, Series 107, Box 4, Dr. Fletcher to Dr. R. C. Montgomery. During the 1950s some Canadian hospitals experimented with total push therapy whereby a random sample of chronic patients were placed in redecorated wards and given intensive care by nurses and staff. Interview, J. D. Griffin.

45 According to a 1944 study by L. S. Penrose, from 1938 to 1944, 285 women and 161 men had received insulin coma therapy. AO, RG 10, Gen. 1–9–4, Series 107, Box 4, Insulin Shock.

46 For a brief discussion of Sakel and Meduna see Elliot S. Valenstein, *Great and Desperate Cures* (New York: Basic Books, 1986) 46–50.

47 AO, RG 10–107, Gen. 1–9–8, February 4, 1939, Dr. N.L. Easton, "Metrazol as used in the treatment of schizophrenia."

48 *The Toronto Star*, 3 November 1937.

49 According to Elliot S. Valenstein "Sakel's theory [on insulin therapy] was so vaguely stated and so impossible to relate to any known—let alone measurable—biological process that it was all but incomprehensible." Valenstein 57.

50 Interview, Dr. J. D. Griffin.

51 Interview, Dr. Patrick G. Lynes.

52 AO, RG 10 Series 107, B. 4, Gen. 1–9–5, MS, "Metrazol as used in the Treatment of Schizophrenia," 2 pages.

53 Canadian National Committee on Mental Hygiene, Bulletin 21, "New Dangers Reported in Metrazol Shock," April 6, 1939.

54 AO, RG 10, Series 107, B. 4, Gen. 1–9–5, May 8, 1939, reports on compression fractures in files concerning a meeting of the American Psychiatric Association, May 9–12, 1939. See also memorandum to Dr. J. Howitt, Superintendent, Ontario Hospital, Toronto from Dr. R. C. Montgomery, Director of the Hospitals Division asking about effect of metrazol on old or incipient tuberculosis, March 31, 1939.

55 CNCMH, Bulletin No. 22 "Recent literature on Metrazol therapy," May 4, 1939 reports on results in New York. AO, RG 10, Series 107, B. 4, Gen. 1–9–5, May 12, 1939, "Metrazol Treatment in Ontario Hospitals."

56 AO, RG 10–107, B. 4, Gen. 1–9–5, May 17, 1939, Dr. N. L. Easton to Dr. R. C. Montgomery.

57 AO, RG 10–107, B. 4, Gen. 1–9–5, May 27, 1939, CNCMH Bulletin No. 24 "Recent Work on Shock Therapy: Compression fractures with Metrazol." The Department of Health suspended metrazol treatments briefly from May 12–17, 1939 while a committee discussed the question of side-effects. However, it unanimously agreed to their resumption with the proviso that all patients be physically sound and that x-rays be taken before and after the treatment and during the subsequent recovery period. AO, RG 10, Series 107, B.4, Gen. 1–9–5, May 12, 1938, "Metrazol Treatment in Ontario Hospitals," and Dr. C. B. Farrar, Director Toronto Psychiatric Hospital to Dr. B. T. McGhie, Deputy Director of Health, May 17, 1939.

58 AO, RG 10, Section 107, Gen. 1–9–4, F.2, June 5, 1945, Dr. J. S. Stewart to Dr. R. C. Montgomery.

59 AO, RG 10, Series 107, Gen. 1–9–4, October, 1949, Division of Medical Statistics, Ontario Department of Health, "Insulin and Metrazol Treatments in Ontario Hospitals: 1937–1941."

60 AO, RG 10, Series 107, Gen. 1–9–8, Metrazol quarterly report, June 1, 1938—December 31, 1943. By 1943, 2,263 patients had been treated with metrazol, although the hospitals at Hamilton and Whitby accounted for 66 percent of the treatments.

61 AO, RG 10, Series 107, Gen. 1–9–8, June 1, 1938—December 31, 1943, Metrazol quarterly report.

62 AO, RG 10, Box 55, HS 7–1, Central Files, June 23, 1943, Dr. R. C. Montgomery to Morrison.

63 AO, RG 10, Series 107, Gen 1–9–4, Box 4, Insulin Shock Therapy. This file contains Penrose's study, "After-Effects of Shock Therapy With Special Reference to Tuberculosis." From 1938 to 1944, 2,222 women and 1,644 men had received insulin, metrazol, electroshock or any combinations of these therapies. Fifty seven women and forty three men had died after therapy.

64 AO, RG 10, Series 107, Gen. 1–9–4, Box 4, April 26, 1945, Insulin Shock, L. S. Penrose to Dr. R. C. Montgomery.

65 AO, RG 10, Series 107, Gen. 1–9–4, Box 4, June 6, 1945, Insulin Shock, R. C. Montgomery to L. S. Penrose.

66 However, Dr. Easton noted that metrazol was "still given occasionally to apathetic schizophrenic patients where electro-shock therapy had failed." AO, RG 10, Series 107, Gen. 1–9–8, Nov. 14, 1950, Dr. N. L. Easton to Dr. R. C. Montgomery.

67 On the history of electroshock, see Norman S. Endler, "The Origins of Electroconvulsive Therapy," *Convulsive Therapy* 4 (1988): 5–23.

68 *The Globe and Mail* 3 November 1943.

69 *The Toronto Star* 9 May 1941.

70 AO, RG 10 B. 104, Gen. E–5-A, Dec. 8, 1964, Electroshock, replies to questionnaire.

71 AO, RG 10, Series 107, Gen. 1–9–8, Dec. 28, 1964, Dr. W. H. Weber, Superintendent, Ontario Hospital, Whitby, to Dr. B. H. McNeel, Chief, Mental Health Branch, Re: Electroconvulsive therapy.

[72] AO, RG 10, Series 107, Gen. 1–9–8, Oct. 4, 1950, Dr. C. H. Lewis, Assistant Director, Hospitals Division to Dr. N. L. Easton, Superintendent. Observing shock therapies at the London institution, Dr. N.L. Easton noted: "I observed approximately seventy-five patients treated during the afternoon. About fifty percent of this number were chronic cases whose treatment went on indefinitely to make them more easily managed." AO, RG 10, Series 107, Gen 1-9-8, Dr. Easton to Dr. Montgomery, October 17, 1950. In December, Dr. Easton noticed that women on the refractory ward were given multiple shock treatments. "Here the patient is given from two to three grand mal seizures at intervals of about one minute. It is felt that the results are better in the chronically disturbed patient than the use of one convulsion per day." AO, RG 10, Series 107, Gen. 1-9-8, Dr. Easton to Dr. Montgomery, December 7, 1950. At the Homewood Sanitarium, a private institution in Guelph, Ontario, patients "received 30 comas" in the first stages of an experiment with electronarcosis. AO, RG 10, B.53, HS 2-1, 1948.

[73] AO, RG 10, Series 107, Gen. 1–9–8, Nov. 6, 1945, Dr. N. L. Easton to Dr. R. C. Montgomery.

[74] AO, RG 10, Series 107, Gen. 1–9–8, n. d., J. J. Geoghegan, "Newer Aspects of Shock Therapies," p. 5.

[75] In 1949, Egas Moniz received the Nobel Prize for medicine for inventing leucotomy. Leucotomy soon became known as lobotomy, a term preferred by the American neurologist and pioneer in psychosurgery, W. J. Freeman.

[76] AO, RG 10, HS S–6, April 25, 1945, Minutes of Superintendents' Conference.

[77] AO, RG 10, Series 107, Gen. 1–9–8, March 5, 1946, Dr. N. L. Easton to Dr. R. C. Montgomery.

[78] AO, RG 10, HS 2–1, Central Files, 1947, anonymous comment on Dr. Cathcart's paper, in files of Ontario Neuropsychiatric Association.

[79] AO, RG 10, B52, HS 2–1, 1945[?], H. K. Moir, M.B. "Electro-shock as an Adjunct in the Treatment of Neuro-syphilis" Ontario Hospital, Toronto. Julius Wagner-Jauregg had used fever treatment for syphilis in the late nineteenth century, and then again during World War I. He later achieved an 80 percent success rate in treating syphilis using a combination of fever therapy and Neosalvarsan. In 1927 he won the Nobel Prize for Medicine for his work. Undoubtedly, fever therapy was an effective treatment for syphilis. See Valenstein, *Great* 30–32.

[80] AO, RG 10, B.52, HS2–1, 1946 [?], J. J. Geoghegan, "Newer Aspects of Shock Therapies" Ontario Hospital, London.

[81] AO, RG 10, Series 107, Gen. 1–9–8, Oct. 3, 1944, Dr. R. C. Montgomery to Dr. K. G. Gray, Assistant Deputy Minister of Health.

[82] AO, RG 10, Series 107, Gen. 1–9–8, October 25, 1950, Dr. N. L. Easton to Dr. R. C. Montgomery. In this same memo, Easton observes that in 1944 he had found 16.8 percent of 434 female patients had incurred spinal fracture after electroshock. See also J. J. Geoghegan, "Newer Aspects of Shock Therapies," p. 4.

[83] AO, RG 10, Series 107, Gen. 1–9–8, Feb. 10, 1947, Offner Electronics Inc. to Dr. R. C. Montgomery.

[84] AO, RG 10, Series 107, Gen. 1–9–8, Mar. 5, 1947, Dr. N.L. Easton to Dr. R. C. Montgomery.

[85] AO, RG 10, Series 107, Gen. 1–9–8, May 1953, "Standards for Electroshock Treatment."

[86] At the Homewood Sanitarium, one of two private asylums in the province, electroshock was used in conjunction with electronarcosis or deep sleep. According to the 18 May 1944 *Toronto Star* electronarcosis "seems literally to rebuild a thinking apparatus in the gray matter." Patients were put to sleep for 8 to 10 minutes with an injection of sodium pentothol and then given a series of electroshocks. Some patients underwent 40 sessions of electronarcosis. The theory was that the sleep plus the shocks would disrupt existing thinking patterns, wipe out bad thoughts or memories and allow the psychiatrist to engage in what was called "mental rebuilding." AO, RG 10, B.53, HS 2-1, 1948, J.J. Geoghegan, "Electronarcosis at the Homewood Sanitarium, Guelph, Ontario." Geoghegan (who moved from London to Homewood) was consistently skeptical about the seriousness of the fractures and critical of the necessity of doing x-rays of electroshock patients. At one point he commented: "No x-rays were taken after electroshock as none of [the patients] complained of backache." Dr. Ewen Cameron of the Allan Memorial Institute of Montreal experimented with multiple shock treatments and electronarcosis in 1945, and it later formed the basis of his 1960 experiments in brain "repatterning" for the American Central Intelligence Agency. For a study of Cameron's career, see Anne Collins, *In the Sleep Room* (Toronto: Lester and Orpen Dennys, 1988). On the inception of deep sleep therapy in North America, see Harold D. Palmer and Francis J. Braceland, "Six Years Experience with Narcosis Therapy in Psychiatry," *American Journal of Psychiatry* 94 (1937): 37–57.

[87] AO, RG 10, Series 107, Gen. 1–9–8, Sept. 26, 1950, Dr. N. L. Easton to Dr. R. C. Montgomery.

[88] AO, RG 10, Series 107, Gen. 1–9–8, Oct. 3, 1958, Dr. Fletcher, Superintendent, Whitby to Dr. R. C. Montgomery.

[89] Quoted in Geoffrey Baruch and Andrew Treacher, *Psychiatry Observed* (London: Routledge & Kegan Paul, 1978) 66–67.

[90] For example, at the Worcester State Hospital in Massachusetts, one of the leading mental hospitals in the United States, an experiment was conducted to determine whether metrazol was effective because of the fear induced by the drug shortly after injection, or by the ensuing convulsions. Toward this end, 20 schizophrenic patients, 4 men and 16 women, were injected with varying amounts of metrazol. "The fear-state produced by this method was quite characteristic. The patient's expression generally became fixed, his face flushed, the pupils sometimes dilated. Breathing became deeper and the pulse more forceful. The patient became obviously tense. Mute patients often began to talk in a frightened manner. Some patients implored someone to come to their aid; more frequently, however, the patient became very quiet." Each patient received 10 injections on successive days. One month then passed and again 10 injections were given. The duration of the fear state varied from a few minutes to, in one case, three hours. At the end of the experiment, the investigator concluded that "'fear' is not an active factor in metrazol therapy." Louis H. Cohen, "Fear in the Metrazol Treatment," *American Journal of Psychiatry* 95 (1939): 1349–1357.

[91] In 1945, Dr. C. E. Hanna, superintendent of the Brockville Hospital wrote to the director of the hospitals division that he agreed with discontinuing metrazol therapy and that he was relying exclusively on electroshock treatments. "Its convenience and absence of drug toxicity, as well as the lessened fear and dread experienced by patients in either Metrazol or Insulin therapy, would to my mind warrant its adoption exclusively." AO, RG 10, Section 107, Gen. 1–9–5, June 6, 1945, Dr. Hanna to Dr. R. C. Montgomery. At a 1947 meeting of the Ontario Neuropsychiatric Association one psychiatrist observed of electroshock: "I am still unable to quite accept with equanimity the reckless daring and abandon with which some investigators throw the switches and press the buttons of this purely empirical yet potentially dangerous therapeutic agent. Human beings are not Guinea pigs...." Discussion of Dr. Cathcart's Paper on Psychotherapy in Manic-Depressive Psychoses," unsigned MS, AO, RG 10 Box 52, HS 2–1, Central Files, Ontario Neuropsychiatric Association.

[92] Dr. C. B. Farrar, superintendent of the Toronto Psychiatric Hospital became editor of the *American Journal of Psychiatry* in July 1931, while Dr. George Stevenson, superintendent at London was President of the American Psychiatric Association from 1940 to 1941. On May 26, 1949, the *Globe* reported that Dr. Abraham Z. Barhash of the American National Committee for Mental Hygiene criticized the indiscriminate use of shock therapy as "neither physiological, nor medical, nor human, nor for that matter, honest."

[93] Oskar Dietholm, "An Historical View of Somatic Treatment in Psychiatry," *American Journal of Psychiatry*, 95 (1939): 1175. Dietholm was not so much concerned with patients' interests or rights as with careless and unscientific use of somatic methods and with trying to put the case for a "psycho-biological" psychiatry. The major conflict was between psycho-biologists and somaticists. In the ensuing discussion Dr. Ewen Cameron, then of the Worcester, Massachusetts Hospital, defended somatic treatments because "these attempts to utilize general medical procedures were healthy evidence of a determination to see psychiatry as one of the medical sciences." Cameron went on to warn that unless psychiatry adopted the techniques of general medicine, "the claims of the lay analyst and of the practicing psychologist would have been easier to vindicate." Although he also insisted that there were theoretical reasons why mental illness had to have a physical basis and thus had to be treated accordingly, for Cameron, somatic techniques were above all an important weapon in psychiatry's fight for professional status. Nonetheless, Dietholm's warning was a clear indication that not all psychiatrists agreed with the indiscriminate use of physical therapies.

[94] AO, RG 10, Series 107,. File 1, B.5, April 25, 1940, Dr. N. L. Easton to Dr. B. T. McGhie. Films continued to be a thorn in the side of the psychiatric profession. In October 1946, Dr. J. D. Griffin of the Canadian National Committee on Mental Hygiene wrote to the provincial censor complaining about negative portrayals of psychiatrists in recent movies: "The public is encouraged to believe that some, if not all, psychiatrists are ruthless, scheming criminals..." AO, RG 10, B. 55, HS 7–1, Oct. 29, 1946, Dr. J. D. Griffin to O. J. Silverthorne, Chairman, Motion Picture Censor Board.

[95] AO, RG 10, B. 55, HS 7–1, May 10, 1940, O. J. Silverthorne, to Dr. B. T. McGhie.

[96] AO, RG 10, B. 55, HS 7–1, November 4, 1946, Dr. J. T. Phair to Dr. Griffin.

[97] In 1954 the provincial solicitor wrote to the director of the mental health division concerning electroshock that "I would not think it would be necessary from a legal

standpoint to secure consent from relatives for this type of treatment." AO, RG 10, B. 115, Gen. P–2–8–1, July 15, 1954.

98 Dr. George Stevenson to Director, Hospitals Division, AO, RG 10, Box 96, Gen. C–24, September 12, 1949. At a meeting of the American Psychiatric Association in Washington D. C., Stevenson participated in a round table discussion on consent to electroshock during which the following colloquy took place: "Dr. Gee, (British Columbia):...'On the application of the admission by relative or friend, whoever assumes the legal responsibility, we have added a little clause whereby the individual gives consent to any form of therapy. Then the relative signs that and it is included in the form.' Dr. Toller (California): 'I wonder how many ask permission from the relative to give hypodermic injections, to give intravenous injections? This could go on to absurdity.' Dr. Stevenson (Ontario): 'That is putting the matter fairly. I think it is more culpable to withhold treatment. We as psychiatrists should see the patient is adequately treated. When shock therapies first came out we were pretty jittery; naturally, we got consent.' " *Better Care in Mental Hospitals*, Proceedings of the 1st Mental Hospital Institute of the American Psychiatric Association, Washington, D.C., April 11–15, 1949, cited in Leonard Roy Frank, ed., *The History of Shock Treatment* (San Francisco: Frank, 1978).

99 AO, RG 10, Series 107, Gen. 1–9–8, February 4, 1938, Dr. T. D. Cumberland to Dr. R. C. Montgomery.

100 AO, RG 10, Gen. C–24, September 27, 1949, Dr. G. Stevenson to C. H. Lewis.

101 AO, RG 10, Series 107, Gen. 1–9–1, April 21, 1948, C. Walker, Provincial Solicitor, to R. C. Montgomery.

102 AO, RG 10, HS 1–2, Box 50, Minutes, Superintendents' Conference, January 23, 1948. In his 1961 testimony before a U.S. Senate Subcommittee hearing, Dr. Manfred Guttmacher stated: "I think one should go to the extreme of always explaining to a patient if he is going to get electroshock why he is going to get it and what it is going to be like and so forth and so on. But as far as getting permission from the patient is concerned, this is not necessary." Testimony before United States Senate Subcommittee, *Constitutional Rights of the Mentally Ill: Part I, Civil Aspects*, U. S. Government Printing Office, Washington D.C., March 28–30, 1961, p. 155, cited in Frank, *Shock*.

103 "We are told that it is foolish to judge Charlemagne or Napoleon or Genghis Khan or Hitler or Stalin for their massacres... Likewise we are told that it is absurd to praise those benefactors of humanity whom the followers of Comte so faithfully celebrated... To this we can only answer that to accept this doctrine is to do violence to the basic notions of our morality, to misrepresent our sense of the past, and to ignore the most general concepts and categories of normal thought." Isaiah Berlin, *Historical Inevitability* (Toronto: Oxford University Press, 1953) 77.

2

Postwar Plans

> When a female patient came in she was always given a bath and had her hair washed. Some of these people had been to hairdressers, but we had to wash their hair and look for nits and things. It was very demoralizing for the patients and it upset me and many others, because as you can imagine you come in and the first thing they do is to take your clothes and you weren't given them back until three days later.
>
> Most often doctors would come and sit and talk with the patient, but seldom would the patients go up to their office. They spent about a week or two weeks on the ward in reception and then they would go to a ward. This was in the days before Largactil. We had lots of violent patients come in and the main treatment would be dry packs. The patient would be nude and you would take a sheet and fold it back and lie them on the sheet and wrap them up like a mummy, the only part that could move would be their head. You'd have to feed them in bed. A lot of them got better in spite of everything; time did it because it was impossible for the psychiatrists to see patients on a regular basis, they had 250 patients each. The tendency was to pay a lot of attention to the newer patients to see who they could help, and the others were in the background. And when they got well enough to get out of the hospital, then families didn't want them, or they had no place to go.
>
> A former psychiatric nurse

During the Second World War the Allied governments began to plan for the postwar period. The western democracies wanted to avoid a repetition of the 1930s when Germany and Italy fell under fascism, France was seriously split between forces of the extreme right and left, and other countries were racked by economic and social difficulties arising out of the Great Depression. Experts in the 1940s warned that if there were widespread unemployment and economic instability after the war, then political instability might follow. In France, the National Resistance Council had drawn up a program of nationalization and comprehensive social security planning. In Great Britain, the 1943 Beveridge Report became a bestseller and set the agenda for social policy for the postwar period. In Canada, the King government began to canvass the various provincial governments concerning health and social welfare policy. These planning exercises were aided by the success of the state in managing the economy and mobilizing manpower for the war effort. For the time being, war planning had mitigated the criticism that state regulation of the economy was bound to fail or to lead to political tyranny.

In these circumstances, and as part of a plan for federal subsidies for health care, the question arose of what role the federal government was to play in mental health care. Until the 1940s, that role had been minimal. Except for federal operation of a few mental hospitals for veterans such as the Westminster Hospital in London, Ontario, the federal government played almost no role in mental health policy. But in 1943, radical changes were afoot. Provincial health authorities were invited to make presentations before the House of Commons Committee on Social Security concerning a proposed national health insurance program. The federal government proposed to give grants-in-aid to the provinces amounting to one-ninth of provincial expenditures on mental hygiene and the care of the mentally ill. In return, the provinces would have to provide free treatment in mental hospitals to all those who required such treatment, establish mental hygiene clinics and increase the number of beds available for the mentally ill, mentally retarded and epileptic. Although Ontario's deputy minister of health B. T. McGhie was receptive to the idea, he and his fellow deputy ministers from the other provinces noted that if the provinces were forced to forgo income from paying patients in the mental hospitals, the proposed federal grant would not compensate them for the lost income. McGhie pointed out that, in fiscal 1942, Ontario collected $1,231,869 from paying patients. This was about 22 percent of total expenditures, better than Manitoba, which had recovered 19 percent, Saskatchewan, which had recovered 7.4 percent, and twice the national average of 10.5 percent.[1] Ontario's total expenditure on mental health for that year was $5,838,950, and one-ninth of that was $648,772. Under the federal plan that would have meant a loss of $583,097.[2] Obviously, the provincial mental health bureaucrats were not happy with this proposal. Before their presentation to the federal committee, McGhie canvassed the provincial deputy ministers and directors of mental health and found that Ontario's ideas on the future of mental health policy were widely shared. After some discussion, the officials agreed that the federal government would have to increase its contribution from one-ninth to 25 percent.

Psychiatry Under Health Insurance

Calling their brief *Psychiatry Under Health Insurance* the provincial mental health authorities set forth the conventional wisdom on mental health policy in the middle 1940s. Mental illness, it was argued, was all-pervasive. "Physicians in private practice have shown that from 20 percent to 70 percent of their patients present psychiatric or mental hygiene issues… It would probably be fair to say that 50 percent of patients visiting doctors' offices are not exclusively cases of physical illness but have psychological problems as well."[3] This rather wild variation in estimates of mental illness was typical of the period and reflected the extremely broad definition of mental illness and the lack of any common reporting standard among general practitioners. The provincial authorities stated that next to the problem of physical well-being, mental illness was the most important health problem of the time. They contended that practically everything—the stability of the family, the health of the community and the success or failure of industry—was influenced by the level of mental health in society. This was in keeping with the views on mental health disseminated by the Canadian National Committee on Mental Hygiene since the 1920s. One reason for dramatizing the pervasiveness and importance of mental illness was related to the demarcation between the mental health and the physical health systems—a separation which mental health professionals deeply resented. As long as medical doctors thought of mental illness as less "serious" than physical illness, then the mental health system and all those associated with it would suffer from public indifference or hostility, low status, low pay, and ultimately, from a lack of political power. Only if the mental health professionals could convince the government and elite decision-makers that mental illness was in fact an illness, if the ordinary general practitioner could be convinced that he should take mental illness seriously and be trained to identify and even treat certain forms of mental illness, and if the public could be convinced that mental health professionals were engaged in approximately the same kind of endeavour as medical doctors, then the gap between psychological and physical medicine might be bridged, with the mental health system reaping the benefits of enhanced status, improved finances and public standing.

This point of view was widely shared in the psychiatric profession. In a 1945 paper, *The Future Organization of the Psychiatric Services*, British psychiatrists, psychologists and medical doctors said "the argument for treating psychiatry in all essential respects like other branches of medicine [was] strong and conclusive…there is everything to be said for making the administrative structure of psychiatry exactly the same in principle and even in major detail as that of other branches of the health services."[4] Since many Canadian psychiatrists served in Great Britain during the war in close association with their British counterparts, their views on integrating mental health and general medicine were widely shared.

It was generally acknowledged in 1943 that ordinary general practitioners were unwilling (and in many cases, unable) to make a diagnosis of mental illness, and that there was a shortage of trained mental health professionals to deal with the problem. It was argued that the medical schools should include courses in psychiatry and in mental health, and that physicians should get some training in mental illness before entering into general practice. The provincial submission noted that one reason for these lacunae was that, in Canada, "psychiatry was the original form of state supported medical care. The relationship between mental institutions and general hospitals has unfortunately never been very close, although it has been improving in recent years. This circumstance has contributed in the past to keep psychiatry and general medicine apart."[5] It also meant that research and education in psychiatry lagged behind physical medicine. In 1937, the Mental Hospital Survey Committee had noted that one of the major disadvantages of the highly centralized Ontario system of mental health administration was that it discouraged innovation or originality in the field.

The Ontario mental health representatives suggested that one means for bridging the gap between physical and psychological medicine was "the establishment of full *psychiatric services in general hospitals*."[6] [their italics] The example cited was that of the Henry Ford Hospital in Detroit which had maintained a psychiatric service since the 1920s. The brief advocated the establishment of psychiatric wards in general hospitals of fifty beds or more. The wards would be for short treatment only, with those who developed prolonged illnesses being directed toward the provincial mental hospitals. Another major theme in the presentation concerned prevention of mental illness. In addition to the usual pleas for better public education in mental hygiene, the travelling mental health clinics were cited as playing an important role in prevention. Ontario proposed that in the future the clinics should be permanently based in "public health centres" where, with a "greatly increased psychiatric staff, including physicians, social workers and psychologists" they would help to keep people in the community who might otherwise end up in a provincial mental hospital. Exactly what form public health centres were supposed to take was not spelled out in the report.

Finally, the large percentage of elderly people in provincial mental hospitals constituted a major problem. In 1943, 17 percent of those admitted to mental institutions in British Columbia were over 70 years of age, while in Ontario 20 percent of admissions were comprised of people over the age of 60. The Ontario brief also recommended that separate hospitals for the elderly mentally ill be created.

With regard to aftercare, the submission first noted a scarcity of trained social service personnel, especially social workers trained in psychiatry, and advocated improved training and recruitment in the profession. Second, it called for an expansion in the boarding out or approved home system. Whereas in California the number of patients boarding out in 1942 was 21 percent of the total on the books of the mental hospitals, in Ontario only 3–4 percent were listed as boarding out. The brief did not spell out the reasons for this radical difference.

Aside from some vague remarks about basing travelling clinics in the community, no attention at all was paid to a problem that had already arisen in Great Britain and the United States and that was beginning to come to the attention of the Ontario authorities: how to deal with mentally ill people who had been returned to the community from the mental hospitals. Certainly the travelling clinics, even if permanently based, could not carry out the function of aftercare since they were mainly directed toward assessment and testing. The proposed psychiatric wards in the general hospital could not perform aftercare functions since they were intended to provide short-term treatment facilities, while the provincial mental hospitals were swamped with patients and had neither the personnel nor the funds to accomplish the task.

Moreover, nothing at all was said about the role of municipal governments which were perennially and universally unwilling to fund or administer social welfare programs. Yet, some way had to be found to reduce the large numbers of chronic and/or elderly patients in the mental hospitals, and to get the municipalities to play a role in providing housing and social welfare services.

Nor was anything said about the future of the large provincial institutions which were geographically and socially isolated from the community. Rather, it was widely assumed that the provinces needed more large mental hospitals. The fact that since the 1920s Dr. Hincks and the CNCMH had advocated smaller regional hospitals linked to university medical departments was ignored.[7]

Little attention was devoted to these important problems because the dominant, overwhelming question was what to do about the terrible overcrowding in provincial mental hospitals. In 1943, overcrowding in Ontario averaged 30 percent. It was estimated that 2,500 additional beds were required for the mentally ill, and 2,000 beds for mentally retarded people.[8] It seemed obvious that if additional resources were made available by the federal government then they should be directed toward a major expansion of hospital bed capacity.

The McGhie Plan

Despite the parliamentary committee's apparent interest and sympathy, little was done in 1943 about either health insurance or mental health matters. Thus, McGhie decided to take the initiative. If the federal government would not act, Ontario would.

On May 8, 1944, McGhie circulated to the superintendents of Ontario's psychiatric hospitals the most radical and innovative proposal for reform ever seen in the history of Ontario's mental health policy.[9] If adopted, it would have led to a complete reorganization of mental health services, the establishment of a community based system and it might have prepared the ground for an aftercare system that could have avoided the problems that occurred three decades later.

McGhie thought of the future of the mental health system in terms of two priorities: vastly increased bed capacity in existing or new mental hospitals and the establishment of a preventive health care system located outside the mental hospitals and modelled along the lines of the existing public health system. McGhie proposed that the province be divided into five mental health districts, and that the total bed requirements be based on a figure of five beds per thousand for the mentally ill and one and one half beds per thousand for mentally retarded people. On this basis he estimated that the province needed an additional 5,332 beds. This meant expanding the St. Thomas hospital from 1,822 to 2,300 beds, (although one superintendent recommended to McGhie that St. Thomas "be increased to three, four or five thousand"), the demolition of most of the mental hospitals in London and the construction there of a 1,500 bed institution for mentally retarded people, the construction of a new 1,150 bed mental hospital in the Sudbury-Parry Sound area and a new mental hospital in the Port Arthur area.[10] In addition, McGhie recommended the establishment of a separate 1,000 bed geriatric hospital for "the old age group," and a 1,000 bed tuberculosis sanitorium in Brampton.

In the same document McGhie included a separate position paper prepared by Dr. George Stevenson, superintendent of the Londonhospitals;London mental hospital, recommending a two-tier system of mental health care, with provincial institutions providing "only standard accommodation" and private "sanitariums" providing "private care." Under this scheme, the province would pay to the private mental hospitals an amount equal to the provincial mental hospital per capita maintenance charges, with the patient or his family paying any additional charges. Thus, the province would provide basic care while private institutions would provide a higher level of care for those who could afford to pay additional fees. Some years later the province did create a two-tier system, but it was exactly the opposite of that proposed by Stevenson. The Homes for Special Care Program of 1964 established a second, lower tier of care for residents of psychiatric and mental retardation institutions who, it was argued, could no longer benefit from active care. Wracked by controversy and scandal since its inception, the Homes for Special Care program provided care at a lower per diem rate than that of the mental hospitals.

At the same time, McGhie proposed reorienting the municipal health services toward prevention rather than control of communicable diseases. "Under this new approach," he wrote,

> the lessening of preventable illness becomes the keystone of our public health arch... Direct reference should... be made to preventive dentistry, nutrition, housing and industrial hygiene. Mental health will be particularly significant from the point of view of our mental health program...[11]

Under the proposed scheme, local boards of health would be replaced with "a compact administrative unit" located in urban municipalities, and serving a population of 30,000 to 35,000. These units would include two physicians, each with some training in psychiatry, a dentist, six to seven public health nurses, two sanitary officers and a personnel officer with training in psychology. The unit would function under the "direction of a unit Board of Health made up of five to seven interested residents appointed by the County and Municipal Councils of the area," with the government appointing one member of the unit. These new boards would come under a regional headquarters which would include a mental health clinic "with a psychiatrist, social worker or nurse." There would be twenty mental health clinics which would "operate from a Regional Headquarters and not necessarily from an existing mental hospital." In conclusion, McGhie added: "It is hoped that the above short outline may assist you in visualizing the manner in which we are attempting to plan a postwar psychiatric service for the entire Province." Unquestionably, McGhie saw the future development of community mental health services through the lens of public health.[12]

McGhie's proposal was the last gasp of a perspective which put public health at the centre of mental health care. Proposals to give public health some role in mental health continued to be put forward until the mid–1960s, but never again would anyone so highly placed in the government argue so strongly and coherently for a preventive public health structure. The problem was that the history of mental health policy militated against its success. In order for a policy to succeed it must have some political support, but aside from personnel in the public health sector, who was there to support McGhie's ideas? The psychiatrists, as will be seen, were desperately trying to get a foothold in the general hospitals where their prestige and salaries would rise. The superintendents and staff of the mental hospitals were still begging for increased funds to deal with overcrowding. It is true that the Canadian National Committee on Mental Hygiene had supported the idea of prevention in the past, but key members of the Committee were still in the armed services, and if the attempt to exclude the Committee from a federal advisory committee some years later is any indication of sentiment in 1944 [see Chapter 5], then there was little sympathy in Ottawa, or later, in Ontario, for the National Committee's position. In the absence of any major public or private interest group fighting for a community-based, preventive mental health system, only political pressure might have brought McGhie's ideas to fruition. But as had been the case for decades, mental health policy was squarely based on the big institutions, and these were seen mainly as sources of jobs or funds for local communities.

In addition, the psychiatrists had a different set of priorities. In 1943, there were 57 psychiatrists from Ontario who had enlisted in the armed forces, and they had prepared their own submission to McGhie.[13] They began with an appeal for increased salaries and compensation which, they argued, "have not been adequate."[14] This was a continuing complaint which had only mitigated during the Depression when jobs were scarce. But in the postwar climate the province would have to raise salaries if it were to draw psychiatrists away from private practice and into government service. The report also proposed that more courses in psychiatry be offered and that clinical teaching be done in general hospital wards. It was suggested that undergraduates spend at least one month at a provincial mental hospital in an observation unit (where individuals were remanded from courts for psychiatric observation) or in a mental health clinic. Further training would be made available after three to five years, there would be exchanges with other state or provincial institutions in Ontario, and additional psychiatric social workers would be trained.

The psychiatrists emphasized that observation units and mental health clinics should not be located in mental hospitals and instead advocated the establishment of observation wards, wards for "acute psychotics" and outpatient clinics in general hospitals, where psychiatrists could treat the mentally ill. Psychiatrists based in the general hospital might double as mental health clinic directors. By contrast, McGhie's sketch of the future shape of psychiatric services said nothing at all about psychiatric units or wards in general hospitals, emphasizing instead the important role of mental health clinics linked with public health in the community. Clearly, the psychiatrists were anxious to expand mental health care into the general hospitals, with themselves as the directing authorities.

One controversial question concerned the location of the mental health clinics. McGhie had proposed they be run from regional health units, but some superintendents felt they should operate from general hospitals, while one superintendent objected to separating the clinic from the provincial hospital because, he felt, it would further isolate it from the community and reinforce the stigma associated with the provincial hospitals. All the superintendents endorsed the proposal set forth in Stevenson's memorandum for establishing psychiatric wards in general hospitals.[15]

However, there were a number of reasons why McGhie's ambitious proposals for reforming Ontario's mental health system came to naught. Probably the most far-seeing and innovative of Ontario's mental health bureaucrats, McGhie's death in 1945 removed a major force for change from the political stage. There was only lukewarm support for community mental health among the medical superintendents and psychiatrists employed in provincial service. There was a change in the Minister of Health in 1946, with Dr. Reginald Vivian giving way, in January 1946 to Russell Kelley. Kelley was an ardent proponent of the psychiatric unit system. Finally, there was the irrefutable fact that institutions were jammed to overcapacity and that if tax dollars were to be spent, it would be easier to defend expenditures on institutions rather than on public health.

The Ontario Health Survey

In the late 1940s and 1950s, it was generally agreed that there was a pressing need for more mental health beds. Institutions were overburdened and the pressure of numbers continued to grow. The 1940 Rowell-Sirois report noted that additional beds were needed, while a national survey of health resources conducted during the war had remarked on bed shortages.[16]

With the establishment of a federal Department of National Health and Welfare in 1944, and the appointment of a chief of the mental health division, the federal government began to play an active role in mental health policy. In 1948, the National Health Grants Program began to direct money toward increasing the stock of mental hospital beds. The Ontario government used federal funds to expand existing institutions or to construct new, large ones.[17] Despite the increase in bed capacity, however, there seemed no relief from the pressure of rising numbers.

One of the requirements of the National Health Grants Program of 1948 was that each province do a survey of its existing health resources, including mental health resources. On September 9, 1948, Minister of Health Dr. Mackinnon Phillips appointed a six-member Ontario Health Survey Committee (OHSC). Upon undertaking its task the OHSC noted: "This study of existing facilities for diagnosis and treatment of mental illness in Ontario, and the inadequacy of those facilities leaves no room for complacency."[18] Because of its critical tone, the Ontario government delayed releasing the report until 1952, so that its findings were already four years old when the report was published.

The OHSC report shows that there had been almost no major changes in the shape of Ontario's mental health system since the 1930s. Despite suggestions that the province reduce the size of mental hospitals, integrate the mental health system with physical medicine by establishing psychiatric wards in general hospitals, extend mental health care into the community through mental health clinics and aftercare services, very little had been done to meet these objectives.[19]

In 1948, the Ontario mental health system remained a hospital centered system. As part of a plan to increase the capacity of existing institutions and to build new ones, the government announced in 1947 that it would construct a 2,400 bed hospital for mentally retarded people at Smith's Falls[20] as well as a new institution in the north.[21] The OHSC noted that on the basis of federal government calculations 11,416 mental hospital beds would have to be added to the existing 13,021. Even then, this would fall short of New York State's bed/population ratio by about 6,000 beds. With regard to mental health clinics and psychiatric wards in general hospitals, the OHSC noted that the situation had hardly changed since 1945, and the province was as far as could be from achieving McGhie's 1944 proposal of establishing "at least" twenty mental health clinics. In 1948, there were four travelling clinics whose staff was supposed to consist of a psychiatrist, psychologist and social worker. At one clinic, however, there was no social worker, one outpatient clinic in the Niagara area was staffed by one part-time psychiatrist, and there was an outpatient department at the Toronto Psychiatric Hospital. Fourteen general hospitals had mental health clinics "limited in that they are usually part of the neuro-psychiatric service of the medical department" and some clinic facilities were scattered around the rest of the province.[22] Despite McGhie's 1943 proposal that mental health clinics be linked to municipal or regional health units, there were only two such clinics in the entire province in 1948. The OHSC also found that of 146 general hospitals in the province only three had separate accommodation for a total of 54 psychiatric patients.

The report noted that a "shortage of trained personnel—traceable to weaknesses in both psychiatric training facilities and the salary scale for such specialists in this province—is an underlying cause of the critical shortcomings in Ontario's mental health program."[23] Ontario mental hospitals had only half the physicians they needed, with a ratio of one physician for every 301 patients, or a total of 53 available for ward duty. From 1935 to 1939, the number of physicians in the mental hospital service had increased, mainly because of the Depression, but then it declined with the war and thereafter remained static. During the period from 1935 to 1949, 91 physicians resigned from the mental health service, not including those who retired or died. In the postwar period, the financial attractions of private practice far outweighed the low salary and poor working conditions in the provincial system. Moreover, there were only 37 psychiatrists in private practice in the province, and 25 of these were located in Toronto. Finally, the Committee found that mental health facilities for children and in the court system were totally inadequate.[24]

The OHSC's recommendations followed the same pattern as those that had been made in the past: beds should be added to the mental hospital system, $500,000 should be given to Ontario universities to train psychiatrists and additional professional personnel, 53 psychiatrists should be added to the medical staffs of the existing hospitals, additional social workers, psychologists, occupational therapists and physiotherapists should be hired, and a special institution for geriatric patients should be constructed. The OHSC also recommended that 31 mental health clinics be established in general hospitals throughout the province, and that psychiatric units be developed in public hospitals. This was a clear departure from Dr. B. T. McGhie's suggestion in 1943 that mental health clinics be established as "public health centres."[25] Only some of these suggestions were followed. Thanks to the federal government's hospital construction grant program, the Department of Health added 4,800 mental hospital beds from 1951 to 1955, and planned to add a further 4,000 to the existing stock.[26] However, beds were added to very large hospitals. By 1955, the gigantic St. Thomas institution had 1,800 patients; the Smith's Falls institution for mentally retarded people, opened in 1951, was intended to house 2,400 patients. In 1955, it was announced that a new hospital in the north at Port Arthur, later Thunder Bay, would house 1,200 people, that construction had begun on a 1,200 bed hospital in North Bay, that there was to be a 700 bed addition at the Hamilton hospital, and 500 bed additions to the Kingston and London institutions.[27]

In the 1950s, therefore, mental health policy chugged along the same tracks that had been laid down in the nineteenth century when the vast majority of funds and personnel were devoted to the large provincial institutions. McGhie's attempt to strike out in the direction of public health had failed. Although most psychiatrists and mental health bureaucrats in the 1950s realized that the mental hospitals could not continue to expand indefinitely and that some alternative would have to be found, they were stymied by the inexorable pressure for new beds. The only major acceptable alternative was to establish psychiatric wards or units in the general hospitals. This appealed to psychiatrists because they believed that psychiatric units would be therapeutically and organizationally beneficial for mentally ill people and because, happily, it suited their professional aspirations to link themselves as closely as possible to general medicine.

Notes

1 AO, RG 10, H.S. 36–2, Appendix 4, May 8, 1943, *Psychiatry Under Health Insurance.*

2 AO, RG 10, B. 76, H.S. 36–1, April 12, 1943, McGhie to Dr. Robert W. MacKay, Medical Superintendent, Nova Scotia Hospitals.

3 *Psychiatry Under Health Insurance*, Draft of Report to be made to the Special Committee on Social Security on May 18, 1943, May 8, 1943.

4 Kathleen Jones, *Mental Health and Social Policy: 1845–1959* (London: Routledge and Kegan Paul, 1960) 148.

5 *Psychiatry Under Health Insurance* 4.

6 *Psychiatry Under Health Insurance* 4. The 1929 Royal Commission on Public Welfare had recommended that: "There ought also to be psychiatric wards and equipment in

the larger General Hospitals." *Report*, (Ontario: Royal Commission on Public Welfare, 1930) 31.

7 Canadian Mental Health Association, *More for the Mind* (Toronto: Canadian Mental Health Association, 1963) 5.

8 AO, RG 10, H. S. 36–2, Appendix, May 10, 1943, Dr. G. Stevenson, "Treatment of Psychopathic Disorders," p. 7.

9 AO, RG 10, Series 107, File HS 1–2, May 8, 1944, McGhie to All Superintendents of Ontario Hospitals.

10 AO, RG 10, B. 50 HS 1–2, May 26, 1944, Dr. T. D. Cumberland, Superintendent, the Ontario Hospital, New Toronto, to Dr. B. T. McGhie.

11 AO, RG 10, Series 107, Box 50, File HS 1–2, 1944, Ontario Department of Health, Office of Deputy Minister, "To All Superintendents of Ontario Hospitals, Municipal Health services."

12 This was the era when mental hygiene linked to public health was assumed by all mental health authorities to be a major weapon in the fight against mental illness. In his report to the Royal Commission on Dominion-Provincial Relations, A. E. Grauer called his section on mental health, "mental hygiene," and he noted: "The importance and ramifications of mental hygiene have only recently been realized. Public health doctors are agreed 'That there is no problem of public health which is more important…'" A. E. Grauer, *Public Health* (Ottawa: Royal Commission on Dominion-Provincial Relations, 1939) 41.

13 Legislative Assembly of Ontario *Debates* March 30, 1950. [Hereafter referred to as *Debates*].

14 AO, RG 10–107, HS 1–2, May 8, 1944, McGhie "To All Superintendents," Appendix, "Future Policy of Psychiatric Services in Ontario."

15 AO, RG 10, B. 50 HS 1–2, Memos to McGhie from Drs. J. R. McGeoch, May 22, 1944; Dr. C. A. Cleland, May 24, 1944; Dr. J. S. Stewart, May 23, 1944; Dr. E. A. Clark, May 13, 1944; Dr. C. M. Crawford, May 25, 1944, Dr. G. Stevenson, May 16, 1944; Dr. S. J. W. Horne, May 18, 1944; Dr. T. D. Cumberland, May 26, 1944; Dr. C. A. McClenahan, May 23, 1944.

16 See Alex Richman, *Psychiatric Care in Canada: Extent and Results* (Ottawa: Royal Commission on Health Services, 1966) 5 and A. E. Grauer 41–49.

17 On the history of the National Health Grants Program see (Ottawa: Royal Commission on Health Services, 1966) 31–46.

18 Ontario Health Survey Committee, *Report* (Ontario Health Survey Committee: Toronto, 1952) 110.

19 In 1930 the Ross Commission recommended that new mental hospitals be built on a cottage system principle. See, Royal Commission on Public Welfare, *Report* (Ontario: Royal Commission on Public Welfare, August 13, 1930) 107.

20 *Debates*, Statement of G. H. Doucet, Minister of Public Works, March 28, 1950, p. B–9.

21 *Debates*, March 31, 1947, p. 669.

[22] OHSC 116.

[23] OHSC 110. In 1988, low salaries and a stressful working environment were blamed for a 26 percent shortfall of psychiatrists in Ontario's mental health system. See "The Missing Shrinks," *Globe and Mail* 8 March 1988.

[24] *Debates*, March 30, 1950, p. DD–6.

[25] AO, RG 10, B. 76, HS 36–1, May 19, 1943, McGhie to Dr. G. F. Amyot, Provincial Health Officer, Victoria, B.C.: "[M]ental health clinics [should] be based on public health centres rather than on the mental hospital."

[26] *Debates*, Statement of Premier Leslie Frost, March 15, 1955, p. 775.

[27] *Debates*, March 10, 1955, p. 1142.

3

Mental Health Clinics and Public Health

> The mental hygiene movement was reaching its peak in the 1950s and 1960s. The thing you wanted to do was to get out into the community and start a mental hygiene movement. We were very naive then, you got out into the community with a team with nurses and went into schools and the community... We came to realize that this didn't work, just by seeing kids at school age didn't prevent mental illness later in life.
>
> Former psychiatric hospital superintendent

B. T. McGhie and the Travelling Clinics

Thanks to efforts of the Canadian National Committee on Mental Hygiene, in the 1930s mental health authorities were convinced that the future of mental health policy lay in improving preventive services. However, one unforseen result of the CNCMH's criticisms of the large mental hospitals had been to lower their prestige in the eyes of the medical profession, thus making it even more difficult to recruit young doctors into psychiatry. This added to an already desperate shortage of psychiatrists willing to work in the provincial mental hospital system. At the same time, Canadian authorities learned that in Europe and the United States, psychopathic hospitals, outpatient clinics in general hospitals and mental health clinics had been established so as to reduce admissions to the large mental hospital.[1] The Ontario Royal Commission on Public Welfare of 1930 had mentioned "the need of preventive work, which is made possible to some extent by outpatient clinics attached to the mental hospitals... a very few cases where mental disease is checked before entrance to the hospital becomes necessary, would save the province enough money to pay for an out-door clinic attached to the hospital."[2] Thus, while the Depression prevented the government from directly attacking the terrible overcrowding in the large hospitals, it did lead to a search for alternatives.

In implementing the mental health clinic program in 1930, B. T. McGhie was following Massachusetts which had established 33 outpatient clinics mandated to provide aftercare, family care and mental hygiene services to specific geographical areas.[3] According to C. R. Myers, a psychologist in the Department of Health in the 1930s, McGhie had visited the Judge Baker Child Guidance Clinic in

Boston with Dr. Clarence Hincks of the Canadian National Committee on Mental Hygiene and had seen first hand the accomplishments of community mental health.[4]

In the spring of 1930, and in the summer and fall of 1931, the Department of Health established six mental health clinics operating out of six of Ontario's mental hospitals. Each clinic team consisted of a psychiatrist, a psychologist and a social worker. The clinic attached to the Toronto Psychiatric Hospital, established in 1925 mainly as a research institution, was stationary and acted as an outpatient clinic. The remaining five clinics were given what eventually turned out to be an impossible task: to travel through their catchment area five days a week providing preventive services through early diagnosis, consultation and education, follow-up services for mental patients discharged from, or on probation from the hospital, and visiting patients in approved boarding homes.[5]

What the travelling clinic teams encountered as they travelled throughout Ontario was a degree of misery and illness that no one seems to have anticipated. From the very beginning their services were overwhelmed, not just by sheer numbers, but because individuals and social agencies brought to the clinic people with every conceivable kind of problem. According to one report: "When first organized there was a marked tendency on the part of the community to refer cases of mental defect to the clinics."[6] In 1939, two percent or 44 cases were brought to the clinics because of "truancy," four percent for "stealing," three percent because of "sex," and two percent because of "incorrigibility." It quickly became clear that there was a crying need in the province for specialized children's services, because by 1936, 78.2 percent of the people seen by the clinics were 21 years of age or under, while 56.5 percent were 13 years or younger.[7] But the province had neither the funds nor the political will to expand services any further, and so the clinic teams soldiered on, increasingly frustrated because of their inability to follow up cases brought to their attention during their flying visits. In 1936, in the midst of the Depression, the deputy minister of health told the superintendents of the Ontario mental hospitals that the primary goal of the clinics was to keep people out of the mental hospitals, since they were "jammed to the doors." He warned them that the "clinics must either justify their existence by limiting admissions to mental hospitals or quit."[8]

By the 1940s the directors of the various mental health clinics were complaining about their difficulties to the Department of Health. In November 1947, the director of the mental health clinic at the Brockville mental hospital stated his "concern" about the "increasing case load." He observed:

> Certain agencies, chiefly the Children's Aid Societies, have come to put a great deal of reliance on the examination of their wards by the clinic. This has resulted in an almost overwhelming number of cases, most numerous of which are probably unmarried mothers, and...a number of overseas guests. The result has been a forced curtailment of the amount of time spent on more psychiatric problems by the clinic psychologist.[9]

Apparently the Children's Aid Societies were requesting that the psychologist attached to the clinic team administer IQ tests to unmarried mothers. After years of propaganda by pressure groups and some members of the medical profession, the belief that unmarried mothers frequently suffered from mental retardation had finally reached rural Ontario communities. Thus, despite their declared intention of working to prevent mental illness and to help care for those who were mentally ill, the travelling clinics found themselves motoring up and down every highway and byway on the province's social problem map. The irony is that there was no proof at all that the travelling clinics helped to reduce the numbers of admissions to the mental hospitals, and some evidence that they helped increase the numbers. For, despite their best efforts to return people to the community for treatment by social agencies and physicians, or to their families, the clinics constantly turned up people who were recommended for institutionalization. Of the 31,688 new cases the clinics saw from 1930 to 1940, 4,521, or 14.2 percent were recommended for commitment in a provincial institution. It is open to question whether these people would have been institutionalized if they had never visited the mental health clinics.

In addition to the mental health clinic program, McGhie established the first approved homes program in the province. The approved homes were patterned after the Scottish boarding-out system whereby mental patients were placed in homes—frequently owned by staff members—near the institution, with the government paying a per diem allowance to the owner.[10] Two kinds of patients were sent to the approved homes: those patients who, it was thought, might be returned to the community but who needed a protected environment to reestablish themselves, and chronic incurables who were harmless but needed supervision. The program began in 1933, and by 1936 there were 392 patients in the various approved boarding homes. By the 1940s the number of patients transferred to boarding homes began to level off. In 1940, there were 550 patients in approved boarding homes, but in 1947, the number had fallen to 467.[11] A variety of reasons seem to account for the fact that the program trod water during the 1940s. One was the sheer difficulty in finding people who were willing to run the approved homes. Despite the fact the government paid a per diem allowance for each patient in the home, it was mainly hospital staff who had the skills and experience necessary to run the homes, and only a limited number of these people were available. In addition, hospitals like Whitby conceived of the approved homes as halfway houses, that is, as residences that could be used temporarily by patients on their way to jobs in the community or to other agencies. Patients who were not expected to move on were returned to the hospital. Since any mental hospital would have only a limited number of people who could function on their own in the community, the pool was quickly used up. Jobs were also scarce and employers were reluctant to take on ex-mental patients. In 1940, Dr. C. A. Buck calculated that one third of those placed in approved homes had returned to hospital, one third had been discharged, and one third remained in the homes.[12] Finally, the war years had limited the funds and personnel available for all programs, not just the approved homes program.

With the departure of most psychiatrists during the war, the clinic program continued, but with reduced staff and responsibilities. However, the population of the large hospitals continued to grow and there seemed no end in sight to the demand for services. After 1945, superintendents, psychiatrists and politicians complained bitterly about overcrowded, understaffed and underfunded mental hospitals, and demanded additional support from government.[13]

Most authorities now agreed that the future of mental health policy lay in prevention and in some form of community care. If only incipient mental illness could be detected, diagnosed and treated in the community, then the problem could be brought under control, fewer people would be committed to the large hospitals, and additional funds could be found to improve conditions. An article on mental health in Canada in the May 1947 issue of *Canadian Forum* noted: "Today community psychiatry—psychiatry dealing with people who are emotionally disturbed but not mentally ill—offers the greatest promise in the entire field of health."[14] In a feature article for the *Globe and Mail*, Dr. J. D. Griffin, General Director of the Canadian Mental Health Association wrote: "As the emphasis in fighting mental illness is placed on the treatment of early cases, it is essential that the battle must leave the hospitals and move out into the community."[15] But what was meant by community care and what form should it take?

Community Care

Generally the term referred indiscriminately to a variety of services including mental health clinics, outpatient clinics in general hospitals, psychiatric units, education programs on mental hygiene in the public schools and to an increased role for psychiatrists in alerting and educating the community about mental illness and mental health. The vagueness about the nature of community care and community psychiatry was a concomitant of the view that mental illness was, as Dr. Griffin put it in 1953, "a breakdown in living."[16] In this view the community became the patient and it was the community that had to be treated.[17] Or, as one expert put it in 1964, "Communities must be seen as personalities."[18]

At this time community care, public health and prevention were all thought of as falling within the same theoretical framework. These links were noted in 1933 by C. E. A. Winslow, professor of public health at Yale University.

> The mental hygiene movement, then, bears the same relation to psychiatry that the public health movement, of which it forms a part, bears to medicine in general. It is an organized community response to a recognized community need; and it lays its prime emphasis on the detection and the control of those incipient maladjustments with which the physician *qua* physician never comes into contact, unless specific community machinery and far-flung educational facilities are provided for the purpose.[19]

However, in Ontario, as in many other jurisdictions in North America, the growth of community mental health services was hardly an "organized community response." Rather, since the end of the nineteenth century, governments and private agencies had established a series of disparate services ranging from child guidance clinics, mental health clinics, and psychopathic hospitals, to outpatient clinics, psychiatric wards or units in general hospitals and other specialized services in the community. These arose in response to specific concerns of the period. The child guidance clinics initially aimed at preventing juvenile delinquency in large urban areas, while later they were used to detect mental retardation. The mental health clinics were aimed at early detection and treatment of mental illness, while outpatient clinics and psychiatric units were intended to treat mentally ill people close to their communities, without having to institutionalize them in the large psychiatric hospitals. It was only after the Second World War that serious thought was given to integrating these services into a community mental health services network. Still, the question was, which services were to be the backbone of community mental health?

In 1955, the Department of Health published a 38-page report on community mental health services. The most complete document on community mental health yet published by the Department, it included a detailed accounting of community mental health services in the province as well as recommendations for the future. The report painted a gloomy picture of community mental health services which were underfunded, maldistributed throughout the province, administered in a bewildering variety of ways, supported financially by the province and the federal government but avoided like the plague by municipalities and lacking a clearly defined mission. The travelling clinics, for example, covered enormous distances, but aside from diagnostic functions, could do nothing in the way of treatment. Indeed, Dr. C. A. Roberts, chief of the mental health division of the federal Department of National Health and Welfare suggested a reappraisal of the travelling clinics, noting that, "I feel that the future contributions by travelling clinics will not be very great."[20]

In 1954, there were 32 mental health clinics in Ontario, five of them attached to the various provincial mental hospitals, and the rest financed and administered in a variety of ways. At this time, $195,220 or 25 percent of the total cost of $765,320 for the various community mental health clinics came from the province, and 64 percent from the federal government.[21] The Department of Health admitted that the Ontario program "is constantly handicapped and is itself a constant source of irritation" to the public and to staff.[22] One reason was because the public wrongly assumed that the province funded the mental health program when in fact it was substantially funded by the federal government. Moreover, the municipalities "have not accepted responsibility for a mental health programme to any significant extent either directly or indirectly." The reason was the local government's suspicion that acknowledging some responsibility for a mental health program might eventually lead them to be saddled with it if the provincial or federal governments pulled out. Most services were "living a hand-to-mouth existence" and there was a general feeling that additional services were required. In "several instances" it was found that clinics had actually spent less than the amount received through federal grants.[23]

There were also continuing complaints about the short duration of their visits and the fact that the travelling clinics were unable to provide more than a cursory service. Certainly, the clinics were unevenly distributed throughout the province. It was estimated that the population of areas not served by the clinics was 937,000, while 365,000 people received only token service. This constituted about 25 percent of Ontario's population. According to the report, "[i]n most areas of Ontario the psychiatric facilities that do exist are spread too thinly and the clinic staffs are constantly pressed for service which they are unable to provide." Although New York State's standard was one clinic team per 50,000 population, the Ontario authorities recommended providing "minimal" service, defined as one clinic team per 100,000 people. This was despite the fact that the provincial regional consultant psychiatrists had concluded that if the standard was one clinic team per 100,000 people, then "the provision of really adequate service by a provincial agency [is] a technical impossibility."[24]

There was also "a lack of facilities for the care of psychotic or seriously disturbed children." The clinics lacked a "clearly defined function" and as a result they were asked by schools and social and welfare agencies to provide services which did not come under the heading of mental health.[25]

In order to deal with these problems, the report recommended that some travelling clinics be converted into outpatient services and given permanent homes in provincial hospitals. At the same time, the number of mental health clinics in urban areas would be increased by 26. A cost-sharing scheme was suggested with the municipal, provincial and federal governments each contributing one-third of the cost.

By August 1956, it appeared that the Department of Health was about to establish a community mental health program under the auspices of local public health units.[26] Because the community program would exclude psychiatric units which would be expected to operate solely within the general hospitals, the psychiatric units would be unable to apply for federal national health grant assistance. This quickly provoked a memo warning that adoption of a community mental health program which excluded psychiatric units would deprive each unit of between $17,000 and $50,000 per year in federal funds.[27]

In May 1957, Dr. H. W. Henderson, director of community mental health wrote to a local medical officer of health that the Department was trying "to formulate a comprehensive program that will foster the development of Community Mental Health Services throughout the Province."[28] Noting that mental health services functioned best when there was some financial contribution from the community, Dr. Henderson proposed that the Department of Health provide the professional staff, while the municipality would "assume all other expenses in establishing and maintaining a service," amounting to one-third of the full cost of the clinic. Henderson also recommended that there be "consultation with the Medical Officer of Health and suitable representatives from the community." He suggested the establishment of a mental health committee of the local board of health, composed of the medical officer of health, the director of the clinic and "three citizens" to deal with activities related to mental health problems. This committee would "assist in the planning and development of adequate services" for the community, including policy formulation for the clinic, obtaining funds and "negotiations for extending services to the courts, schools and other agencies in the community." The committee would also review annually the activities of the clinic, submit a statement of expenditures to the director of community mental health services, submit a report on services, an account of the budget and proposals for operations for the following year. Yet, compared to B. T. McGhie's earlier sketch of a community mental health system integrated with public health, Henderson's proposal for community participation in the mental health clinic system was a minor administrative reform.

Moreover, by July 1957, it became clear that the clinics would be relocated in the provincial psychiatric hospitals, that community mental health services would be provided mainly by the psychiatric units and that community clinics would be established where services could not be provided by either the psychiatric or the general hospitals. Dr. Henderson observed to Dr. B. H. McNeel, the chief of the mental health branch, that the provincial mental hospitals were expected to assume responsibility for community mental health services in the province "so far as this is possible." Community mental health clinics would be established "in collaboration with the municipal or county health authorities" in those rural and urban areas which could not be served by clinics based in the provincial mental hospitals.[29] By this time as well, the mental health branch had changed its mind about putting the local mental health committee under the board of health. Rather, the mental health committee would be an autonomous body with representation from the board of health, and with its members chosen by the director of the clinic and the medical officer of health, subject to the approval of the Department of Health. Since the clinic director was chosen by the Department of Health, this meant an assertion of departmental influence over the local mental health committee. Nor was it just over the local mental health clinics that the mental health division wished to exercise its authority, for in October 1957, the director of community mental health services advised the chief of the mental health division that "the community services provided by an Ontario Hospital are the direct concern and responsibility of the director of community mental health services."[30] According to Dr. Henderson, "matters of policy and function of these Clinics could best be determined in terms of the overall plan rather than the local situation." Thus, "policy with respect to the development of services in any area" would be determined by the provincial Department of Health in Toronto, not by local officials *in situ*. However, there was one problem with these plans. As Dr. Henderson noted in October 1957: "At the present time we are unable to proceed with our plans for the establishment of additional community mental health services because of the shortage of professional staff."

The issue was put on December 6, 1962 in the form of three questions to the chief of the mental health branch (the Department of Health changed mental health from division to branch to division a number of times from the 1940s to the 1980s) by the director of community mental health:

> Should any new Provincial Mental Health Clinics be established, other than those located in a Provincial Hospital? In an effort to encourage the development of services in public general hospitals, should preference be given to the establishment of a local service under the administrative responsibility of a general hospital rather than a public health department or a public health unit? If we are to abandon the policy of Provincial services in the ratio of one clinic team per 100,000 population, should we not attempt to formulate a more equitable basis for financial support to a local hospital assuming this responsibility?[31]

There is no record of Dr. McNeel's answer. A few weeks later, however, Dr. Henderson sent his "Proposed Revision of Provincial Policy" to the deputy minster. Henderson suggested that Health help the general hospitals establish psychiatric outpatient services to provide diagnostic and treatment services to the areas served by the hospital. This policy, would "limit the outpatient services maintained and administered by the Provincial Department of Health to those facilities located in Ontario Hospitals."[32] In a confidential memo to the deputy minister, Henderson expanded on the shortcomings of the clinics. There were 24 clinics, but they were "spread unevenly throughout the province" with most concentrated in the large urban centres. Moreover, "[t]he volume of service provided is inadequate and poorly distributed," while it was difficult to find sufficient staff to increase the volume of service. The clinics could not offer the "range of diagnostic and treatment services required to provide continuity of care," while establishing additional clinics would mean "setting up an increasing number of isolated outpatient facilities." Finally, "[i]t would be impractical and undesirable for the province to establish and operate comprehensive psychiatric centres in all of the larger communities" since this would mean establishing more institutions "which would perpetuate the separation and distinction between facilities for the diagnosis and treatment of psychiatric disorders from those established for other health needs."[33] Clearly, the idea of community based mental health clinics was to be abandoned, with the clinics being integrated into the provincial mental hospitals and the general hospitals. No more mental health clinics would be established as part of local public health departments and the existing clinics were to be wound up. Local services were to be transferred to the general hospitals by expanding the functions of the psychiatric units to include outpatient services, there was to be an increase in the number of units and the province would help to subsidize the newly-established outpatient units.

However, there was some resistance to the idea of locating community mental health services either in the provincial psychiatric hospitals or in general hospital psychiatric units. The New Democratic Party was particularly critical of the policy, and along with some public health units across the province, it fought to reestablish and expand the role of public health units in mental health. But the curious form the debate took casts some light on why the Department of Health never established links between public health units and community mental health services.

Public Health and the Tuberculosis Paradigm

One of the major historical tasks—and successes—of public health had been in dealing with tuberculosis. Not surprisingly, discussions about the future role of public health often reverted to the experience with tuberculosis. Because mental illness had been fully incorporated into a medical model of care, both public health authorities and medical doctors laid claim to the treatment of mental illness, with the public health authorities often comparing mental illness to tuberculosis. By 1934, it was a matter of course for the president of the Ontario Health Officers' Association to include mental health clinics, travelling chest clinics for the identification and treatment of tuberculosis, and cancer clinics in the armamentarium of public health.[34] In 1945, the superintendent of the London Asylum drew a remarkable analogy between mental illness and tuberculosis:

> In the same way that every contact with a case of active tuberculosis is examined by a tuberculosis clinic so in my opinion every child and adult in contact with a frankly mentally ill person should be examined by a mental health clinic. Mental illnesses are, like tuberculosis, always due to exposure to adverse influences and that old superstition, defective inheritance, need be no more regarded than in the case of tuberculosis.[35]

Of course, few authorities thought of mental illness as a communicable disease, but unquestionably some people saw both tuberculosis and mental health as diseases which were caused by a bad environment and could be prevented by improving that environment. Since the public health service was the centre of education and prevention in health matters, it was naturally assumed it would play a major role in education and prevention in mental health.

In 1952, Minister of Health Dr. Mackinnon Phillips told the legislature,

> mental illness is absolutely no different from physical illnesses... we are going to be able to defeat mental illness the same as we have practically defeated tuberculosis. When we think that fifty years ago tuberculosis...was considered an incurable disease, there was no specific treatment—all they did was really get rest, sunshine and good food. At that time they had a mortality rate of one hundred per one hundred thousand people. Today our mortality rate in Ontario is thirteen last year... If we are going to attack this mental health program...if we are going to attack this, we must attack it first at the level of the community with the family doctor being the main person.[36]

In 1960, during a panel discussion of mental health and public health, the director of the children's outpatient department at the Toronto Psychiatric Hospital drew an analogy between the requirements of good physical health and good mental health. In the first case, he said, one needed "a wholesome physical environment...proper sanitation, pure food, adequate diet and protection from exposure to pathological conditions." For good mental health one needed "a wholesome emotional environment...a pathological emotional environment can warp a personality and destroy it, as effectively as tuberculosis can destroy the lung tissue."[37] In that same discussion, the director of the Victorian Order of Nurses said of the public health nurse that:

> she is doing exactly the same type of work [in treating patients with mental illness] as she is doing with persons suspected of tuberculosis or returning home following treatment of tuberculosis. She tries to get the patient under medical care and in the second instance she tries to support the patient and his family following treatment. Her aim is the same whether the diagnosis is tuberculosis or mental illness, that is, to assist the patient to take his place in the community once again.[38]

Thus, in addition to education, identification and diagnosis, public health had an important role to play in follow-up and aftercare in mental illness.[39]

In April 1966, Stephen Lewis of the NDP attacked the Minister of Health for the decision to exclude public health from any major role in community mental health. Lewis observed:

> Everything is consolidating into one single scheme. We begin with a supposed variety. There are the Ontario hospitals; there are the Ontario hospitals with outpatient departments, there are the psychiatric wings, there are the psychiatric wings with outpatient departments which are called euphemistically, "community mental health clinics," there are community mental health clinics which are genuinely in the community, that is, separate from the hospital but they are gradually being pulled into the bosom of the hospital, there is an inexorable tide pulling them along; and there are these new psychiatric hospitals. All of that, I suggest, represents the systematic destruction of the community emphasis in mental health...Everything becomes hospital-oriented.[40]

Lewis went on to argue that *More for the Mind* [See Chapter 5] was "dominated by...psychiatrists [who] set the pattern."[41] Moreover, he stated:

> There is a tremendous resource available; it is flouted daily. Public health wants to help, public health is rejected. Public health nurses could be stationed permanently in Ontario hospitals. Mental health clinics could be attached to public health units. The entire aftercare service could be rejuvenated and the readmission rate could drop, but all this depends on a little ministerial initiative, and so far we have not had a tittle of evidence that the hon. Minister is so inclined.[42]

Lewis also raised the question of public health's "fixation over tuberculosis" and the power of the "pretty formidable TB lobby" and he suggested that public health should play an important role in dealing with non-communicable chronic diseases.[43] A few days later Lewis again criticized the government for the lack of an aftercare program for ex-mental patients, to which Minister of Health Dr. Matthew Dymond replied:

> Many patients do not need the services of a public health nurse when they return to their homes. Others do not want it, and we must respect their wishes, and have no right to give out information concerning a patient's illness, or his personal affairs, without his knowledge and consent. I believe this was likened or compared with a programme in tuberculosis. There is no comparison whatso-

ever. Tuberculosis is a communicable disease which can constitute a very serious and severe hazard to the public health. Mental illness is not a communicable disease and it does not constitute, necessarily, a hazard to the public health.[44]

However, the problem was not that the supporters of public health had misconceived the nature of mental illness; rather, the debate hinged on different ideas each side had of the role public health should play in providing mental health services. Public health supporters argued that it could provide educational, diagnostic, follow-up and aftercare services. But Dr. Dymond believed that public health should deal mainly with communicable diseases—which mental illness was not. Although everyone admitted mental illness was a disease, psychiatrists argued it was the kind of disease best treated by medical doctors in a hospital setting. For the Department of Health, therefore, public health was irrelevant to, and not equipped to deal with mental illness. According to Dr. Dymond, "if a family wants the services of the public health authorities, it may have them…But others require more help than a public health nurse could be expected to provide and arrangements are being made for continuing treatment under the care of the family doctor, or local clinic, or the hospital clinic."[45]

The two sides in the debate were talking past each other: the supporters of public health emphasized the important social service functions public health could perform through aftercare and follow-up for ex-mental patients, the opponents emphasized the medical nature of mental illness and the necessity of dealing with mentally ill people in a hospital setting.

The Lost Battle—Public Health and Community Mental Health

Public health unit authorities were particularly opposed to the policy of transferring mental health clinics from the local public health units to general hospitals. The reason was simple: the province did not have enough clinics to serve the province and it was not even meeting the criterion of one clinic per 100,000 people. For example, in 1964, the Department of Health decided to relocate the mental health clinic that operated out of the provincial mental hospital in Hamilton, but which spent four days a month at the local health unit, to the general hospital in the city of Brantford. However, the general hospital was unwilling to provide space for the clinic. This meant that Brantford would no longer be served by a mental health clinic, even for the minimum four days a month, and people would have to travel to Hamilton, about twenty miles away, to visit a psychiatrist.

In December 1963, the medical officer of health for Brantford wrote to the director of community mental health: "With our Minister, Dr. M. B. Dymond being so enthusiastic about expanding mental health facilities; and with the increasing number of patients seeking aid through our own Clinic it never occurred to us that mental health would ever exclude Public Health Services."[46] The medical officer of health also noted that after public health nurses had been asked to participate in an aftercare program for patients discharged from the St.

Thomas provincial mental hospital, the program had been "very effective." Dr. Henderson replied that there "is no intention or desire in our planning to exclude Public Health from activity in the mental health field."[47] A week later, the medical officer of health wrote to Henderson approving his decision to locate mental health clinics in general hospitals, but expressing concern that "public health agencies will be excluded. As a general rule hospitals object very strenuously to any activity which is combined with those of health units. Most of the hospitals feel...that this is step in the direction of socialized medicine." Two days later, Dr. Henderson noted that he had visited the medical officer of health in Brantford and the superintendent of the Brantford General Hospital. For about three years, he observed, there had been plans to construct a building adjacent to the hospital to house the county health unit. The building was to include office space for a psychiatrist and three psychologists. However, Henderson opposed this plan as "undesirable and impractical. In view of the direction and planning for Community Psychiatric Centres, support of such a service in this location would be contrary to the basic principle of identifying local services with general hospitals."[48] Or, as the Minister of Health put it on February 24, 1964, "our policy is to encourage the establishment of the mental health clinic as a part of the service provided by the general hospital."[49]

While the legislature was debating the question, within the Department of Health the executive director of the public health division, Dr. Gordon Martin, was arguing for the establishment of public health units throughout the province which would draw staff from the provincial psychiatric hospitals and provide psychological assessments, counselling and follow-up of discharged patients.[50] But Dr. Henderson was opposed to developing links between public health and mental health and in this he was supported by most psychiatrists and by the Minister of Health. Ultimately, the victory over public health was formally inscribed in the Mental Health Act of 1967. Whereas the Mental Health Act of 1954 had stated that the Minister of Health "shall promote and encourage the establishment and co-ordination of facilities for the accumulation and dissemination of information relating to mental health, and advise and assist local boards, medical officers of health, public hospitals and other persons and institutions in all matters pertaining to mental health," thanks to the director of community mental health, this section disappeared in the 1967 Act. It was not until 1985, in regulations formulated under the Health Protection and Promotion Act, 1983, that boards of health were assigned specific responsibilities in the promotion of mental health and the provision of community mental health services.[51]

Why did public health lose the battle to provide mental health services?

Dr. B. H. McNeel, formerly chief of the mental health branch, said that the idea of linking public health and community mental health "just faded away."[52] Certainly the Tyhurst Committee, whose report *More for the Mind* appeared in 1963, opposed linking the mental health clinics and public health departments, and instead recommended relocating the clinics in general hospitals as outpatient departments.[53] On the other hand, *More for the Mind* was in favour of establishing community mental health councils linked to both public health and the psychiatric unit systems and charged with integrating and coordinating psychiatric services within a community or region. This was different from Dr. Henderson's proposal to establish a community mental health board whose job it was to link the mental health clinics with the rest of the community.

Ironically, its success in the fight against tuberculosis hindered public health in its attempt to play a role in mental health policy. Public health authorities drew false analogies between tuberculosis and mental illness, and they raised false expectations about their ability to deal with mental illness. As Dr. Dymond pointed out, tuberculosis and mental illness were not analogous. Moreover, although improved public health measures had helped reduce the rate of tuberculosis, mental illness continued to grow by leaps and bounds. Whereas the BCG vaccine had been discovered in 1926 and was widely administered in Canada after the Second World War, in the early 1950s psychiatrists still depended for treatment on heroic therapies such as psychosurgery or electroshock. Thus, public health might help identify cases of mental illness, but could do little in the way of care. Moreover, the vagueness, the tautological nature of a concept like a "pathological emotional environment" gave no clear indications of what specific measures public health authorities might take to deal with mental illness. Not even the idea of prevention escaped criticism. In 1961, the U.S. Joint Commission on Mental Illness and Health stated that the parallel between preventing mental illness and preventing physical illness was inexact, and it quoted one expert who said: "Our hopes of preventing mental illness by mental health education and child guidance clinics have been disappointed, and there is no convincing evidence that anyone has ever been kept out of the state hospital by such measures."[54]

In addition, by the mid–1950s the neuroleptic drugs had come on the scene. Drug therapy fit perfectly into the medical model of mental health care, and although it would have been hypothetically possible to prescribe and administer these drugs through mental health clinics, the general hospital setting was available and logical. Moreover, new theories that mental illness was caused by a chemical imbalance in the brain dealt a severe blow to previous assumptions that better education or mental hygiene might prevent mental illness. All this tended to undermine justifications for the mental health clinics and to call into question the role public health could play in preventing mental illness. At the same time, the effectiveness of the new drugs confirmed psychiatrists in their belief that the most effective locus for treatment was in psychiatric hospitals or in psychiatric units. Finally, working in public health units held few attractions for psychiatrists who preferred the more "professional" (and more lucrative) environment of a general hospital psychiatric unit. No wonder then, that in the 1960s the director of community mental health services told Dr. Martin, executive director of the public health division of the Department of Health, that in mental health there was no such thing as primary care, only secondary and tertiary care.[55]

Clearly the weight of professional opinion was opposed to giving public health a role in mental health services. In 1966, Dr. D. G. McKerracher, reporting for the Royal Commission on Health Services, noted that in the eight provinces where the deputy minister of public health was put in charge of provincial psychiatric hospitals and mental health clinics, "public health administrators have not known what to make of their huge—and to them indigestible—mental health program." In addition to administrative problems, there was another, even more formidable obstacle.

> [A]lways faintly suspicious of public health departments anyway, family doctors tend to be cool towards provincially employed psychiatrists. Although the public's view of psychiatry and of mental health is improving, this improvement probably results more from psychiatry's closer contact with general hospitals, and with general physicians than from its attachment to public health services.[56]

McKerracher also found "most public health officers and public health nurses have had little to do with psychiatric care."[57] In this way, the search for professional status which was to be found in the closest possible identification with general medicine and general hospitals led psychiatrists away from public health and the community and into a medical and hospital based model of care. In the 1950s and 1960s, when it became apparent that psychiatrists would resist any links with public health and that mental illness and tuberculosis were not analogous, no good argument could be found for granting public health a major role in mental health policy.

Thus, mental health policy in Ontario was to continue down the road toward a medical model, with the psychiatric units expected to provide hospital as well as community care services. Public health had been eliminated from playing any role in mental health policy.

Of course, the decision had its advantages. Since municipalities were reluctant to contribute one-third of the expenses of the mental health clinics, and since, if they had been established in the community the Department of Health would have had to bear the administrative costs of centralized control plus one-third of the funding costs, establishing the clinics in the general hospitals saved money, administrative costs, and obviated the necessity of pressuring the municipalities for a financial contribution. By the mid–1960s, therefore, the travelling clinics had disappeared, the mental health clinics had been relocated in psychiatric hospitals or absorbed into the psychiatric unit system, and, in Ontario at least, the term community mental health care was understood as referring almost exclusively to the psychiatric units in general hospitals.

Could the Department of Health have acted forcefully in linking community mental health and public health? Certainly the policy would have encountered resistance, although how much is hard to say. According to Dr. B. H. McNeel, not all public health nurses or local medical officers of health in public health looked favourably on community mental health.[58] On the other hand, Dr. Gordon Martin, ex-director of community public health thinks public health would have willingly taken on the burden.[59] Perhaps if public health authorities had realized that the one area in which they could play a role—aftercare and follow-up of ex-patients—would in the late 1970s and 1980s emerge as the major problem in mental health policy, they might have made a better case. But the Department of Health defined the role of public health too narrowly in terms of education and assessment, while the problems of ex-patients in the community were not yet serious enough to provoke authorities into looking for better ways to deliver community services. Hypothetically, the Department of Health might have established a network of community mental health boards with representation from public health, mental health and the community. At the very minimum such boards would have alerted the provincial authorities to the impact of deinstitutionalization on the community at a very early stage in the process. A system linking public health and community mental health services might also have provided aftercare services for ex-patients or support services to mentally ill people in the community, while the psychiatric units could have devoted themselves to emergency care, short-term inpatient services, as well as to the diagnostic and educational services taken over from the clinics. Whether the government would have responded by providing housing or counselling services is impossible to say, but the problem might have been raised at least two decades earlier than was actually the case.

Even at this stage, forging some link between public and community mental health was not beyond the power of the Minister. The Department of Health's failure to pursue the public health–community mental health link was not due to fear of confronting resistance from the community, nor to the inherent preference of democracies for incremental rather than overall, coherent planning.[60] Rather, it was due to the disinterest of the psychiatric profession, the lack of any pressure groups fighting for a connection between public health and community mental health, changing ideas on the causes of mental illness, and the fact that such a move would have required an additional expenditure of funds. Under these circumstances, and given the enormous weight of opinion in favour of the psychiatric units, perhaps any attempt to establish some kind of community mental health care system was doomed from the start.

Notes

1 Gerald Grob, *Mental Illness and American Society, 1875–1940* (Princeton: Princeton UP, 1983) 165–166.

2 *Report of the Royal Commission on Public Welfare* 31.

3 Grob 239.

4 Simmons *Asylum* 126–127.

5 The 63rd *Annual Report* of the Inspector of Prisons and Public Charities states that mental hygiene clinics were to be established in the various Ontario Hospitals as part

of their "responsibility in the public health field" and as part of the attempt to prevent mental illness. Ontario, *Sessional Papers* Vol. 63, Pt. IV, No. 15, 1931, p. 3.

6 AO, RG 10, Series 107, Nov. 1, 1938, McGhie to Eric Silk, Attorney General's Department.

7 Department of Health, 69th *Annual Report* of the Hospital Division, upon the Ontario Hospitals for the Mentally Ill, Mentally Subnormal and Epileptic, 1937.

8 AO, RG 10, 20-A–1, July 24, 1936, Minutes, Superintendent's Conference, Deputy Minister J. T. Phair.

9 AO, RG 10, 20-A–1, November 27, 1940, Dr. D. G. McKerracher, Director, Mental Health Clinic, Brockville to Dr. C.S.Tennant, Superintendent, Brockville, copy to B. T. McGhie, Deputy Minister of Health.

10 Simmons *Asylum* 129.

11 Department of Health, *Annual Reports*, 1933–1947.

12 C. A. Buck, "Rehabilitation of the Mentally Ill," *Canadian Journal of Public Health* 31 (1940): 65.

13 In April 1948, Dr. G. Stogdill, chief of the mental health division of the federal Department of National Health and Welfare sent to Dr. R. C. Montgomery, director of the hospitals division of the Ontario Department of Health a copy of a highly critical report on public psychiatric hospitals conducted by the Group for the Advancement of Psychiatry. See AO, RG 10, B. 78, April 30, 1948, G. Stogdill to R. C. Montgomery. Among the numerous critical articles on the state of mental hospitals, see for example the article by D. M. LeBourdais, "Our Shameful Mental Hospitals," *Canadian Forum* 27 (1948): 226–227, and "Mental Health Experts Say Hospitals Packed," *The Globe and Mail* 10 November 1953.

14 Bill Bird, "Mental Health in Canada," *Canadian Forum* 27 (1947): 34.

15 *Globe and Mail* 16 December 1953.

16 *The Globe and Mail* 12 and 16 May 1953.

17 See H. Warren Dunham who refers to "the conception...that the community is the patient, and consequently the necessity arises to develop techniques that can be used in treating the community." H. Warren Dunham, "Community Psychiatry: The Newest Therapeutic Bandwagon," *Current Issues in Psychiatry*, ed. Jason Aronson (New York· Science House, 1967) 293.

18 "[T]here is no *general* [author's italics] mental health problem. Communities must be seen as personalities..." J. R. Newbrough, "A Movement in Search of a Theory," article originally published in 1964 and reprinted in Arthur J. Bindman and Allen D. Spiegel, *Perspectives in Community Mental Health* (Chicago: Aldine Publishing Co., 1969) 77.

19 Quoted in Ascanio M. Rossi, "Some Pre-World War II Antecedents of Community Mental Health Theory and Practice," in Bindman and Spiegel 23.

20 AO, RG 10, B. 157, M–3, June 5, 1953, Dr. C. A. Roberts to Dr. R. C. Montgomery.

[21] AO, RG 10, B. 115, Gen P–2–8–2, n.d. [1955?], "Report on Community Mental Health Services."

[22] "Report on Community Mental Health Services," p. 7.

[23] "Report on Community Mental Health Services," p. 3.

[24] "Report on Community Mental Health Services," pp. 10 and 13.

[25] "Report on Community Mental Health Services," p. 5.

[26] AO, RG 10, B.157, HS M–3, August 29, 1956, Dr. B. McNeel to J. T. Phair.

[27] AO, RG 10, B. 157, HS M–3, "Effect of Policy Re Psychiatric Units." Unsigned and undated, probably from Dr. H. W. Henderson.

[28] AO, RG 10–108, May 16, 1957, Henderson to Dr. C. D. Farquharson, Medical Office of Health, Scarborough.

[29] AO, RG 10–108, July 19, 1957, Henderson to McNeel, "Organization of Community Mental Health Clinics."

[30] AO, RG 10, Series 107, October 25, 1957, Henderson to McNeel.

[31] AO, RG 10, Series 5, December 6, 1962, Henderson to McNeel.

[32] AO, RG 10, Series 5, B. 119, January 17, 1963, Henderson to Dr. Brown, "Community Mental Health Services—Proposed Revision of Provincial Policy."

[33] AO, RG 10 Series 5 B. 119, April 23, 1963, Dr. H. W. Henderson to Dr. Brown.

[34] James J. McCann, "Some Public Health Activities and Needs in Ontario," *Canadian Journal of Public Health* 25 (1934): 257.

[35] AO, RG 10, B. 55, HS 5–1, Mar. 31, 1945, Superintendent, Ontario Hospital London to Director, Hospitals Division.

[36] *Debates*, March 4, 1952, p. G–3.

[37] Edward J. Rosen, M.D. "The Changing Attitude of the Community Toward Mental Health," *Canadian Journal of Public Health* 51 (1960): 361–362.

[38] Bernice Seeds, "The Public Health Nurse," in *Canadian Journal of Public Health* 51 (1960): 363.

[39] On the role of public health in the battle against tuberculosis, see George Jasper Wherrett, *The Miracle of the Empty Beds* (Toronto: University of Toronto, 1977) 197–209.

[40] *Debates*, April 27, 1966, p. 2731.

[41] *Debates* 2731.

[42] *Debates* 2753.

[43] *Debates* 2753 and 2755.

[44] *Debates*, May 2, 1966.

[45] *Debates* 2920.

[46] AO, RG 10, Series 108, December 9, 1963, E. Aenid Dunton, Medical Officer of Health, Brant County Health Unit to Henderson.

[47] AO, RG 10, Series 108, December 10, 1963, Henderson to Dunton.

[48] AO, RG 10–108, Henderson to file, December 18, 1963.

[49] *Debates*, February 24, 1964, p. 879.

[50] Interview, Dr. Gordon Martin.

[51] See Ministry of Health, *Mandatory Health Programs and Services*, Guidelines (Post Phase I), pp. 32–34, November, 1985.

[52] Interview, Dr. B. H. McNeel.

[53] *More for the Mind* 97.

[54] Joint Commission on Mental Illness and Health, *Action for Mental Health* (New York: Basic Books, 1961) 70–71.

[55] Interview, Dr. Gordon Martin.

[56] D. G. McKerracher, *Trends in Psychiatric Care* (Ottawa: Royal Commission on Health Services, 1966) 10.

[57] McKerracher 10.

[58] Interview, Dr. B. H. McNeel.

[59] Interview, Dr. Gordon Martin.

[60] "For a democracy like the United States, the commitment to incremental change is not surprising...Political democracy is often endangered by nonincremental change..." David Braybrooke and Charles Lindblom, *A Strategy of Decision* (New York: The Free Press, 1963) 73.

4

The Psychiatric Unit System

> In many parts of the U.S. and Canada, the mental hospital continues to be considered by many as the facility where selected types of patients can and should be treated; in these places, the general hospital psychiatric division emerges as an adjunctive element to mental hospital care and a two-tier system of psychiatric care has emerged.
>
> Dr. Alex Richman and P. Harris, 1984

> We're getting schizophrenics, manic depressives, all the psychotic and severe personality disorders. We've had a recent increase in psychosomatic disorders. You're not looking any more at minor disorders.
>
> Director of Inpatient Services, Psychiatric Unit

The Origins of the Psychiatric Unit System

In 1970, for the first time in Ontario's history, more people were admitted to the psychiatric units of general hospitals and to community psychiatric hospitals than were admitted to the ten provincial psychiatric hospitals. The psychiatric unit system had become the second major leg in Ontario's unbalanced tripod of mental health services. Yet, the development of the psychiatric unit system can only be understood if it is seen against the background of more than a hundred and fifty years of asylum history.

Michel Foucault has pointed out how changing perceptions of madness directly influenced treatment policies. Thus, it was not until the nineteenth century when madness had been stripped of its metaphysical associations with religion and morality and defined as a disease, that the way had been cleared for the integration of mentally and physically ill people in the same institution.[1] At the same time, the physician emerged as the dominant and legitimate treatment authority. According to Foucault: "With the new status of the medical personage, the deepest meaning of confinement is abolished: mental disease, with the meanings we now give it, is made possible."[2] In the United States the transformation of medical education and the desire of psychiatrists to work with their medical colleagues, the growth of the mental hygiene movement and its interest in prevention, and the increasing tendency of psychiatrists to think in terms of treating patients in the community all helped prepare the ground.[3] And wherever the custodial institution had sprung up, the enormous pressure of numbers and the desire of psychiatrists to treat middle and upper-class patients led to a search for alternatives to the asylum system.

In 1869, John Langmuir, the inspector of prisons, asylums and public charities remarked that "more than three-fourths of the present population of our Asylums, as well as those now seeking admission to them, are of the indigent or non-paying class whose condition in life before becoming insane utterly unfits them to appreciate architectural beauty or expensive embellishments..."[4] Noting that only 73 out of 1,030 asylum "inmates" were paying patients, Langmuir stated, "surely it is time that something was done for those who, although more fortunate in circumstances, have been so long neglected in their mental affliction."[5] To remedy this situation a ward had been set apart in the Rockwood asylum for "such female patients as are able to pay for the extra attendance and comforts that will through this means be placed at their disposal." In 1873, Dr. Henry Landor, superintendent of the London Asylum recommended that a separate institution be established for paying patients. "They and their relatives would then see that they had something different from the non-paying in their accommodation, and in all their surroundings and the relations of one class to the other, and to the asylum authorities would be improved."[6] Moreover, the prospect of committing their dependents to a better class of asylum would prompt reluctant relatives to seek cures at an earlier stage of the disease than was currently the case. By 1880, Langmuir noted that there were no private asylums in Ontario but that accommodation for paying patients at the Toronto Lunatic Asylum had been "increased and greatly improved" and this "obviates the necessity, except for personal reasons, of sending the insane of the better class of the community to a foreign asylum."[7] Despite attempts to make the asylum more attractive to the middle classes, the vast majority of patients in Ontario lunatic asylums belonged to the working or lower middle classes, or were farmers, agricultural workers or unemployed.

Unable to attract large numbers of middle class people to public institutions, desperately seeking some means to reduce overcrowding and to prevent mental illness before it became chronic, and eager to provide a setting whereby medical students might become acquainted with psychiatry, nineteenth century mental health authorities began to treat mentally ill people outside the asylum setting. In 1897, for example, Dr. Walter Channing opened an outpatient clinic for mentally ill people at the Boston Dispensary.[8] A few years later, a department of psychiatry was opened and a psychiatric unit established at the Albany, New York Hospital.[9] In 1916, Dr. Good of the English Oxford County and City Mental Hospital observed that patients who were reluctant to be treated in a mental hospital might be willing to go to a general hospital "because they are not afraid of being locked up there or specially labelled."[10] In 1910, Dr. Albert W. Ferris of New York advocated the establishment of psychopathic wards in general hospitals as "the most important link in the chain; a most essential agency for the early protection and conservation of the recently developed or the recently discovered case of mental impairment."[11] From 1906 to 1925, the Toronto Nervous Ward, a psychiatric ward headed by Dr. Campbell Myers, was located in the Toronto General Hospital.[12] In 1918, the CNCMH complimented the government of Manitoba for establishing a psychopathic ward in the Winnipeg General Hospital while, in its 1919 Mental Hygiene Survey of British Columbia, it advocated the establishment of psychopathic wards in general hospitals.[13] In 1923 a division of neuropsychiatry was established at the Henry Ford Hospital in Detroit, Michigan. A psychiatrist gave his full time to carefully planting nervous and mental patients among the other patients in the hospital. No barred windows, no locked doors, no segregation, not even separation of the sexes was permitted. The idea seems to have been successful from the very beginning.[14] And, in 1925, the Toronto Psychiatric Hospital was established, with Dr. C. B. Farrar as its head.[15]

For psychiatrists, the advantages of specialized psychopathic hospitals and of psychiatric wards or units in general hospitals seemed obvious. They could deal with incipient signs of insanity at a time when they were treatable, thereby reducing the numbers who had to be committed to large hospitals. They could accept voluntary patients thereby avoiding the necessity of legal commitment to an institution.[16] If properly equipped, psychopathic hospitals could do valuable research similar to research in physical medicine in the general hospitals.[17] Equally important, specialized psychiatric facilities in general hospitals would appeal to the middle classes who tended to avoid public institutions. After all, the low status and incomes of psychiatrists compared to the rest of the medical profession is only partly explained by the problematical nature of psychiatry. A good deal derives from the fact that the vast majority of mentally ill people in large institutions are, and have always been, of low socioeconomic status. Thus, psychiatrists could only benefit from their links with general hospitals.

By the mid–1940s, therefore, separate provision for mentally ill people either in psychopathic hospitals or in special wards or units in general hospitals was an accepted idea. In 1943, before the federal Special Committee on Social Security, Ontario and the other provinces supported the establishment of psychiatric wards in general hospitals "for short treatment only; prolonged illnesses would be cared for in mental hospitals."[18] Even before that, however, as early as 1940, the medical officer of health at Windsor had applied to the Department of Health for the establishment of a psychiatric unit, but nothing came of it.[19]

In their 1944 statement on the future policy of psychiatric services, Ontario psychiatrists in the armed forces had recommended the establishment in the major urban centres of wards in general hospitals for acute psychotics, that "neurotics and mild psychotics should be cared for in general wards or outpatient clinics,"[20] and that "the teaching of clinical psychiatry take place in general hospital wards."[21] The superintendent of the London hospital stated that,

> the best work in psychiatric research and the advancement of the care of the mentally ill can be done to better advantage in the close association with a general hospital than with a separate institution. I think the best way of bringing

psychiatric viewpoints into general medicine is through the general hospital and not by the establishment of separate psychiatric hospitals.[22]

At a 1945 meeting of the provincial health directors in Ottawa the question of establishing psychiatric wards in general hospitals came up, and it was noted that architects recommended that 10 percent of bed capacity of general hospitals over 200 beds should be set aside for psychiatric wards.[23] On March 13, 1945, Minister of Health R. P. Vivian announced a "program for the treatment of early mental disturbances in general hospitals." In order to determine exactly what such a program would entail, a delegation of mental health authorities from Ontario travelled to Montreal in the fall of 1945 to look at the Allan Memorial Hospital established by Dr. D. E. Cameron, Chairman of Psychiatry at McGill and Head of the Department of Psychiatry at the Royal Victoria general hospital.[24]

Administratively a branch of the Royal Victoria Hospital, but located in a nearby building, the Allan Memorial was financed by a $30,000 grant from the Rockefeller Foundation and by a matching grant from the province of Quebec. Admission to the hospital was voluntary, there were no locked wards, and there was bed accommodation for 17 men and 36 women. Allan Memorial was used as a teaching and research centre and was staffed by hospital interns. The Allan carefully selected its patients, rejecting alcoholics, for example, because it was thought they could not benefit by therapy. In his discussions with the delegation, Dr. Cameron suggested that a psychiatric unit should not be larger than 100 beds, and discussed with them his proposal to use the Allan as a day hospital with patients returning home to sleep at night. Present also was Dr. Barrero, director of the psychiatric hospital in Albany, New York. He told the Ontario delegation that the Albany general hospital had an outpatient department and a closed unit of 45 beds, and that mental patients were treated on the general wards of the hospital.

The Ontario delegation was obviously impressed, because Dr. Montgomery noted that similar hospitals to the Allan might be set up as wings at the Kingston and London general hospitals. Montgomery also speculated about the possibility of getting funds from the Rockefeller Foundation.[25] The psychiatric unit idea also got valuable support from Dr. C. Hincks of the CNCMH who suggested in a speech to the Ontario Neuropsychiatric Association that:

> A most desirable forward step would be for general hospitals to assume increased psychiatric responsibility in accordance with plans that might be approved and supported financially by provincial governments. Psychiatric wards for 24 hour and for day care, together with psychiatric clinics, manned in the main by part-time psychiatrists who would receive remuneration—such facilities are needed across Canada for the early treatment of psychoses and for the intensive treatment of the neuroses.[26]

A few months later Hincks stated that the "mental hospital as we have known it in the past [is] more or less obsolete," and he suggested as an alternative the establishment of psychiatric "divisions" in general hospitals or "self-contained active treatment units attached to mental hospitals."[27]

It was also thought that psychiatric units in general hospitals would alleviate the enormous demands put on the travelling mental health clinics. At a meeting of mental health clinics directors and consultant psychiatrists in 1948, Dr. Brillinger of the Hamilton mental health clinic reported that "there were so many requests for his services there is difficulty organizing his time to cover the area." Those present at the meeting recommended to the director of the hospitals division that "special psychiatric wards be established in the larger General Hospitals."[28]

Despite the apparent consensus surrounding the establishment of a psychiatric unit system, the Department of Health moved slowly. In their 1948 survey the Ontario Hospital Survey Committee found only three psychiatric units with 54 beds in the province. One unit at the Ottawa Civic Hospital had nine beds but, according to the OHSC "the facilities are far from ideal."[29] A second 13-bed unit for female patients was located at the Victoria Hospital in London and, in July 1949, the Wellesley division of the Toronto General Hospital established a 32-bed unit staffed by two psychiatrists funded by federal mental health grants administered by the province. The OHSC visited hospitals in Massachusetts and New York where psychiatric units were being developed and it recommended the establishment of psychiatric units in Ontario general hospitals with funding from both the province and the federal government.[30] The survey committee also noted that nine of the 37 private psychiatrists responding to questionnaires recommended the establishment of "adequate in- and outpatient psychiatric facilities in a general hospital."[31]

In 1948, the Ontario Health Survey Committee found that because of the lack of outside examination facilities, people suspected of mental illness were held in jail until an examination could take place. The select committee on reform institutions urged hospitals to establish the units to "keep people out of jails and institutions."[32] Although some psychiatric units seem to have established examination rooms or secure rooms for violent patients, C. A. Roberts, chief of the federal government's mental health division, criticized this move during a visit to Ontario in the summer of 1953: "It does not appear wise to have locked wards...It does not appear desirable for psychiatric units to admit for care patients who are not compatible with the general hospital environment."[33]

A 1955 Department of Health report on community mental health services noted that in Europe there was a "trend to bringing treatment of the mentally ill close to the community." One option was to establish moderately sized regional mental hospitals. Another was to increase the number of psychiatric units which had been established in general hospitals "to supplement the inpatient services" of the large psychiatric hospitals. As justification for the units, the report mentions a "survey" indicating that a "significant number of patients" who had been treated in the psychiatric units might otherwise have gone to the psychiatric hospitals.[34]

It was not until the federal government became actively involved in promoting, and, most important, in helping to finance the program, that Ontario's psychiatric unit system finally got under way. Under the aegis of Dr. G. D. W. Cameron, deputy minister of the Department of National Health and Welfare, and later under Dr. C. A. Roberts, the federal government held meetings of the provincial mental health directors and, in 1947, established an advisory committee on mental health, composed of fifteen members including Dr. R. C. Montgomery, director of the hospitals division of the Ontario Department of Health, and Dr. Ewen Cameron of the Allan Memorial Hospital in Montreal. Since Cameron was an ardent proponent of the psychiatric unit concept, Montgomery was leaning in that direction, and most psychiatrists were in favour, it is not surprising that both the advisory committee and the provincial mental health directors supported the psychiatric unit program. In the summer of 1948, a subcommittee of the federal advisory group on mental health noted that "attention should be given to the establishment of psychiatric services in general hospitals."[35] A few years later the fifth meeting of the advisory group focused on reports on the development of psychiatric wards in different provinces.[36] In the early 1950s, the federal government offered the provinces $1,500 for chronic beds in general hospitals, and it agreed to include beds in psychiatric units of general hospitals under that definition. Thus, in the fall of 1951, after federal grants for beds in psychiatric units were assured, the government of Ontario announced that it would provide an additional $8,500 per bed to general hospitals to establish psychiatric units.[37] At this time, it was assumed that the federal government would share in the costs of maintenance.[38] One year later, the Ontario Department of Health was anticipating that "most if not all of the personnel of such units, will be financed through Federal Health Grants on application of the Province."[39] In December 1952, Dr. C. A. Roberts, wrote to Dr. Montgomery stating that the federal government was considering extending grants specifically for mental health beds in the general hospitals.[40] Apparently the provincial mental health authorities were quite optimistic about funding and political support for the psychiatric units, because in February 1954, Dr. Montgomery wrote to the Minister of Health, Dr. Mackinnon Phillips accepting Phillips' recommendation that the Department of Health plan for a maximum of 1,000 psychiatric unit beds.[41]

Psychiatrists and the Psychiatric Unit System

Despite objections in the mental health literature, the psychiatric community enthusiastically supported the psychiatric unit concept.[42] Such an association would confirm the prevailing paradigm of mental illness as akin to physical illness which was best treated in a hospital setting; it would help to raise the prestige of psychiatry and of psychiatrists and this, in turn, would provide an argument for better remuneration.[43] Unlike the psychiatric hospitals where they were employed exclusively on a salaried basis, individual psychiatrists in general hospitals could combine private practice with hospital work as well as working in a more congenial, prestigious and professionally exciting atmosphere than in the psychiatric institutions.

There were other attractions as well. Federal cost-sharing funds could be obtained for mental health beds and for psychiatric services in the general hospitals and enterprising hospitals could even obtain federal funds for operating expenses.[44] And there was always the hope that with the federal government becoming increasingly involved in the financing of the health care system, additional federal funds would become available for mental health needs. It was also expected that the units would benefit from whatever government largesse happened to rain down on the general hospital sector.

None, or few of these advantages held for the policy of establishing community mental health centres as either independent entities or as part of the public health service. Public health had always suffered from underfunding.[45] Psychiatrists would be unable to share the prestige of working in general hospitals alongside specialists. There were fears as well that community mental health centres might eventually stigmatize patients and staff in the same way as the large mental hospitals. Unless the province were to establish independent community mental health centres fully funded by the provincial government, linking mental health and public health would immediately create funding problems because local communities were reluctant to contribute to local public health units. Moreover, municipalities were fearful that if they committed themselves to supporting outside initiatives, then at some future date when the provincial or federal government might decide to withdraw financial support, they would be stuck with full responsibility. The 1955 Department of Health report on community mental health noted the fear that "if the municipality were to acknowledge the program by even a token contribution it would eventually be 'saddled' with the whole program."[46]

Given the promise of federal funds, the enthusiastic support of the psychiatric community, the hope of stemming the rising tide of commitments to the large institutions, and the full support of the Minister of Health, it was full steam ahead for the psychiatric unit program. After Mackinnon Phillips wrote to him about the psychiatric units, Premier Leslie Frost replied that there was "a great deal to be said for this [the establishment of psychiatric units] and he approved the plan 'in principle.'"[47] In the summer of 1952, Dr. Phillips wrote to Premier Frost referring to "our discussions" on psychiatric units. "May I say that I became convinced some considerable time ago that one of the most important approaches to our tremendous problem of mental illness was the development of a program involving the early recognition of the symptoms of mental illness, and provision for early treatment other than in a mental hospital." Dr. Phillips explained that after looking at the results of the unit program at St. Catharines and after conversations with Dr. Aldwyn Stokes, Professor of Psychiatry at the University of Toronto, he believed that the psychiatric units helped to stem the flow of people to the mental hospitals. Moreover,

> it is safe to say in my opinion, that apart from the value of this service from a humanitarian point of view, its importance in the economic field is tremendous... Incidentally, it is anticipated that the cost, if not all of the personnel of such units, will be financed through Federal Health Grants on application of the Province.[48]

Later that summer, Dr. Phillips wrote to the director of the hospitals division saying that he was "very anxious" to establish psychiatric units in Peterborough and in Women's College Hospital in Toronto.[49] By the end of the year, the Department of Health published a news release on "early therapy" and the psychiatric units. The release put the establishment of psychiatric units in the context of the "development of a community approach to mental illness." According to the Minister of Health, the units would allow for early and adequate treatment of mental illness in general hospitals, thus obviating admission to a mental hospital.[50]

Although one of the major attractions of the program for Ontario authorities was the federal contribution, financing of the psychiatric units was complicated. The psychiatric units were "maintained chiefly by grants from the Federal Government under the National Health Grants scheme," but financing was distributed in an incoherent fashion with some hospitals applying on their own initiative to the federal government for funds which the Department of Health administered but which the hospitals added to provincial contributions, while others depended entirely on the province for support.[51] One major factor retarding the development of the scheme was a lack of "available personnel."[52]

However, the 1955 report recommended that additional psychiatric units be established and suggested that by 1956, 351 psychiatric unit beds should be available. In fact, it was not until 1958 that that figure was reached. It was also expected in 1955 that the maximum number of psychiatric unit beds would be 630. That figure was reached in 1965 and was quickly surpassed in 1966.

The question of financing remained a thorny one. Initially it was expected that the psychiatric units would be financed on a cost-sharing basis with local communities contributing one-third and the province and the federal government sharing the remaining two-thirds.[53] When it became apparent in 1955 that the federal government was unwilling to make a permanent commitment to provide grants for general hospital psychiatric services, the general hospitals turned to the Department of Health. However, Health stated that it would not replace the federal funds. According to the chief of the mental health division, the problem was that "no definite philosophy had been developed; the hospitals were encouraged to build psychiatric units, which, in some instances, were operated by members of the staff of the Department of Health, and in others by psychiatrists employed by the hospital."[54] In the end, the psychiatric units were financed from within the hospitals which, by 1959, were financed through the Hospital Insurance and Diagnostic Services Act.

Psychiatric Units and the Mental Hygiene Model

The psychiatric units were established when the prevention of mental illness was an important element in provincial mental health policy. Through programs in schools and in the community, the mental hygiene movement laid heavy emphasis on educating the public to view mental illness as a disease like any other disease, one that could be cured if promptly and properly treated. Since it was assumed that early treatment of mental illness improved the chances of recovery, the psychiatric units fit nicely into the mental hygiene paradigm. Establishing psychiatric units in general hospitals in the province would realize the goal of early identification and treatment of mental illness thus mitigating the severity of the disease and reducing the numbers of mentally ill people who had to be committed to the psychiatric hospitals. But the beauty of the psychiatric unit program was that it also fit into new theories about chemical imbalances causing mental illness. As the drug revolution of the 1950s took hold and new theories on brain chemistry developed, psychiatrists could argue that the most appropriate locus for treatment was in a general hospital setting. In 1952, the Minister of Health said: "The psychiatric units are going to serve many purposes. The main purpose is that a great number of the patients who may have later to go on to a mental institution are going to be treated in their own communities. We are going to have early diagnosis and treatment at the community level."[55] A few years later, these hopes seem to have been borne out when psychiatric unit directors estimated that from 33–50 percent of their patients might have been institutionalized if they had not sought help at a psychiatric unit.[56]

However, the medical staff of the general hospitals were not as enthusiastic about the psychiatric units as the mental health division. Dr. H. W. Henderson noted that there were no medical reasons why the size of psychiatric units was limited to between 20–40 beds but that the figure was a compromise between the general hospitals which wanted to keep the psychiatric units small, and the psychiatrists who wanted to get as many beds as possible.[57] In some hospitals the medical staff ignored the psychiatrists or were openly hostile to them, and there was constant bickering between the psychiatric units and the hospital administration, with the psychiatric unit personnel accusing the administration of short-changing them in the disbursement of funds.

Within the Department of Health, financing and administrative difficulties with the psychiatric unit program led the chief of the mental health division to consider establishing a community mental health network outside the general hospital. In 1956, he proposed to the deputy minister of health that the Department of Health might establish community mental health services linked to local health units or health departments. Local communities would be asked to provide buildings and to contribute to administrative costs. It was suggested that "the Province should not undertake to provide support for Psychiatric Units other than the usual per diem grant given to hospitals for all services." In these circumstances, the units would not be allowed to apply separately for federal grants.[58]

By 1959, in a complete reversal of the previous conventional wisdom, the Department of Health reported that the psychiatric units were not necessarily helping to reduce the intake of the provincial hospitals. Dr. H. W. Henderson wrote to his chief, B. H. McNeel, that despite the assumption that the psychiatric units helped reduce admissions to mental hospitals "there are to my knowledge no figures to indicate their effectiveness in achieving this objective." Henderson further noted that the psychiatric units had a high turnover rate, with the majority of patients returned to their homes within three to four weeks, but that they also had a high readmission rate. As for the fact that only a small percentage of the psychiatric unit patients were transferred to the mental hospital, Henderson surmised that the psychiatric units may have been serving "different types of patients."

This did not lead Dr. Henderson to advocate establishing a community mental health system outside the hospital along the lines of McNeel's tentative proposal of 1956. Rather, he argued that the defects in the psychiatric unit system only served to highlight the continued importance of the large mental hospital. "With our present knowledge, it is debatable whether the general hospital service can or should attempt to replace the mental hospital."[59] According to Henderson, mental health services in Ontario would continue to center around the large mental hospital, which would be the "focal point in the planning and development of services" providing outpatient, day and night care, examination units and even "such open ward service as a psychiatric unit."

Still, the chief of the mental health division was ambivalent about the psychiatric unit program. In 1959, Dr. McNeel stated that: "The Department of Health never has accepted psychiatric units in hospitals as a government responsibility."[60] But this apparent lack of support was probably a maneuver by the Department of Health to extract funds from other departments. Thus, at a meeting between officials from the Department of Health and the Ontario Hospital Services Commission, it was agreed that the Hospital Insurance Commission would pay the operating costs of the psychiatric units, while the Department of Health would pay the salary of the psychiatrists. This resolved the problem of financing, and, more importantly, confirmed the province in its policy of placing the psychiatric units in general hospitals, rather than establishing community mental health centres which would be independent or integrated with community health centres. In the early 1950s it was not clear whether the federal government would continue subsidizing the psychiatric units nor, if so, at what level of funding. By 1959, when Ontario implemented the Hospital Insurance and Diagnostic Services program, there was an enormous financial incentive to continue with the psychiatric units. In 1977 the funding arrangements under the Hospital Insurance and Diagnostic Services Act were amended to block financing under the Established Programs Financing Act.[61] Thus, federal funds were no longer specifically directed toward health programs so that the prospect of federal cost-sharing funds was no longer an incentive for the establishment of psychiatric units in the general hospitals.[62]

According to one former official in the mental health bureaucracy,

> there was a natural pressure on the planners in the province to shift resources from an area that was 100 percent provincially funded to an area that was at least 50 percent funded by the federal government. So this was one of several pressures on the planners in the late 1960s and early 1970s to expand psychiatric units and shrink the size of provincial hospitals. Planners used to talk about this periodically when I was privy to one of their meetings, they talked about the fact that the ideal would be to close mental hospitals and expand psychiatric units to do things the mental hospitals did, because among other things, it would mean they could be cost-shared. I think the feds would have balked if it had gone the whole way, but it never did.[63]

During this time the Tyhurst Committee (See Chapter 5) was elaborating a position which would place the psychiatric unit at the center of community mental health services, while the United States Joint Commission on Mental Health and Illness had recommended in 1961 that every community general hospital of 100 beds or more establish a psychiatric unit.[64] In 1962, psychiatric units got another boost from the Canadian Psychiatric Association which recommended that "all general hospitals of over 200 beds should have an established psychiatric division."[65] Of course, the fact that Dr. B. H. McNeel, chief of the mental health division, was at this time a member of the Tyhurst Commission gave added impetus to the establishment of the psychiatric unit system.[66]

A New Model for Community Care—The Psychiatric Units.

By 1963, the year of publication of *More for the Mind*, the die was cast. Nineteen psychiatric units with 591 beds had been established. No more was heard about establishing a community mental health network outside the general hospital system, and no one proposed linking such a network with public health. The Department of Health had decided that the psychiatric units would form the core of community mental health care in the province. The phrase "community mental health" would henceforth refer to psychiatric units in the general hospitals. Although some general hospitals had already established psychiatric outpatient facilities aided by federal health grant funds, the idea was to supplement this with provincial funds which would come through the Ontario Hospital Services Commission.[67] On February 26, 1963, Minister of Health Matthew Dymond announced to the legislature that "increasing emphasis will be put upon the establishment of community mental health clinics."[68] In this context, "community mental health clinics" could have referred either to mental health clinics or to psychiatric units in the general hospitals, but a year later Dr. Dymond stated that the mental health clinics would be integrated into the general hospitals "as part of the service provided by the general hospital."[69]

In 1966, Dr. H. W. Henderson became executive director of the mental health division. A strong proponent of the psychiatric unit system, he opposed any links with public health. He rejected the idea that local public health units should themselves employ psychiatrists, psychologists or child care workers, and he

Table 4.1
Psychiatric Units

Year	*No. of units*	*Beds*	*Year*	*No. of units*	*Beds*
1954	6	125	1969	37	1,238
1955	7	156	1970	42	1,351
1956		257	1971	43	1,502
1957		257	1972	43	1,492
1958		351	1973		1,502
1959		351	1974	49	1,712
1960	13	431	1975	45	1,735
1961	14	457	1976	53	1,798
1962	17	545	1977/78	57	2,144 (15 mths)
1963	19	591	1978/79	59	
1964	20	620	1979/80	59	2,224
1965	22	662	1980/81	63	2,197
1966	24	725	1981/82	60	2,155
1967	26	804	1982/83	62*	
1968	33	1,077	1983/84	63	

* Bed capacity not included after 1982/83
[Source: *Annual Reports*, Psychiatric Units and Community Psychiatric Hospitals, Ministry of Health, 1954–1983/84]

objected to the "practice of nurses and school officials referring a child to a psychiatric service." Rather, he argued, the parents and the family doctor should be consulted before a decision was made to contact a psychiatrist. Dr. Henderson quoted President John F. Kennedy "ideally the [community health] center could be located at an appropriate general hospital."[70] In fact, the 1963 Community Mental Health Centers Act left open to individual states to decide whether the centres should be associated with general hospitals or established independently of them.[71]

During the 1950s and 1960s a hidden revolution had occurred in Ontario's mental health system. In 1955, there were seven psychiatric units; in 1960, there were 13; in 1965 there were 22; and in 1970, 42. By 1970, for the first time, combined admissions to the 42 psychiatric units and six community psychiatric hospitals including the Clarke Institute exceeded admissions to all the provincial psychiatric hospitals.[72] But it was clear that the provincial psychiatric hospitals and the psychiatric units were catering to different populations. During the late 1950s and 1960s between 26–30 percent of those admitted to the provincial hospitals suffered from schizophrenia as compared to 12–13 percent of those admitted to the psychiatric units. Whereas between 40–47 percent of those admitted to the hospitals were diagnosed as suffering from psychoneurotic disorders, the comparable figure for the psychiatric units was between 10–15 percent. Obviously, the psychiatric hospitals were caring for more serious cases of mental illness than the psychiatric units. In addition, per capita, although not total, expenditures on the psychiatric units were greater than for the provincial hospitals. In 1965, for example, the per diem cost of providing psychiatric care in the units was $34.69, as compared to $21.68 for short term care, and $14.69 for long term care in the provincial hospitals. Insofar as expenditures are directly correlated with quality of care, then the psychiatric units were providing a higher level of care than the psychiatric hospitals.[73]

Thus, the policy of establishing psychiatric units had worked—if by "worked" one means that more people were seeking help at the general hospitals than at the provincial psychiatric hospitals. By the 1960s, the provincial mental health system rested on two large and one extremely small pillar: the provincial psychiatric hospitals and the psychiatric units on the one side, heavily overbalancing the tiny community and aftercare program on the other.

Incremental Politics

How did the psychiatric unit program come about? According to Dr. Dymond:

> My recollection is that the establishment of the psychiatric units in the general hospitals came about largely as a result of discussions concerning medicare...there was no intention on the part of the federal government to do anything toward financing psychiatric hospitals...however there was agreement that the federal government would assist in the financing of psychogeriatric units, short-term psychiatric care in general hospitals, but without changing their policy in respect of government-operated psychiatric hospitals. It was more the evolution of political policy than any real health care policy.[74]

The decisions which led to the psychiatric unit program fit perfectly Braybrooke and Lindblom's definition of incremental politics.

> It is decision-making through small or incremental moves on particular problems rather than through a comprehensive reform program. It is also endless; it takes the form of an indefinite sequence of policy moves. Moreover, it is exploratory in that the goals of policy-making continue to change as new experience with policy throws light on what is possible and desirable...it is also better described as moving *away* from known social ills rather than as moving *toward* a known and relatively stable goal [their italics].[75]

As is often the case in the history of social policy, a major policy innovation resulted from the slow accretion of minor decisions. Only when viewed in retrospect does the psychiatric unit system seem, falsely as it turns out, to have come about as a result of coherent policy planning. In fact, there was no planning: there was no clear statement of goals or objectives to be achieved and no research into alternatives. The Department of Health did not consult in any formal way with outside bodies such as the CNCMH. The public was not consulted at all. Once the program got under way, there was no discussion concerning links between the psychiatric units and the provincial psychiatric hospitals, nor of links with community services outside the hospital system. The psychiatric unit program came about incrementally as a response to existing problems and not as part of a grand design for reform of the mental health system.

The fact that the mental health bureaucracy, from the Minister of Health on down, was staffed by medical doctors and psychiatrists biased the case in favour of the psychiatric unit system. On every possible ground—status, salaries, prestige, and relationships with other medical professions—the psychiatric unit system was the preferred alternative of the psychiatric profession. The medical model of mental illness militated in favour of treating mental illness within general hospitals. In a 1966 confidential report, an interdepartmental committee on emotionally disturbed children noted that interest groups had expressed concern "about the Mental Health Branch's policy of locating psychiatric services in public general hospitals without at the same time developing community mental health services."[76] But by then community mental health had become a dead issue. At the end of the 1960s, the Department of Health was still plodding onward, solving day-to-day problems, unwilling and possibly unable to formulate a long-term policy to meet provincial mental health needs. Very soon, however, it was to find that incremental decision-making sometimes created more problems than it solved.

Notes

1 "At the end of the nineteenth century...we find that prodigious postulate which no medicine had yet dared formulate: that madness, after all, was only madness." Michel Foucault, *Madness and Civilization* (New York: Vintage Books, 1973) 277.

2 Foucault 270.

3 On the establishment of psychiatric wards in general hospitals in the United States see Gerald Grob, *Mental Illness and American Society, 1875–1940* (Princeton: Princeton UP, 1983) 236–243.

4 Ontario Sessional Papers, *Second Report of the Inspector of Asylums, Prisons &c. for Ontario*, 2, No. 4 (1869): 25.

5 *Second Report* 27.

6 Ontario Sessional Papers, *Report of the Medical Superintendent of the London Lunatic Asylum* 5, Pt. 1 (1873) 157.

7 Ontario Sessional Papers 13, Pt. 2 (1880) 3.

8 Grob 238ff.

9 *More for the Mind* 85.

10 Quoted in Kathleen Jones, *Mental Health and Social Policy, 1845–1959* (London: Routledge and Kegan Paul, 1960) 124.

[11] Quoted in Grob 241.

[12] C. K. Clarke, "The Story of the Toronto General Hospital Psychiatric Clinic," *Canadian Journal of Mental Hygiene* 1 (1919–20): 30–37. A recent study of the ward is: Susan Roxburgh, "An Investigation of Neurasthenia: Patients of the Toronto General Hospital Nervous Ward, 1907–1924." Unpublished essay, University of Toronto, Toronto, 1989.

[13] Richman 53ff.

[14] Although some general hospitals had established separate wards for mental patients, most of these were daytime wards only or were housed in separate day hospitals annexed to the general hospital. In 1939, Canada counted four psychiatric wards in general hospitals, while out of 4,309 general hospitals in the United States, 112 had accommodation for mental patients. However, all but one of these departments were physically detached from the general hospital and located in annexes. In Western Europe, psychiatric services in general hospitals were also a rarity. Thomas J. Heldt, "Psychiatric Services in General Hospitals," *American Journal of Psychiatry* 95 (1939): 865.

[15] Aldwyn B. Stokes, "The Toronto Psychiatric Hospital: 1926–66," *Canadian Psychiatric Association Journal* 12 (1967): 521–23.

[16] Grob 136–143.

[17] Grob 126ff. In 1931, the Ontario Department of Health established the Neuro-Pathological and Research Division at the Banting Institute. The department seems to have devoted itself mainly to conducting autopsies and to preparing slides for students. See Ontario *Sessional Papers* 71, Pt. 14, No. 15 (1939): 20.

[18] Canada, House of Commons Special Committee on Social Security, May 18, 1943, p. 321.

[19] AO, RG 10, B. 157, HS M–3, June 21, 1951, Dr. R. C. Montgomery, Director Hospitals Division to Dr. Mackinnon Phillips, Minister of Health, Re: psychiatric requirements, Windsor, Ont.

[20] AO, RG 10–50, May 1944, "Future Policy of Psychiatric Services made by a committee of psychiatrists in the Armed Services," p. 6.

[21] "Future Policy" 2.

[22] AO, RG 10–50, HS 1–2, May 16, 1944, Superintendent, London Hospital to McGhie.

[23] AO, RG 10, 20-A–1, April 25, 1945, Appendix "B," Conference of Provincial Medical Directors.

[24] AO, RG 10, B. 157, HS M–3, October 20, 1945, R. C. Montgomery to "Fyle" Re: Allan Memorial Hospital, Montreal. In the 1980s it was revealed that while under contract from the American Central Intelligence Agency, Dr. Cameron had engaged in experiments designed to replicate brainwashing techniques. Patients were given LSD, electroshock treatment and a variety of chemical agents. Of course, the Ontario delegation visited Cameron nearly two decades before he was to begin working for the CIA, but in his memo Montgomery noted that insulin, adrenalin, electroconvulsive therapy and narcosynthesis were among the techniques Cameron used at the Allan Institute. The delegation that visited the Allan Memorial was composed of Dr. J. T.

Phair, the deputy minister of health, Dr. C. R. Myers, the director of mental health clinics, G. N. Williams, the provincial solicitor and Dr. R. C. Montgomery, the director of the hospitals division.

25 Montgomery to "Fyle."

26 AO, RG 10, HS 2–1, 1947, C. M. Hincks, "The Further Development of Mental Hospitals and Community Psychiatric Work in Canada."

27 Clarence M. Hincks, "Conserving Mental Health in Canada," *Canadian Journal of Public Health* 38 (1947): 317 and 321.

28 AO, RG 10, Series 107, Gen. 16–14, January 2, 1948, R. C. Montgomery, Director, Hospitals Division Re: MH Clinic Directors and Consultant Psychiatrists, to File.

29 Ontario Hospital Survey Commission 133.

30 OHSC 140. According to Dr. Aldwyn Stokes, Professor of Psychiatry at the University of Toronto and director of the Toronto Psychiatric Hospital during this time, "the consequence of the Ontario Health Survey Report was the establishment of Departmental policy on psychiatric units in General Hospitals." AO, RG 10, B. 157, HS M–3, September 8, 1955, Aldwyn Stokes, Director, Toronto Psychiatric Hospital to Dr. B. H. McNeel, Department of Health.

31 OHSC 154.

32 *The Globe and Mail* 30 September 1953.

33 AO, RG 10, B. 157, HS M–3, June 5, 1953, Dr. C. A. Roberts to Dr. R. C. Montgomery.

34 AO, RG 10, Series 107, Gen. 16–14, n.d. [1955?] "Report on Community Mental Health Services."

35 AO, RG 10, B.78, June 28–30,1948, "Minutes of the Second Meeting of the Advisory Committee on Mental Health."

36 AO, RG 10, B.78, January 22–23, 1951, "Minutes of the Fifth Meeting of the Advisory Committee on Mental Health."

37 *Debates*, Mackinnon Phillips, Minister of Health, March 4, 1952, G–8.

38 AO, RG 10, B. 157, HS M–3, June 21, 1951, Montgomery to Dr. Mackinnon Phillips: "I am attaching herewith copy of a letter…from the Honourable Paul Martin in which it is suggested that some suitable arrangements might be made for the sharing of the cost of operation of the psychiatric ward."

39 AO, RG 10, B. 157, HS M–3, July 22, 1952, Phillips to Hon. L. M. Frost.

40 AO, RG 10, B. 157, HS M–3, confidential letter from Roberts to Montgomery, December 3, 1952.

41 AO, RG 10, B. 157, HS M–3, February 8, 1954, Montgomery to Phillips.

42 In September 1953, the expert committee on mental health of the World Health Organization published a highly critical report stating that: "Too often the psychiatric hospital does not do its best job by imitating the general hospital… Patients are expected to be in bed and nurses are expected to be engaged in activities which resemble general nursing." The committee also pointed to another characteristic of

psychiatric units which was "very detrimental" to the community mental hospital especially if the former were the only way for getting into the latter. The expectation was that the psychiatric unit would treat patients who could quickly be returned to the community, while turning over to the mental hospital "those patients who are grossly disturbed, chronic, or of apparently bad prognosis." The ultimate result would be to turn the mental hospital into a "madhouse." WHO, Technical Report Series, No. 73, *The Community Mental Hospital*, Third Report of the Expert Committee on Mental Health (1953) 25. In 1958, Dr. F. S. Lawson, director of the psychiatric services branch of the Saskatchewan Department of Health opposed the psychiatric unit plan because the small size of the units would not be sufficient to cope with existing and future needs, the cost of establishing units in general hospitals was about forty percent greater than the cost of an equivalent bed in a "small mental hospital," the large mental hospitals would become a repository for chronic, accentuating the stigma attached to them and lowering staff morale, and, finally, because the units would tap a new source of patients rather than alleviating the burden on the existing hospitals. Instead Lawson recommended, and Saskatchewan planned to build, "eight small mental hospitals" housing no more than 400 patients each, and located near general hospitals. F. S. Lawson, "Mental Hospitals: Their Size and Function," *Canadian Journal of Public Health* 49 (1958): 191–192.

43 It also provided them with an opportunity to impress their medical colleagues with their skills. According to Dr. C. A. Roberts: "We now have the ability to deal with psychiatric emergencies on a medical basis and the image of psychiatrists held by other physicians and by the public in general may well be more related to the care provided for psychiatric emergencies than to any other aspects of our role in society." C. A. Roberts, "Psychiatry at the Crossroads," *Canadian Psychiatric Association Journal* 10 (1965): 449.

44 According to Lee Soderstrom: "The ability to share the cost of these services [psychiatric units in general hospitals] with the federal government...provided the provincial governments with a financial incentive to shift the locus of patient care from psychiatric institutions to general hospitals." *The Canadian Health System* (London: C. Helms, 1978) 145.

45 Interview, Dr. Gordon Martin.

46 "Report on Community Mental Health Services," 7.

47 AO, RG 10, B. 157, HS M–3, July 10, 1952, letter from Leslie Frost to Dr. Phillips.

48 AO, RG 10, B. 157, HS M–3, July 22, 1952, Dr. Mackinnon Phillips, Minister of Health to Hon. L. M. Frost, Prime Minister and Provincial Treasurer.

49 AO, RG 10, B. 157, H5 M–3, August 25, 1952, Dr. M. Phillips, Minister of Health, to Dr. R. C. Montgomery, Director Hospitals Division.

50 AO, RG 10, B. 157, HS M–3, December 31, 1952, News Release, Department of Health.

51 In 1955, the Report on Community Mental Health Services estimated that of total expenditures on community mental health services of $765,320, $570,100 came from the federal government.

52 "Report on Community Mental Health Services," 3.

[53] "Report on Community Mental Health Services," Appendix B.

[54] AO, RG 10, B. 157, HS M–3, May 26, 1959, "Report of Meeting Re Psychiatric Units in Public General Hospitals."

[55] *Debates*, March 27, 1952, p. BB–5.

[56] AO, RG 10, B. 157, HS M–3, January 18, 1955, C. A. Buck, Inspector of Hospitals to Mackinnon Phillips.

[57] AO, RG 10, B. 157, HS M–3, October 25, 1967, H. W. Henderson, "Changing Responsibility for Psychiatric Care—The General Hospital's New Role," address to the Ontario Hospital Association Annual Meeting.

[58] AO, RG 10, B. 157, HS M–3, August 29, 1956, Dr. B. H. McNeel, Director, Community Mental Health to J. T. Phair, Deputy Minister of Health.

[59] AO, RG 10, B. 157, HS M–3, January 5, 1959, H. W. Henderson to B. H. McNeel.

[60] AO, RG 10, B. 157, HS M–3, May 26, 1959, "Report of Meeting re: Psychiatric Units in the Public General Hospitals in Ontario."

[61] The Federal-Provincial Fiscal Arrangements and Established Programs Financing Act, 1977 came into effect on April 1, 1977.

[62] According to Stephen Dreezer, Executive Director, Institutional Division, Ministry of Health in telephone discussion, November 4, 1987.

[63] Interview, Dr. John Deadman.

[64] Joint Commission on Mental Health and Illness, *Action for Mental Health* (New York: Basic Books, 1961) 265.

[65] A. Richman, *Psychiatric Care in Canada: Extent and Results* (Ottawa: Royal Commission on Health Services, 1966) 55–56.

[66] In an interview Dr. McNeel recalled that some members of the Committee thought the psychiatric units might even replace the large mental hospitals, an opinion which Dr. McNeel did not share.

[67] AO, RG 10, Series 5, B. 19, July 25, 1963, "Report to the Treasury Board," unsigned memo.

[68] *Debates*, February 26, 1963, p. 1129.

[69] *Debates*, February 24, 1964, p. 879.

[70] H. W. Henderson, "Community Mental Health—Administrative Implications, *Public Health* 57 (1966): 145–152.

[71] See US 88th Congress US, Public Law 88–164, October 31, 1963, "Mental Retardation Facilities and Community Mental Health Centers Construction Act of 1963," Title II, Section 203, para. (2). In the end, most community mental health centres were either established independently of, or affiliated to hospitals. Few took the form of psychiatric units in general hospitals. See Alex Richman and Pamela Harris, "General Hospital Psychiatry: Are its Roles and Functions Adjunctive or Pivotal?" *General Hospital Psychiatry* 7 (1985): 258–266.

[72] See Table 4–1. AO, RG 10–108, November 4, 1971, Keith Kerns, Mental Health Statistics Branch to H. W. Henderson.

[73] AO, RG 10–108, May 7, 1969, W. Bain, Senior Economist, Hospital Operations Analysis, Statistical Research Division, Ontario Hospital Services Committee to H. W. Henderson. For figures on hospitals see RG 10–108, B. 18, "Census Tabulations and Cost Estimates: Hospital Care of Mentally Ill and Mentally Retarded, 1965–1970."

[74] Interview, Dr. Matthew B. Dymond.

[75] David Braybrooke and Charles E. Lindblom, *A Strategy of Decision* (New York: Free Press, 1963) 71.

[76] AO, RG 10–108, B. 12, March, 1966, "Report of the Interdepartmental Committee on Emotionally Disturbed Children," 22.

PART II: 1960–1970

5

The 1960s—An Era of Change

> This report represents five years of a committee representing eight psychiatrists... This report...does not attempt to include reference to the whole field of mental health as defined by the psychologist, the sociologist, the educationist or social worker.
>
> *More for the Mind*, 1963

> Psychologists, biologists, sociologists, nurses, occupational therapists, welfare experts, mental health educators, pediatricians, clergymen and other members of the mental health professions, and leaders from other groups with a professional or a public interest in the mental health movement joined with the psychiatrists.
>
> *Action for Mental Health*, 1961

Reforming Mental Health Care: Ontario and the United States

During the 1950s and 1960s, the contrast could not have been greater between what was happening in mental health policy in Canada and the United States. In Canada in 1946, after a series of informal meetings with representatives from the provincial governments, the federal government convened the first meeting of provincial mental health directors. In October 1947, it declared its intention of creating a 15-member mental health advisory committee composed of representatives from the federal and provincial mental health bureaucracies. But while the United States federal government and the National Institute of Mental Health sought wide political support by including a variety of interest groups on mental health bodies, the Ontario authorities pressured the Canadian federal government to exclude representatives of the Canadian National Committee on Mental Hygiene from the advisory council. Three months before a conference of the provincial medical health directors was to begin, Dr. J. T. Phair, deputy minister of the Department of Health of Ontario, wrote Dr. G. D. W. Cameron, deputy minister of the federal Department of National Health and Welfare:

> I note that representation from the National Committee for Mental Hygiene is to be limited to one representative [at the Conference]. You will recall that at the November meeting of the Council last year, I spoke strongly regarding what was obviously a domination of the conference last year by the representatives of the

Committee who were present... As far as I am concerned...no voluntary agency which is basically promotional in character, should have any place in a gathering of this type beyond whatever contribution they are in a position to make to a specific item or items in the program. Every Director in this Service in the province, is much more intimately aware of the difficulties which present [*sic*] in those aspects of the Service which are not adequately being cared for, than a representative of a voluntary agency.[1]

In reply, the chief of the federal mental health division Dr. C. G. Stogdill wrote to Phair about "the place of the voluntary agency in consultation with government officials...There is no disagreement here with the principle you expressed." Stogdill went on to point out that only one representative from the CNCMH would be present during the general meeting, while, "[i]n connection with the Advisory Committee on Mental Health, it is not our intention to appoint representatives from any voluntary agency on it."[2] In this way, the federal and provincial mental health bureaucracies ensured that no dissenting voices would be heard on the advisory committee and that its deliberations would represent the views of the medical doctors who staffed the provincial mental health divisions and the psychiatrists who were their consultants.

But, while Ontario was heading in one direction, the United States was heading in another. From the very beginning, the movement to change mental health policy in the United States was national in scope, community care in orientation, and heterogeneous in composition. The story of how the National Institute of Mental Health (NIMH) came to dominate American mental health care politics from 1945 to the 1970s has been told a number of times, but the differences between what happened in the United States and Ontario are worth noting.[3]

In 1945, Surgeon-General Thomas Parran of the U.S. Public Health Service asked Robert Felix, assistant chief of the hospital division, to sketch a national mental health program. Felix then met with the chief psychiatrists of the military service, all of them members of the Group for the Advancement of Psychiatry and all of them in favour of improving community care. Together they worked on a bill which led to the National Mental Health Act of 1946, creating the NIMH. Initially created as a research, training and educational organization, the NIMH rapidly became an extremely wealthy (ultimately, the fourth wealthiest institute in the United States) and very powerful pressure group.[4] Led by Felix and ably assisted by lobbyist Mike Gorman, the NIMH directed its activities toward a major reform of the state mental hospitals. According to Gorman: "My hidden agenda was to break the back of the state mental hospital system."[5] Part of the plan was to prepare the nation for a national mental health program. By assiduously cultivating professional, interest group and political constituencies, the NIMH was able to marshall enough support to get Congress to pass the Mental Health Study Act of 1955. The Act led to the appointment of a 45-member Joint Commission on Mental Health and Illness, 25 of whom had medical degrees, while the remaining 20 came from diverse fields such as social work, psychology, and law. However, neither the commission report of 1961 nor the

Community Mental Health Centers Act, 1963 stipulated that community care necessarily meant independent, free-standing, community mental health clinics. In fact, until the passage of the Act, the phrase "community care" was broadly applied to any structure or facility which was established independent of the state mental hospital. The terms of the 1963 Act left it up to the individual states to decide what kind of facility was to be constructed. By 1978, of the 675 community mental health centres, 19 percent were general-hospital based, 3 percent were mental hospital-based, 2 percent private psychiatric hospital-based, 64 percent were hospital affiliated, and 12 percent were free-standing.[6] There is, of course, an enormous amount of controversy over the community mental health centres, but clearly the United States made a start toward establishing a system of community-based services long before most countries. However, it was difficult to break the ties that bound psychiatrists to hospitals and to establish community services that were truly independent. In 1982, one group of critics observed that:

> Community centers are often located within general hospitals or very nearly, and the hospitals often have few if any contacts with the community the center is supposed to serve. A high proportion of staff time is devoted to the treatment of inpatients and inpatients account for a high percentage of the center's clientele...two more signs that in essential respects the centers are no different from traditional hospitals.[7]

While the United States was building the National Institute on Mental Health into one of the most powerful pressure groups within the federal bureaucracy, and laying the groundwork for a major extension of community mental health services in free-standing clinics and in general hospitals, there was no analogous development in Canada.[8] Rather, the federal government turned its attention to increasing hospital bed capacity, with the result that the number of hospital beds in Canada increased drastically, from 1948 to 1962, with a per capita ratio 10 times greater than the number in the United States.[9] Of the total funds disbursed during this period, approximately 53 percent was spent on mental hospitals, primarily on mental hospital beds, 23 percent on clinics and 13 percent on training. In Ontario, 47 percent of mental health expenditures were devoted to mental institutions, 26.3 percent to training, 13.4 percent to research, 7.1 percent to outpatient and community clinics, 4.5 percent to psychiatric units in general hospitals and 1.7 percent to other services.

But were these expenditures disbursed according to an overall plan? In one sense they were since the federal government, in cooperation with the provinces, decided that the bulk of expenditures should be devoted to mental hospital construction and that most of the remainder should go to educational and training purposes. But if the concept of planning implies examining a wide range of alternatives, choosing a limited number of objectives, specifying the means to achieve these objectives, and presenting the plan as an integrated, coherent package, then no planning took place. Moreover, there was no evaluation of existing programs, another crucial component of any realistic plan. Although the federal government certainly kept track of provincial expenditures, thereby ensuring that monies were spent on specific program objectives, that was as far as it went. Moreover, there was nothing at the federal or provincial level in Canada that resembled the NIMH with its network of individuals and agencies researching, evaluating, and monitoring mental health services, or providing an array of experimental or pilot projects. The federal government did establish a mental health division when it created the Department of National Health and Welfare, and its advisory committee of provincial mental health directors did have some influence on policy in the late 1940s and 1950s, but its influence waned and, ultimately, the provincial governments took over direction of mental health policy.[10] It is true that as part of the federal grants program, each province had been required to conduct a provincial health survey, including a survey of mental health needs, but, as Dr. Alex Richman points out:

> The failure to implement recommendations made by the provincial health surveys regarding mental health services were discussed in 1955 by the National Scientific Planning Council of the Canadian Mental Health Association [the successor to the Canadian National Committee on Mental Hygiene].[11]

A number of reasons were adduced for this failure: lack of funds, conflict between the various parties concerned with mental health delivery and services, lack of "clearly defined premises" for specific policies, negative public attitudes toward mental health expenditures and lack of trained personnel.

Moreover, the center of gravity of Ontario's mental health care system still rested squarely on the large institutions. In 1956, for example, there were 13,600 patients in residence in mental hospitals (excluding 4,643 residents of the hospitals for mentally retarded people), while there were 257 beds in the seven psychiatric units.[12] As well, expenditures for operating expenses were devoted mainly to the large institutions. In 1955/56 the province spent $23,406,082 on mental hospitals, compared to $97,919 for the psychiatric units. The actual expenditure on the psychiatric units for that year totalled $266,301, but $168,382 of that sum came from federal health grants.

More for the Mind

Because the mental health surveys had little impact on provincial policies, members of the professional advisory committee of the CMHA decided to influence policy by writing their own report. In 1955, the CMHA had established the Committee on Psychiatric Services, the so-called Tyhurst Committee. The link between the Tyhurst Committee and the Ontario Department of Health bureaucracy was personified by the presence of Dr. B. H. McNeel, chief of the mental division of the Department of Health on the Tyhurst Committee. In addition to McNeel, the members of the Committee were Dr. F. S. Lawson, who in 1958 was director of psychiatric services for the Saskatchewan Department of Public Health, Dr. C. A. Roberts, formerly the chief of the mental health division for the National Department of Health and Welfare, Dr. J. D. Griffin, general director of the Canadian Mental Health Association, and Dr. J. S. Tyhurst, professor of psychiatry at the University of British Columbia. The Committee's report, *More for the Mind*, was published in 1963.[13]

Originally, the Tyhurst committee was called the Committee on Psychiatric Services, then it renamed itself the Committee on Mental Health Services, and finally, in 1962, reverted to its original name. Although the Committee was chosen by the CMHA, that same pressure group whose members the Ontario deputy minister of health had argued should be prevented from serving on the advisory committee to the federal government in 1947, the CMHA in turn seemed completely indifferent to, or perhaps unconscious of the possibility that other professional bodies concerned with mental health such as psychologists, social workers, nurses or mental health staff might have something of value to add to their deliberations. This was brought to the committee's attention in January 1962, and the committee responded by agreeing to deal "only with treatment for the mentally ill"...and to change its name from Committee on Mental Health Services back to the original name, the Committee on Psychiatric Services.[14] Thus, while the American Joint Commission on Mental Health and Mental Illness invited the participation of mental health pressure groups and professional organizations, the Tyhurst Committee relied almost entirely on the narrow circle of psychiatrists, medical doctors and mental health decision-makers who had traditionally dominated mental health policy in Ontario.

In 1957, while the Committee was sitting, the federal Hospital Insurance and Diagnostic Services Act was passed, providing federal cost-sharing funds for general hospitals, but excluding mental hospitals. By depriving the provinces of funds for mental hospitals, the federal government hoped to encourage the provinces to devote more mental health expenditures to psychiatric units and community care.[15] According to the Tyhurst Committee, however, this was a "serious blow" to the developing trend of treating mental illness from a "medical approach." The result was to impel the Tyhurst Committee to emphasize even more the medical model of mental illness and to press for an integration of mental illness and medical care systems.

The Tyhurst Committee touched on all aspects of mental health policy, from treatment modalities through institutions and services in the community, to mental and general hospitals. Given the composition of the committee, it is not surprising that everything was viewed from a psychiatric perspective and that the medical model provided the framework for analysis. "In all instances...mental illness is regarded as a disorder or breakdown of living requiring psychiatric treatment. In this field the medically qualified psychiatrist was the acknowledged senior authority."[16] The report stressed that the psychiatrist had to play the central role in the treatment of mental illness, and that the mental health care system had to be integrated with the medical care system. The committee emphasized, in bold type, that: "Mental illness should be dealt with in the same organizational, administrative and professional framework as physical illness." The report went on to say: "This belief is the keynote of all recommendations made by the Committee on Psychiatric Services and a pivotal point on which all arguments rest."[17]

In page after page the impression given was of a profession that was misunderstood, undervalued and under-rewarded. The Tyhurst Report was a *cri de coeur*, a cry of outrage against unjust and unfair criticism and, at the same time, an attempt to stake a claim to vast tracts of medical territory over which the psychiatrist would rule supreme. This is evident from the defensive tone of its first few pages. For example, because the 1957 federal Hospital Insurance and Diagnostic Act excluded mental patients from benefits available to general hospital patients, "the mental health worker, especially the psychiatrist, seemed to be designated...as different and less worthy than other medical personnel."[18] Because general medicine had not yet accepted the idea that mental illness was a disease, "[t]he status of physicians who have made a career of the specialty of psychiatry...seems to have suffered in comparison with other specialities." Not loath to apply the techniques of psychoanalysis to psychiatrists themselves, the committee suggested that this might explain the attitudes of "defensiveness and aggressiveness" by psychiatrists.[19]

The solution was to reveal the truth to the medical and political community, to show them that mental illness was everywhere and that it was the psychiatrist, above all, who was best equipped to deal with it. This was an imperialist view of psychiatry with a vengeance. According to the committee:

> Mental health transcends medical concern with sickness and health. It relates to the whole spectrum of organized social living. It has to do not only with spotting and treating children with mental health problems in the school, but with the whole fabric of the school itself. It has to do not only with the neurotic and character disorders of adults in the community, but with their marital, occupational and social needs."[20]

After this, one might well ask whether there was any role left for psychologists, social workers, nurses, policemen, or politicians. The answer is that there wasn't—as long as the psychiatrist was present to diagnose, to guide treatment and to take the final decision. The logic was inexorable. First, it was asserted that mental illness was a medical problem and that mentally ill people were medical patients. According to the Tyhurst Committee: "It must be emphasized that the mental patient is a medical patient."[21] Next, it was asserted that the psychiatrist was peculiarly suited to deal with mental illness because of "the nature of his training in both medicine and in the biological, psychological and sociological aspects of mental health."[22]

Finally, it was argued that because modern psychiatry relied on the clinical team consisting of a psychiatrist, psychologist, nurse and/or social worker, it followed that the psychiatrist "is the person with medical authority and final responsibility for the clinical team's activities."[23] Thus, whether in large provincial hospitals, psychiatric units in general hospitals, schools, correctional institutions or elsewhere, wherever psychiatric services were available, the psychiatrist led while psychologists, social workers and nurses followed. Once one accepted the premises, the conclusion was inevitable. The psychiatrist must play a dominant role in the mental health system.[24]

Moreover, the Committee asserted that psychiatric authority extended beyond the boundaries of medical treatment of the mentally ill because administrative matters were linked to medical problems. After all, if "all aspects of hospital and psychiatric service—budget, personnel policy, plant development, maintenance, etc.—have therapeutic implications which bear directly on patient care," then "it is certain that for psychiatric hospitals administration should be in the hands of medical-psychiatric administrators." Even the details of budgetary decisions could not be trusted to non-psychiatric personnel. "The profound therapeutic implications of budgetary decisions are not generally appreciated; the specific allocation of funds...should be a matter for medical policy rather than decision by a business manager who may have no knowledge of the therapeutic issues involved. The psychiatrist should have final responsibility and authority."[25]

In strongly arguing for an organizational integration of psychiatric and medical services, the committee criticized provincial governments for establishing large and isolated psychiatric hospitals. "Political considerations rather than the health needs of the mentally ill frequently influence the development of hospitals and other services... Yet, for reasons which are often obscure, most provincial hospitals in Canada are attempting to care for 1,000 to 5,000 or more patients."[26] As an alternative, the report recommended that no more large hospitals or additions to large hospitals be established, that "no community inpatient service exceed 300 beds" and that, wherever feasible, psychiatric units be established in general hospitals.[27] For the Tyhurst Committee, the psychiatric unit was the wave of the future since "the bulk of all mentally ill patients requiring treatment in hospital will be cared for in such a setting."[28] However, the committee admitted that there were differences between psychiatric wards and medical wards, and since mental patients "must not be expected to be 'sick' in bed," it might be advisable to establish the psychiatric unit adjoining, but separate from, the general hospital. Still, it was important that the mentally ill be covered by the penumbra of physical illness. Where new psychiatric hospitals were constructed the Tyhurst Committee recommended that they be established adjacent to, or preferably as wings of, general hospitals.[29]

The psychiatric units in general hospitals were to be the focal point of community care, and the psychiatrists who ran them would play a major role in determining mental health policy in the community. They would be the leaders of the "psychiatric teams" which would establish links to agencies in the community concerned with mental health, they would shape aftercare policy, and they would be the dominant authorities in the mental health hierarchy which, at its lower rungs, would be staffed by social workers, public health workers, and other professionals and volunteers. Discharged patients, it was assumed, would be cared for by a network of services dominated by psychiatrists or medical doctors.

Clearly, the Tyhurst Committee envisaged the future of mental health policy in terms of a major reorientation toward the psychiatric unit system. Sociologist David MacLennan has argued that: "Since the early decades of the twentieth century, the professionalization of psychiatry was linked to a move away from the asylum." He explains this desire to raise the status of the profession as one of the factors behind the Tyhurst Report's attempt to carve out a major role for psychiatry in community mental health.[30] Certainly, in the 1960s, both the government and the psychiatric profession defined community mental health policy in terms of a medical model of care based on the psychiatric unit and dominated by psychiatrists.

The committee advanced five reasons why psychiatric units should be located in or near the general hospital: to provide treatment "close to the patient's place of residence...and to help the hospital to fulfill its functions of all-round services to the community"; to "recognize the psychiatric patient as a medical patient"; to enrich the "understanding of psychiatry" and improve the training of medical staff regarding the mentally ill; to "better the technique of the psychiatrist through contact with his colleagues in other services"; and to promote "public acceptance of psychiatry."[31] However, the first reason was a tautology since it assumed that only when a hospital had a psychiatric unit did it perform an all-round service to the community, while the remaining three had more to do with advancing the cause of psychiatry than with the specific needs of the mentally ill. Only the fifth reason having to do with the reduction of stigma was directed toward the specific needs of the mentally ill. Nor was it clear why psychiatric units should be located in, or adjacent to the general hospitals. The Committee reiterated its claim that mental illness was a medical problem which had to be treated in a medical, that is, a hospital setting, but in stating that mental patients needed different structures and treatment modalities than the physically ill, the whole rationale for integrating psychiatric units with general hospitals was called into question.

More for the Mind devoted an entire chapter to "The Community" and it predicted that there would be a shift from hospital care to "community psychiatric services."[32] Community care would take place in a variety of settings, with the mental hospital, psychiatric unit, community clinic, general practitioner and psychiatrist all playing a role. "In recent years there has been an increasing emphasis on the community orientation of psychiatry. It is recognized that the patient's illness began in the community and that, although during a phase of it he may need hospital care, he will return to the community when hospital treatment is over." But what constituted community care? According to the Committee "a wide range of psychiatric services at the local level is necessary," including inpatient hospital services and the facilities of "the small regional hospital." However, the Committee predicted that there would be a shift away from inpatient services and toward "community psychiatric services..."[33] Exactly what those community services were was never specified, but for the Tyhurst Committee, the psychiatric units and regional psychiatric hospitals were thought to comprise the bulk of any future community system. The notion of establishing mental health clinics associated with public health departments was briefly mentioned only to be immediately rejected because "at present there is a swing of professional opinion in favour of attaching all mental health clinics to general or pediatric hospitals as specialized outpatient departments."[34] In fact, when the Tyhurst Committee turned its attention to community care, the report became vague on the one hand, and sweepingly broad on the other. There was one specific reference to a "community clinic" but otherwise it was left to the reader's imagination to determine exactly which structures were to provide community care.[35] At the same time, one authority on community care was quoted approvingly for contending that "it is sounder to think of the community as one comprehensive agency for its people."[36] The "community" included practically every conceivable institution: "public health, education, social work, public safety, industry, the church, recreation, the court and other agencies." But even here, the psychiatrist was the dominant figure. In discussing the question of rehabilitation, for example, the Committee emphasized "the importance of the role of the medical practitioner... Rehabilitation should be a medical prescription by the physician caring for the patient."[37] Even when the patient was no longer in an acute stage and had returned to the community, it was up to the psychiatrist to determine the specific mode of rehabilitation and to monitor the patient's progress in the community.

Despite the paucity of services that would actually be located in the community as opposed to the mental hospital or psychiatric unit, *More for the Mind* envisioned mental health councils organized on a community and regional basis with strong links to both the local mental hospital and to the public health department.

> What is needed is a council widely representative of the community agencies and services having a mental health interest, the specific psychiatric services including the hospitals, the medical officer of health, the local medical society and the lay public. An executive committee of the council comprising the key health and psychiatric personnel is essential.[38]

But since "[t]he function of the co-ordination of psychiatric services was a medical responsibility," it was not surprising that "it is essential" that the executive committee of the council include "key health and psychiatric personnel." The next level of organization of services after the local community was to be the region. Here Tyhurst favoured a private board consisting of "professional persons from the medical and health services, persons in the community professionally concerned with mental health and lay representatives."[39] Tyhurst also complained that there was an absence of long term planning and that services had been established on a "haphazard basis... Political considerations rather than the health needs of the mentally ill" influenced policy. The provinces had, for political reasons, built large, remote and understaffed institutions. There were marked differences in salary between physicians in general hospitals and those in provincial service in psychiatric institutions. Finally, because of central administrative and funding control, there was no reason for local communities to interest themselves in mental health policy nor any modalities for them to get involved in the administration of the system.

The solution to these problems was clear: the federal government should extend the benefits of cost-sharing hospital and medical insurance to psychiatric institutions and to mental patients but abjure administrative control over the system. The committee noted that "[r]ecommendations had been made that conditions attached to the National Health Grant program be reduced or eliminated and that the provinces be given authority over their administration."[40] The committee also recommended that "the provinces should no longer employ psychiatrists on a full-time salaried basis," rather psychiatrists should "diversify" their activities, working in a variety of settings, part-time in private practice, part-time for the community or the province.[41] Smaller, regional hospitals should be constructed and the number of psychiatric units increased. Provincial governments were to divest themselves of the responsibility for the direct management of the mental hospital system and turn them over to the same kind of autonomous local boards which ran the general hospitals.[42] Even the financing of the mental health system was to be taken away from provincial departments of health and handed over to provincial hospital insurance authorities supplemented by provincial welfare agencies and other funding bodies.[43]

The Political Environment and *More for the Mind*

The Tyhurst Committee's recommendations were directed toward reducing the role of the federal and provincial government in the administration of the mental health system and to the creation of a layer of semi-autonomous administrative bodies at the local and regional level, representative of the mental health community but heavily biased toward psychiatrists. In contrasting the 1961 Report of the U.S. Joint Commission on Mental Illness with the Tyhurst Report, one critic observed: "The Joint Commission is friendly toward government and wants an increase in psychiatric services run by government. The Canadian Mental Health Association is basically anti-government and wants a reduction in government services, although not, of course, a reduction in government funds."[44] To a certain extent this was true, but the Joint Commission was merely reflecting the traditional American practice of trying to win state support for federal policies by promising the states an increased role and increased funding in proposed legislation. After all, supporters of the community mental health centres had to fight a battle, which they finally won, against the American Medical Association, which opposed federal government funding for mental health center staff. Moreover, both the financing and administration of the community mental health centers in the United States came from a number of private and public sources.[45] There were additional differences between the U.S. Joint Commission and the Tyhurst Committee. The Joint Commission emerged out of a resolution of the U.S. Congress to conduct a major survey of mental health services and policy in the United States. The National Institute of Mental Health was directed to appoint committee members and to supervise the study. It was generally expected that the outcome of such a study would be proposals for major legislation on mental health. By contrast, the Tyhurst committee was appointed by the Canadian Mental Health Association, a private interest group. Although most of the committee members had served the federal or provincial governments in one capacity or another, the committee spoke only for the CMHA—not for the federal government nor for any provincial government. Since, unlike the Joint Committee, the Tyhurst committee was not a creature of government, it was entirely open to government whether or not to respond to the committee's recommendations.

In advocating divestment of the provincial hospitals to private boards, in suggesting that psychiatrists be paid on a sessional basis—for time spent in patient care, rather than on a fully salaried basis by government—and in arguing for disengagement of the government from the task of direct management of the mental health system, the Tyhurst committee consistently argued for the full autonomy of the psychiatric profession. However, it would be a mistake to assume from this that psychiatrists were mainly interested in gouging the system for the largest financial reward or that they were completely opposed to national hospital or health insurance—for they were not. Rather, Tyhurst expressed the views of a profession that wanted on the one hand to work with government, but on the other hand deeply resented the fact that, historically, it had less influence over the shape of the mental health system than it thought it deserved.

The major impact of the Tyhurst Report on mental health policy in Ontario was to legitimize policies that were under way. Although Dr. Dymond had decided that no more large hospitals should be constructed, and although the psychiatric unit program had been in operation for a number of years, *More for the Mind* provided the psychiatric imprimatur for provincial mental health policy.[46] In 1983, Dr. C. A. Roberts observed that *More for the Mind* "was an attempt to outline understandable principles which could serve as a basis for the future development of services and…a rationale which would continue to sustain the services."[47] In an interview in 1986, he said: "If you read the Tyhurst report, we took the approach that integration was the thing, we were prepared to sacrifice certain community opportunities to integrate with the health side. I don't know if it's better or worse."[48]

Although many policies advocated by *More for the Mind* were already underway when the report was published, a number of recommendations were ignored. The psychiatric hospitals were not divested to community boards, community mental health councils were not established, psychiatrists working in the psychiatric hospitals continued to be paid on a salaried basis, and the government retained firm control over the financing and administration of the system.

Nonetheless, both the composition of the Tyhurst Committee and the tenor of the report reflect the self-confidence of the psychiatric profession at the end of the 1950s and the beginning of the 1960s. This was an era when, as Arnold A. Rogow pointed out for the United States: "In their role as part-time doctors and consultants to corporations, government, the armed forces, universities, labor unions, neighborhood mental health centers, and other agencies, the nation's psychiatrists also deal with a significant portion of the estimated 10 percent of Americans who are suffering from some form of mental illness."[49] But in claiming authority over such a broad area, psychiatry risked losing its credibility. In 1961, this had evoked a warning from the U.S. Joint Commission on Mental Illness and Health: "[I]t would pay a great dividend, if the profession were to be cautioned against overvaluing, overreaching and overselling itself, and, in general, against assuming attitudes of omniscience or superiority that are neither becoming nor soundly based."[50] However, neither in Canada nor Ontario, was there any sign of self-consciousness about the possibility of the psychiatric profession overreaching the boundaries of its authority. Given that the Tyhurst Committee had, wittingly or unwittingly, eliminated from its ranks non-medical groups or professions, it had insulated itself from internal dissent. D. B. Coates argued that the Tyhurst Committee represented the elite of Canadian psychiatry, pointing out that the members of the Tyhurst Committee were the major opinion leaders in the field, and were often called upon by government for advice or to fill major civil service positions. According to Coates this elite played a major role in shaping provincial and federal government policies and influenced "the restructuring of psychiatric services around private practice, general hospital and medical integration and the ideology that mental illness is identical with physical illness."[51]

More for the Mind did little to prepare either psychiatry or government for the problems they were to encounter in the 1970s and 1980s. Whereas psychiatrists were intent on carving a niche for themselves in the hospital system and in improving their professional position and prestige, and whereas governments were desperately attempting to control rising mental health care costs, the plight of ex-mental patients soon loomed as one of the most formidable problems mental health authorities had ever faced.

Notes

1 AO, RG 10, B–78, July 22, 1947, J. T. Phair to Dr. G. D. W. Cameron, Deputy Minister of National Health.

2 AO, RG 10, B–78, September 12, 1947, C. G. Stogdill, Chief, Mental Health Division, Department of National Health and Welfare to J. T. Phair.

3 Henry A. Foley and Steven S. Sharfstein, *Madness and Government* (Washington, D.C.: American Psychiatric Press, 1983); David A. Rochefort, "Origins of the 'Third Psychiatric Revolution' The Community Mental Health Centres Act of 1963," *Journal of Health Politics, Policy and Law,* 9 (1984): 1–31; and, for a critical comment, see Franklin D. Chu and Sharland Trotter, *The Madness Establishment* (Grossman Publishers: New York, 1974).

4 Foley and Sharfstein 20ff.

5 Foley and Sharfstein 23.

6 Alex Richman and Pamela Harris, "General Hospital Psychiatry: Are its Roles and Functions Adjunctive or Pivotal?" *General Hospital Psychiatry* 7 (1985): 258–266.

7 Robert Castel, Françoise Castel, and Anne Lovelle, *The Psychiatric Society* (New York: Columbia UP, 1982) 137.

8 In 1945, Dr. Clarence Hincks of the CNCMH had suggested that a "National Institute of Human Behavior or Humanics" dedicated to training and research in mental health be established at the University of Toronto and at McGill University, but nothing ever came of the idea. See J. D. Griffin, *Mental Health—Canada: The Chronicle of a National Voluntary Movement, the Canadian Mental Health Association, 1918–1980*, ms. 1981: 230.

9 Richman, *Psychiatric Care in Canada* 10.

10 According to Dr. C. A. Roberts: "The early Advisory Committee meetings were called with enthusiasm, and an impression of active involvement in the planning and implementation of necessary improvements and expansion of mental health services developed. During more recent years the effect of the Federal Mental Health Division has been much less noticeable." Dr. C. A. Roberts, "Major Changes in the Administration of Psychiatric Services in Canada," *Canadian Psychiatric Association Journal* 11 (1966): 230–231.

11 Richman, *Psychiatric Care* 7.

12 See Table 4–1.

13 For the best critique of the report see Clyde Marshall,"'More for the Mind': A Review and Comparison," *The Canadian Psychiatric Journal*, 9 (1964): 3–18.

14 *More for the Mind* i. In "'More for the Mind' Twenty Years Later, the Canadian Experience," a speech delivered in Toronto on May 25, 1983, Dr. C. A. Roberts noted: "While many other professional groups and individuals were consulted it will be noted that the committee consisted entirely of psychiatrists and that they were all male! No one even thought of or mentioned the possibility of including other professions or females to say nothing of the native population, our French speaking compatriots or other minority groups," p. 15.

15 Roberts, "More for the Mind," 15. Roberts says that Dr. D. G. McKerracher made this argument.

16 *More for the Mind* ii.

17 *More for the Mind* 38.

18 *More for the Mind* 3.

19 *More for the Mind* 13.

20 *More for the Mind* 205.

21 *More for the Mind* 39, 82, and 86.

22 *More for the Mind* 151.

23 *More for the Mind* 146.

[24] "The third level of service—the psychiatric services proper—consists of the psychiatrist and the members of his team working in a number of settings...Mental illness is a multifactorial affair requiring the assistance of professionals such as the psychologist, the nurse and the social worker." *More for the Mind* 68.

[25] *More for the Mind* 152–153.

[26] *More for the Mind* 27.

[27] One psychologist argued that the Tyhurst Committee had no evidence that smaller hospitals, or community care were better for psychiatric patients than the large hospital. See W. H. Coons, "Mental Health Services in Canada: Some Comments on One Aspect of the 'Tyhurst Report'," *The Canadian Psychologist*, 3a (1962): 88–93.

[28] *More for the Mind* 87.

[29] *More for the Mind* 42.

[30] David MacLennan, "Deinstitutionalization in Canada: The Intellectual and Social Context in Historical Perspective," Paper read at the annual meeting of the Canadian Sociology and Anthropology Association, Winnipeg, June 1986, p. 39.

[31] *More for the Mind* 86.

[32] *More for the Mind* 55.

[33] *More for the Mind* 55.

[34] *More for the Mind* 97.

[35] *More for the Mind* 59.

[36] Warren C. Lawson quoted in *More for the Mind* 60.

[37] *More for the Mind* 71 and 76.

[38] *More for the Mind* 63.

[39] *More for the Mind* 64 and 197.

[40] *More for the Mind* 202.

[41] *More for the Mind* 157.

[42] The report suggested "placing the responsibility for these hospitals, as for general hospitals, in the hands of the local community. Mental hospitals should be reconstituted under corporate boards of management... They should become public hospitals authorized to care for a variety of illnesses and their administration and organization should be essentially the same as that of general hospitals." *More for the Mind* 26–27, and 42.

[43] *More for the Mind* 198.

[44] Clyde Marshall, "More for the Mind: A Review and Comparison," *Canadian Psychiatric Association Journal* 9 (1964): 17.

[45] Foley and Sharfstein 39–81.

[46] According to Dr. B. H. McNeel, Dr. Dymond, the Minister of Health, accepted many of Tyhurst's recommendations and incorporated them into policy. Interview, Dr. McNeel.

[47] C. A. Roberts 14.

[48] Interview, Dr. C. A. Roberts.

[49] Arnold A. Rogow, *The Psychiatrists* (New York: Dell Publishing Co., 1970) 15.

[50] Joint Commission on Mental Illness and Health, *Action for Mental Health* (New York: Basic Books, 1961) 280.

[51] D. B. Coates, "Is There a Power Elite in Canadian Psychiatry?" *Canadian Psychiatric Association Journal* 14 (1969): 207.

6

The Dymond Era

> I discovered some terrible patronage things where only certain people got the orders because they were members of the governing party, and because the business administrators of the institution were political appointments. But they said, "I'm the boss, you stay over there."
>
> Former psychiatric hospital superintendent

Dr. Dymond's Magna Carta

In December 1958, Dr. Mackinnon Phillips was replaced as Minister of Health by Dr. Matthew Dymond. According to Dr. Dymond:

> One of the first things that met me when I went into the Ministry was a great concern among my staff about the state of our provision for the mentally disturbed. The psychotropic drugs had just begun to come in. We had chlorpromazine and we had largactil and we had one or two others. At last medicine seemed to feel that something could be done for the mentally disturbed.[1]

Immediately upon assuming his position Dr. Dymond was presented with a proposal for reform of the mental health system.[2] Drafted within the Department of Health by Dr. B. H. McNeel, chief of the mental health division, and signed by both Dr. Dymond and the deputy minister of health, it first appeared in January 1959 under the title "Proposed Revision of Mental Health Program in Ontario." The following month, on February 11, 1959, Dr. Dymond presented it to the legislature. He did not consult with the medical superintendents of the large mental hospitals prior to introducing his program.[3]

Dr. Dymond's Blueprint, or as some called it, "Magna Carta," was derived almost completely from the Tyhurst Committee, and every one of Dr. Dymond's recommendations can be found in *More for the Mindd*. He began with a remarkable criticism of Ontario's record in mental health policy.

> Suffice it to say, briefly, that our entire attitude, and again I point out this has been a general attitude, has been to start at the wrong end of the problem... We want to try now to completely reverse the old order, to begin treatment where it should begin—at the home level and direct that treatment toward keeping the patient in, or at least near, his home community.[4]

Despite this attack on the existing system, Dr. Dymond's speech was a curious amalgam of the old and the new. On the one hand, he had been converted to the idea that large institutions were a thing of the past, on the other, the government had committed itself to build new, large hospitals, and was still under pressure to fill gaps, such as a short-fall of 1,000 beds in the Toronto area.[5] Thus, Dr. Dymond stated: "We may still find it necessary to have apparently large institutions, but what I do hope—and what we plan at the present time—is that we will not have the huge mausoleum-like structures with great numbers of beds piled row on row in them, as has been the thinking over the past 50 or 60 years."[6] To mitigate the problems of the large institutions, Dr. Dymond proposed a unit system of organization: each hospital would be divided into units—mini-hospitals—of between 250 and 300 beds, each with its own staff. However, Dr. Dymond's staff was aware that the opposition might pounce on the apparent contradiction between his promise to curtail the construction of larger hospitals and to establish a regional hospital network, and the actual policy of planning additional large hospitals and adding new wings to existing structures. Thus, the chief of the mental health branch advised Dr. Dymond to cite the plans to establish two new hospitals and a new hospital for the mentally retarded at Cedar Springs as "progressive steps toward providing regional services. The additions to the other large hospitals which appear to contradict this principal [*sic*] can be interpreted as steps toward the replacement of obsolete accommodation except in the case of Brockville which cannot be explained away on this basis."[7]

Dr. Dymond's speech was greeted with some skepticism by the press. The Toronto *Globe and Mail* said that the new plan was "not a change…its value is chiefly a practical one: where previous extensions of service were haphazard they will now be controlled. It marks, in fact, the first time the Government has stated a firm policy on a mental health program."[8] *The Globe and Mail* noted that despite the attempt to move away from the large provincial hospital, short of blowing them up, the ten large institutions could only be reorganized through the unit system proposed by Dr. Dymond. However, confused signals came from the government. On May 20, 1959, the Owen Sound *Sun-Times* quoted Premier Leslie Frost as announcing the construction of three 1,000-bed hospitals. In November 1959, Dr. Dymond told the superintendent's conference that "[t]he Goderich Hospital is going to be another 1,200-bed institution and have to admit complete failure in this regard, but too many commitments had been made. But at least they will be in separate 300-bed units."[9] Dr. Dymond also admitted that a small institution had been planned for Grey County, "but here again commitments were made and [he] may not be able to abide by the 300-bed limit." Unable to reverse existing commitments, Dr. Dymond's strategy was to reduce the size of projected hospitals. In 1961, he announced the construction of two new regional mental hospitals in Goderich and Owen Sound at 300 beds each.[10] The Cedar Springs institution for the mentally retarded had initially been planned with a capacity of 2,000, but Dr. Dymond scaled down the building so that Cedar Springs never held more than 1,000 people.[11] In 1962, he stated that 150-bed hospitals were better than 300-bed hospitals. "[A] year ago we stated certain localities would have to build a hospital of at least 300 beds In the short space of a year we have revised our thinking...and accept the fact that possibly a hospital half that size will do the job, and that we should branch out into other areas rather than sticking to the idea of institutional or in-hospital care."[12] In 1964, Dr. Dymond had to announce the construction of two 300-bed hospitals in northern Ontario, at Timmins and Sault-Ste. Marie.[13] However, by the 1960s, the decline in the number of long-stay patients in Ontario's mental hospitals prompted Dr. Dymond to predict that, just as had been the case with tuberculosis hospitals in the 1950s, the continuing decline in the mental hospital population would obviate the necessity for constructing additional institutions, while making it easier to treat those still in care.[14]

By this time, the Liberals and the NDP were questioning the policy of building large mental hospitals and pointing out the contradiction between Dymond's preference for small hospitals and the Department of Public Works' penchant for building large institutions.[15] On February 12, 1960, in support of his contention that no more large mental hospitals or additions to large hospitals be built, Liberal James Trotter quoted from a World Health Organization Report recommending that the maximum size for a mental hospital should be 500 beds. According to Trotter, the problem was that the hospitals were constructed by the Department of Public Works which, he said, "seems to be having control of this...and it would seem for the record to suit their own purposes."[16] However, the opposition parties inconsistently criticized the government for building large institutions and then demanded that mental hospitals be constructed in members' ridings. Since 1960, Bernard Newman, the Liberal member for Windsor had been pressuring Dymond to establish a mental hospital in the city because, as he pointed out, mentally ill people from the Windsor region who needed hospitalization had to be admitted to the provincial facility in St. Thomas, about 120 miles away. Although Dr. Dymond had promised in 1960 that a mental hospital would be built in Windsor, he later changed his mind and delayed the decision. In 1965, he decided instead to establish psychiatric units in the various general hospitals in the region. But the Liberals continued to press for the establishment of a 300 bed hospital.[17] Although he made no specific suggestions about how to meet the problem, NDP spokesman Stephen Lewis noted in 1965 that Metro Toronto was 1,000 mental hospital beds short of what was required based on accepted bed-ratio standards.[18]

Dr. Dymond also made important changes in another area. For years, the Department of Public Works had been criticized for designing institutions for the mentally ill and mentally retarded that were completely out of keeping with current thinking on architectural design. In 1958, at a superintendent's conference, Dr. Cumberland observed that "many new buildings were using old designs planned for ideas about mental patients long since abolished."[19] Stories were told of architects using thirty year old plans to design mental retardation institutions in the 1950s, or of using the same set of plans for institutions across the province regardless of geographical location or the type of patient to be served.[20] Dymond put a stop to this practice by asking private architect John

Parkin to design the Clarke Institute, opening to competition the design of provincial mental and mental retardation institutions, and establishing an architectural committee including members of the mental health service. He also authorized the establishment of the Thistletown centre for emotionally disturbed children, increased resources for training for psychiatrists and nurses and announced new initiatives in the field of mental retardation policy.

Another important decision was taken during Dr. Dymond's tenure—although perhaps it should be characterized as a non-decision. This concerned the question of divesting the government of its responsibility for the provincial psychiatric hospitals.

Since at least 1963, the government had been advised to divest itself of direct responsibility for the operation of the provincial psychiatric hospitals, and to turn them over to public boards to be operated along the same lines as the general hospitals. *More for the Mind* suggested,

> placing the responsibility for these hospitals, as for general hospitals, in the hands of the local community. Mental hospitals should be reconstituted under corporate boards of management... They should become public hospitals authorized to care for a variety of illnesses and their administration and organization should be essentially the same as that of general hospitals.[21]

The attitude of the Minister of Health toward divestment was, however, unclear. In the summer of 1967, a Progressive Conservative MPP, A. M. Pritchard, criticized the "over-centralization" in the organization of the mental hospitals and requested that "immediately steps be taken to create local boards of governors and hospital organizations to whom mental hospitals would be turned over for operation."[22] At the conclusion of her speech Ms. Pritchard observed: "I must say, Mr. Speaker, the hon. Minister is in complete accord with this statement." Whether or not Dr. Dymond was in fact in agreement is unclear. In 1979, *Agenda for Action* noted that in 1964 Dr. Dymond had proposed to transfer responsibility for the provincial hospitals to the community. However no evidence of this can be found, and in an interview in 1988 Dr. Dymond not only denied he had made such a statement, he claimed he was always utterly opposed to divestment. Some of the confusion might arise from the fact that, in 1967, Dr. Dymond stated that he favoured community boards running children's institutions.[23]

In addition to questions about overcrowding, the opposition parties also noted differences between the salaries of attendants in the mental hospitals and provincial employees in other institutions. In 1962, Liberal James Trotter observed that attendants in mental hospitals received lower salaries than guards in the Toronto Don Jail.[24] Three years later he noted that attendants received lower incomes than welfare recipients.[25] Dr. Dymond's response was to note that salaries of provincial employees were out of his jurisdiction because they were handled by the provincial civil service commission.

The NDP criticized the government for the shortfall in the number of psychiatrists in the provincial institutions. On the basis of American ratios, Stephen Lewis calculated in 1965 that Ontario lacked 44 psychiatrists in provincial institutions and that the province was short of psychologists, social workers and welfare workers. Lewis also accused the government of never having done any kind of manpower survey to assess current and future needs.[26] Dymond's response was to argue that public service psychiatrists were lacking everywhere in North America, not just in Ontario.

The Politics of Institution-Building

For more than 100 years, governments in Ontario—and elsewhere—used public institutions (mental hospitals, jails, detention centres, and hospitals) to garner political support. The most egregious example was the construction of the vast St. Thomas mental institution in an isolated rural area which was part of Premier Mitchell Hepburn's constituency, and on land he owned. In 1950, Progressive Conservative MPP H. A. Reynolds from Leeds suggested that the "old theory" that mental hospitals should not have more than 1,200 beds was "in discard" and he suggested that the government build larger hospitals for 5,000 to 6,000 patients. Reynolds made this point in the course of a speech proposing an expansion of the Brockville mental hospital located in his constituency.[27] Even the Minister of Health's statement that "the answer to our mental health problem today is not going ahead and building bigger and better hospitals" did not put an end to the construction of large institutions.[28] Millions of dollars continued to be invested in buildings which were too large, poorly-located and ill-designed.

Typically, the establishment of a hospital, an institution for the mentally ill or the mentally retarded, a prison or any other public institution occurred only when the pressure of numbers became overwhelming, and/or a major scandal or tragedy forced government to act. But governments then turned the compulsion of statistics about overcrowding or of public opinion into an opportunity to create jobs and to inject government funds into local economies. Those aspects of policy concerning patient care—treatment modalities, the environment in which patients lived, community programs, rehabilitation or recreational programs—were of little consequence. Decisions about the size and location of mental hospitals were used by the Premier and the Cabinet to reward loyal constituencies or to garner political support in shaky ones; psychiatrists in the Department of Health had to fight tooth and nail to get the Minister and Cabinet to lay down policies which were in keeping with current ideas on the best way to treat mental illness. Of course, by itself this kind of decision-making is the very stuff of politics, and all other things being equal, is harmless. But in the case of mental health policy *ceteris paribus* has never held. Since there was no contravening force to defend the interests of mentally ill people or to rouse public opposition to these policies, the best interests of mentally ill people were often ignored. This is why enormous, ugly and inhumane provincial institutions were established in isolated rural areas or in areas of low employment or depressed economic condition. From the construction of the early lunatic asylums to postwar plans for enormous human warehouses, the Department of Public Works thought in terms of hospitals whose size, design and location could not be justified in terms of any therapeutic rationale whatsoever. The main objectives of government policy were to provide employment, to win political support—and to spend no more than was necessary to achieve these objectives. Since nothing was to be gained by making any attempt at creativity in architecture, and since the hospitals were to be built as cheaply as possible they tended to look alike. A former head of the mental health division states that institutions were considered to be local industries with everyone trying to get one in their area. "One of the problems was getting services properly located because the government would make political commitments to build a hospital somewhere. Mackinnon Phillips planned to build a 2,400 bed hospital in Owen Sound, the member from Goderich worked on Leslie Frost for years and finally got him committed to build a 2,400 bed hospital in Goderich, but these were two peripheral places." This mental health bureaucrat recounts how he was asked to speak to a meeting of local mayors in North Bay knowing full well that "their impression was that here was a new industry that would hire a lot of people, so I started talking and said it isn't what the mental hospitals can do for you it's what you can do for the mental hospital…but it was this business of the political pressure and the attitude that this was just an industry."[29] In 1969, NDP MPP Morton Shulman stated that among the reasons for establishing mental retardation institutions was the desire, "in part to satisfy demands to locate employment opportunities in under-developed areas in order to provide jobs and income for the surrounding communities."[30] In 1970, NDP MPP William Ferrier accused the government of establishing a $6.5 million facility in the northern Ontario town of South Porcupine in 1963 because of "political reasons," that is, to create jobs and inject money into the local economy. Ferrier claimed that staff were never consulted about the planning of the building and that it was much too large for the area. The result was that it was never used to capacity, and it was extremely difficult to attract medical and psychiatric staff to the area. "So we have a half-used facility on our hands that cost the province $6.5 million because political opportunism took precedence over sound health care planning."[31] According to a former high civil servant from the Department of Health, the location of the Timmins institution was determined by "economic" considerations, it "was somebody's land."[32] This same point was made in 1976 by Liberal MPP John K. Riddell who stated that "[psychiatric hospitals] have been rated right up there with prisons as job-creating institutions to be located in loyal ridings. The prisons came from the feds; the hospitals from their provincial brothers."[33] The Minister of Health, who was present, did not contradict him. A 1966 interdepartmental report on emotionally disturbed children noted that institutions had been built with no apparent reference to the availability of manpower in region.[34]

According to a former Minister of Health, "it was just the way politics used to run in those days, people used to think that it was really great if you were a local member and you were a member of the government party and you could get a big public works built in your constituency. Take Cedar Springs as a good example, once it was decided that southwestern Ontario was an area that needed to be served, there would have been a battle to see whose constituency it could go in."[35]

According to this Minister, when Leslie Frost was Premier from 1949 to 1961, the Department of Health would decide which part of the province needed a new institution. Once the general area had been chosen, discussions might take place in Cabinet about the exact constituency in which to locate the institution, but Frost himself would make the final decision. At this point the Department of Public Works would be notified and construction would begin. Once the institutions were constructed, and only then, the mental health bureaucracy came on the scene. Until the late 1950s, the mental health bureaucracy had little influence over the location, size or design of the mental institutions. Thus they took over institutions which many of them felt were unsuited to the needs of mentally ill people or to the objectives of the mental health system. Yet, because the system had functioned this way since the middle of the nineteenth century, the mental health authorities had to accept the institutions as they were and to try to tailor their policies to fit the structures.

Transinstitutionalization in the 1960s

Despite the fact that Dr. Dymond's 1959 major statement on mental health occasioned a good deal of comment, one passage went unremarked, although it was to have major consequences. Dr. Dymond said: "I want to say very emphatically that the mental hospital will not be considered as an institution for custodial care."[36] According to Dr. Dymond there were about 12,000 patients in the "chronic, more or less hopeless category, including approximately 6,500 mental defectives."[37] These patients were to be removed from the institution and,

> placed in a wing or cottages of the present structures for the time being where they will be cared for in pleasant and comfortable surroundings. The ultimate objective is that they will be separated completely from the hospital setting and placed in a special type of institution where they will live in a homelike atmosphere and be given the care necessary for them, but will not occupy the time of highly trained specialists.[38]

Although no one used the term at the time, these chronic patients were about to undergo what in the 1960s became known as "transinstitutionalization"—the transfer of large numbers of mentally ill people, most of them elderly, from psychiatric hospitals to private nursing or residential homes. This policy was adopted throughout North America as a desperate response to the enormous numbers of elderly people who crammed psychiatric hospitals, but who, it was argued, could not benefit from active care. Although the term was new, transinstitutionalization was the latest attempt to deal with a very old problem.

From their inception in the early nineteenth century, mental hospitals became repositories for large numbers of elderly people who, although not necessarily mentally ill, had no other place to go in the community. Because there was no legislation providing for the establishment of poorhouses or other institutions for aged people in Upper Canada, the early asylum superintendents began to complain that local communities were fobbing off large numbers of people who were not mentally ill onto the provincial asylum system.

In the 1920s, there was some discussion about establishing a separate hospital for elderly people, but the idea was dropped.[39] In 1937, the Mental Hospital Survey Committee noted that as life expectancy increased, there was a "distinct increase in the number of cases due to the bodily changes of later life."[40] Whereas, in the past, senile old people would have remained in the community or been placed in "almshouses," the public now demanded that they be granted admission to mental hospitals.

Certainly the numbers of elderly people in the provincial psychiatric hospital system posed difficult problems for the superintendents and the government. In 1937, 22.3 percent of those admitted to all provincial psychiatric hospitals were 55 years of age and over, and they comprised 27 percent of the total hospital population. Ten years later, in 1947, patients aged 55 and above comprised 33 percent of total admissions and 32 percent of the population in residence.

The problem of elderly people in the mental hospitals was raised when the federal House of Commons Committee on Social Security met with the provincial mental health representatives in 1943. The provincial representatives noted that the number of people above the age of 60 was gradually increasing, and they proposed that "separate facilities at existing provincial hospitals or otherwise be provided for the treatment of elderly people and for research investigation into their health problems."[41] A year later, deputy minister B. T. McGhie proposed the establishment of a separate hospital or group of hospitals under the administrative control of the mental hospitals branch of the Department of Health. He also suggested that the medical staff of such an institution would, "if possible" have some postgraduate education in geriatrics.[42] The superintendents were generally favourable to McGhie's idea for a separate institution for elderly patients. However, one superintendent, Dr. D. R. Fletcher of the Ontario Hospital at Whitby suggested that they be treated in smaller institutions as close as possible to their own homes.[43]

The question of whether to accommodate elderly people in the provincial psychiatric hospitals or to build separate accommodation came up frequently in discussions among the asylum superintendents. In the summer of 1944, Dr. Stevenson suggested that a separate hospital be constructed for "geriatrics." Dr. Fletcher noted that he did not like to certify "old people unless necessary," while Dr. Farrar of the Toronto Psychiatric Hospital noted that the question of geriatrics had recently "come to the fore" and he predicted further developments in the field as had been the case with pediatrics.[44] Other superintendents disagreed, arguing that services for the elderly should be attached to mental hospitals, while Dr. Clarke warned that if hospitals for old people were attached to county homes they would be neglected and would not receive medical attention.

The topic continued to be raised in different quarters. At a meeting of the Ontario Neuropsychiatric Association in 1947, Dr. Clarence M. Hincks proposed the establishment of a mental hospital for the elderly "organised on the basis of an institute for geriatrics," with a research capability and with close links to the local community where the hospital would be located.[45] At a 1949 superintendents' conference it was noted that whereas in 1938, patients 65 and over comprised 11.9 percent of first admissions to the provincial psychiatric hospitals, ten years later they comprised 23.3 percent, and it was estimated that of the 2,861 first admissions, 40 percent did not require mental hospital care.[46] Once again there was a discussion of alternatives to mental hospitals ranging from separate accommodation to the establishment of separate wings for the elderly on the grounds of mental hospitals. That same year, MPP W. H. Temple of the Cooperative Commonwealth Federation (the precursor of the New Democratic Party) raised the question of elderly people in institutions. He stated that he had been struck by the number of elderly people at the Ontario Hospital in Toronto who were "in reality old-age pensioners...waiting for death." Temple argued that these people should not be in a mental hospital and he proposed that Ontario follow the example of British Columbia which had established seven 200-bed buildings for the elderly.[47]

For the next six years the topic of elderly people in the mental hospitals languished, but in early spring 1955, Minister of Health Dr. Mackinnon Phillips announced that elderly people would be transferred from the provincial psychiatric hospitals to infirmaries which were being built as part of our "aged homes."[48] According to Phillips, the province would pay half the capital cost of the infirmary with the municipality expected to pay the rest. He noted that there had been a sharp rise in the percentage of people 65 and over in mental hospitals, from about 6 percent in 1945 to around 20 percent in 1955. The expectation was that about 50 percent could be transferred to the infirmaries.[49]

But the policy failed. Most municipalities were reluctant to expend the necessary funds to establish the homes and, in those cases where they were established, they were almost immediately filled to capacity. By the late, 1950s, therefore, the Department of Health cast around for another alternative—and thought they had found one whose major attraction was that it promised to tap cost-sharing funds from the federal government.

This possibility had been first raised in 1948, when at a superintendents' conference, Dr. Stevenson of the London mental hospital suggested that 300 or 400 bed "special units in connection with certain existing mental hospitals" designated exclusively for use by elderly people might be eligible for grants under the federal Hospital Construction Grant Program. But the federal government would not agree, and so in the late 1950s the province sought some other means to elicit federal funds. The Department of Health decided to approach the federal government through the Ministry of Welfare after it learned that Prince Edward Island had obtained Unemployment Assistance funds by discharging from large institutions elderly people who could no longer benefit from active treatment and housing them in separate infirmaries. However, Ontario was reluctant to incur the expenses involved in establishing separate institutions, and, moreover, under federal regulations, the homes for the aged could not take any transfers from the provincial psychiatric hospitals. In this situation the Department hit on the idea of trying to satisfy federal requirements by establishing separate administrative units within the mental hospitals called "rehabilitation units." This explains the passing reference in Dr. Dymond's 1959 "Proposed Revision" document to discussions with the Ontario Hospital Services Commission and the Department of Welfare, regarding the transfer of "suitable patients" from psychiatric hospitals to accommodation that would "be provided by rental, purchase or building."[50] In fact, this was a major policy move whereby the Department would eventually transfer to alternate accommodation 12,000 patients from the psychiatric hospitals and mental retardation facilities.[51]

The Department of Health then entered into conversations with Dr. J. Willard, the federal deputy minister of welfare, to learn how Ontario might qualify for federal funds. At a December 15, 1960 meeting, officials from Ontario's Department of Health including deputy minister of health Dr. W. G. Brown, described the rehabilitation program to Dr. Willard. Dr. Willard pointed out that in order for the federal government to provide aid under the Unemployment Assistance Act the administration of the units had to be moved from Health to Welfare:

> any person who could respond to any form of therapy was not to be contained in this "infirmary." The Infirmary had to comply with all the general standards laid down concerning overcrowding, etc. An intake policy had to be adopted to insure that the above requirements were maintained...to insure that it was a domiciliary and not a treatment institution...the inhabitants had to be decertified.[52]

Dr. Willard warned the Ontario authorities that they would "want to be assured that the Province of Ontario would not just be shifting patients from one ward to another simply to pick up money since the Treasury people would wonder why the Department of Health was running a domiciliary institution which ordinarily was run by the Department of Welfare." In fact, this is exactly what the Department of Health tried to do. Rather than establishing separate institutions for the elderly, the Department of Health told the superintendents of the provincial psychiatric hospitals to establish separate wards or units in their institutions for the reception of elderly patients who could no longer benefit from active treatment. These were to be formally discharged as hospital patients, re-labelled as residents and kept in the separate units until such time as accommodation could be found. According to the deputy minister of health there was a possibility that the federal government might agree to participate in such a plan. In any case, "we are proceeding with this process since by doing so we cannot possibly be worse off than we are at the present time and have the prospect of collecting some revenue or maintenance and more important getting some empty beds." After Dr. Willard laid down the federal government's conditions, Dr. Dymond asked the superintendents to conduct a census of their institutions to determine which patients were chronic and which were eligible for active treatment, and then establish administratively separate wards or units in the institutions. The deputy minister of health explained that these people would be

Table 6.1: Residential Units in Ontario Hospitals

Year	*Numbers in Unit*
1961	1,234
1962	3,466
1963	3,465
1964	3,460
1965	2,879
1966	2,621
1967	3,071
1968	2,385
1969	2,082
1970	1,663
1971	1,158
1972	721

[Source: Ontario, Ministry of Health, *Mental Hospital Statisitcs*]

decertified and considered as temporarily lodged in the hospital "pending placement, if possible, in the community."[53] Eventually, it was hoped, Ontario would be eligible for federal funds for residents in the rehabilitation units. (Initially they were called rehabilitation units, but because the patients could not benefit from active treatment the term was changed to residential units.) For the next few years, Dr. Dymond prodded the sometimes reluctant superintendents to identify the chronic patients and set up organizationally distinct, but institutionally contiguous residential units.[54] On July 1, 1961, the process of discharging patients from the mental hospital and admitting them to the residential units began. During the year, 951 mental hospital beds were reclassified but Dr. Dymond was dissatisfied and he chided the superintendents saying that "action to date has not come up to my expectations... If we cannot discharge the patients who *should* [his italics] be discharged to other accommodation in the community, then at least we can identify them, and allocate to them suitable accommodation in our institutions until we can find or arrange community provision for their care. We can then say *this* is hospital and *that* is residence [his italics]."[55] The creation of the residential units did have one major consequence: it led to an apparent decline in the patient population in the provincial mental hospitals. Until 1959, the number of patients in Ontario's provincial mental institutions had continued to rise: in 1959, there were 13,773 patients on the books, in 1960 there were 13,619. But in 1961, there were 12,695; in 1962, 11,232; and in 1963, 10,851. This drop of more than 20 percent in three years was due almost solely to the transfer of the chronic population to the residential units.

By March 1962, nine residential units housing 3,466 residents had been established at the provincial psychiatric hospitals. By this time, however, the Department of Health realized that the residential unit program would not succeed in attracting federal funds and that the province would have to conform to federal guidelines and discharge the residents into separate accommodation. The Department of Health then decided to discharge patients from the residential units to existing nursing homes under the newly-created Homes for Special Care Program. The costs of residents in the homes for special care were then indirectly subsidized by the federal government to the extent they were eligible for federally cost-shared provincial social welfare funds.

Thus, there was a double transfer: patients were transferred within the institution from regular wards to the residential units, and then from the units to the homes for special care. Each year from 1961 to 1969, an average of 600 patients was reclassified and transferred within the institution to the residential units, while at the same time there was a continual transfer of patients from the residential units to the homes for special care. In 1964, there were 3,460 elderly people in the residential units, but from that point on the numbers declined as transfers to the homes for special care increased. From September 1964 to December 31, 1969, 10,875 people of all ages were admitted to the homes for special care from all provincial facilities, that is, mental hospitals, facilities for the retarded and from the residential units. In 1972, the executive director of the mental health division pointed out that psychiatric hospitals had been allocated 4,300 nursing home beds and 1,200 residential beds for a total of 5,500 beds in the Homes for Special Care Program.[56] The Department of Health justified the program as moving people back into the "community" and into a "homelike atmosphere."[57] But, over the years critics argued that far from returning people to the community, the homes for special care were frequently located in isolated rural settings, or, if in urban areas, far from transportation or shopping facilities, that the residents hardly left the homes, and that conditions in the homes were sometimes very poor and the staff often indifferent. The program was also notoriously understaffed. While in 1967 there were 35 staff workers available to inspect the homes for special care, the number fell to 29 in 1970. At that time there were 719 homes in the province. As NDP MPP M. Makarchuk put it in 1970: "In most cases in most of these homes there is absolutely nothing for them to do. They vegetate."[58] In 1973, the director of the psychiatric hospitals branch wrote to the general manager of the direct services division of the Ministry of Health that the large numbers of psychiatric patients discharged to the community were imposing a heavy burden on municipal finances while at the same time "[s]ome of the lodging homes are often considered quite unsuitable...the group lodging homes are nothing more or less than an extension of the hospital ward system since the patients are in no way in the community, but move peripatetically between day care and a fairly closely supervised group lodging home where they meet nobody else but other patients."[59]

The Politics of Transinstitutionalization

Unquestionably, provincial policy toward elderly mentally ill people was influenced by a variety of factors. From the very inception of psychiatric hospitals, the percentage of elderly people had increased. By the mid–1950s, when the residential unit program got under way, patients aged 65 and over comprised about 20 percent of the population of Ontario's facilities for the mentally ill and mentally retarded, and about 25 percent of the patient population of the mental hospitals alone. Many of these elderly people did not need to be in a mental hospital in the first place. The provincial psychiatric hospitals were being used as places of refuge, or as dumping grounds for elderly people who might have survived outside the institution if their families, relatives, or the community had been able or willing to help them. Naturally, the Department of Health desperately wanted to reduce the proportion of older mentally ill patients in the provincial psychiatric hospitals. However, the interests of the elderly people themselves were far from paramount. When the residential unit program got under way no one suggested, as B. T. McGhie and Clarence Hincks had some twenty years before, that separate institutions for the elderly be established and staffed by people with specialist training in geriatrics. The whole issue of geriatric training, having been raised in the 1940s, quietly disappeared from the scene. Nor was any serious attempt made to ensure that rehabilitation programs were available for elderly people in the residential units or in the homes for special care. In his highly critical 1966 Report on Ontario Mental Health Services, Dr. C. A. Roberts commented on the fact that the residential units had been established because of "administrative pressures" rather than to meet "the needs of the patients."[60] Although there was a good deal of talk about returning people to the community, the main goal was find some kind of program that would attract federal funds and would free mental hospital beds for more acute cases. The residential unit was supposed to achieve those goals. Although patients in the psychiatric hospitals were not charged for maintenance nor were they eligible for welfare funds, once de-certified and transferred to the residential units, they were charged for maintenance if they or their immediate families could afford it, or if they were eligible for provincial welfare funds. Moreover, expenses for people in the residential units were substantially below those of patients in the hospital. In 1962, the daily per capita cost for patients at the London psychiatric hospital was $5.5621, compared to $1.8404 for residents in the residential unit. At Toronto the daily per capita cost for the hospital was $7.6252, while for the residential unit the per capita cost was $2.6444. Expenditures on salaries were generally three to five times larger in the hospital than in the residential units because so many fewer staff were employed to care for residents in the units. Disproportionately more was also spent for hospital patients on "books, magazines and papers," and for "occupational therapy supplies."[61] As a 1963 unsigned memo to the Minister of Health notes: "The extent of this operation has now reached the point where we are talking about [saving] more than $1 million a year, which you know is of very great interest to the Treasury Board."[62] In an early 1967 memo proposing expenditure cuts, the deputy minister of health noted a reduction for the fiscal year 1967/68 of $5.5 million to the Homes for Special Care Program, between $500,000 to $1.5 million to special centres for emotionally disturbed children, about $1 million from mental retardation institutions, and other reductions totalling about $23 million. He hoped that with "recoveries" of $5 million from residents in the Homes for Special Care Program, plus reimbursements through the federal Canada Assistance Plan, revenues would amount to about $25 million—providing the government with a $2 million surplus.

Two conclusions can be derived from this memo: first, the Progressive Conservatives were quite willing to reduce the government's contribution to health policy as long as it could get compensation from the consumers and from the federal government, and second, the deputy minister counted on making a small profit in the transaction. There is nothing in the memo to indicate whether this profit would have gone into general revenues, been returned to the Department of Health to reduce its expenses, or been used for existing or new health programs.[63] The policy implications behind this memo are all the more interesting in the light of a 1970 statement from Dr. H. W. Henderson, the executive director of the mental health division. In a progress report for that year, Dr. Henderson noted that programs "relying entirely on provincial funds have been in a more difficult position than others drawing funds from additional sources."[64] Dr. Henderson was referring to the fact that the provincial hospital insurance program was cost-shared with the federal government whereas expenses for the provincial mental hospitals and most mental health expenses were funded almost exclusively by the provincial government. He also observed that the general hospitals were able to expand services despite rising costs because of the "increased revenue from the Federal Government." Apparently the Department of Health did not intend to use Canada Assistance Plan funding to improve or expand mental health services, but rather as a means for reducing provincial expenditures in mental health.[65]

One reason for the different policies toward the general hospital and mental hospital systems had to do with different administrative structures. Although the government certainly was interested in reducing provincial expenditures, the general hospital boards were not completely dependent on government financing because they could appeal to the community for funds. Moreover, they commonly exceeded their budgets and then used their political clout in the community to force the Department of Health to meet their deficit. But the psychiatric hospitals did not enjoy the same community political support as the general hospitals. In these circumstances, the government found it much easier to restrain expenditures in the mental health area than in the general hospital sector.

In 1968, Minister of Health Dr. M. B. Dymond announced that by the end of 1967, 5,745 people had been discharged from the mental hospitals to the homes for special care. He characterized this transfer as "an important development of community services," although he revealed the real object of the program in the very next sentence when he added: "The province expects to make substantial claims against the Canada assistance plan for the support of this programme."[66] Dr. Dymond also criticized Saskatchewan unfairly for its "overly ambitious" program of deinstitutionalization. "They have been more anxious to reduce the hospital's population or perhaps to present a better set of statistics, I do not know which, I think they are serious in their attempts to get more people out of the hospital but we believe that they have discharged them too early. We are trying to be a little bit more cautious and yet stay within good medical practice."[67] In view of C. A. Roberts comments that he could see little difference in the way patients in the hospital and residents in the residential units were treated, and the fact that the residential units were merely an administratively different part of the mental hospital, then the Minister's implication that the residential units were either medically justified or had anything to do with community care was misleading.[68]

Transferring patients to the residential units was also intended to help subsidize a planned expansion of outpatient and aftercare facilities in psychiatric hospitals and psychiatric units. This was made quite clear in a July 1972 submission to Cabinet from the Department of Health. The Department sought Cabinet approval for transferring 2,000 psychiatric patients to nursing and residential homes within the Homes for Special Care Program, and 2,000 "retardates" to residential units in the mental hospitals.[69] The Department estimated that an expansion of outpatient and aftercare services over the next four years would cost $15.7 million, but this would be reduced to $6.8 million if the recommended transfers were made. In justifying this request the Department argued there would be a "large" improvement in the quality of life of mentally retarded and mentally ill people as well as "reprivatization of health care by $5.7 million in 1973/74 rising to $12.7 million in 1976/77. This would produce a marked employment effect." It is not clear where the figures for "reprivatization" came from, although they may have been based on some estimate of the profits that would accrue to the private nursing and residential homes which would receive the discharged psychiatric patients.

Substantial costs savings were to be achieved by transferring mental patients to nursing or residential homes because the annual cost of maintaining a patient in a psychiatric hospital in 1972/73 was $7,670 as compared to $4,562.50 in a nursing home and $2,372.50 in a residential home. But these savings were not due entirely to the putative efficiency of the privately run nursing and residential homes, rather, there was evidence that the economies resulted from a lower level of care than that provided in the mental hospitals.[70] Even Minister of Health Thomas Wells admitted this in 1970: "Let us realize that these are not treatment facilities, these are residential homes. These people have basically been discharged from the institution and moved into the home, presumably because they have no family, no one else who wishes to take them, and yet we feel that there is a chance for them to go back out into the community."[71]

Clearly the government aimed to reduce provincial expenditure by manipulating federal government cost-sharing regulations and by letting the social costs of caring for chronic patients fall on the private sector. In 1971, the Committee on Government Productivity suggested that ministries "contract for program delivery with agencies both inside and outside the government... Widely applied," the report says "this concept could result in significant reprivatization... Its primary advantages would be greater flexibility and access to sources previously untapped." In justifying this proposal, the Department of Health noted that it was "in line with" the COGP recommendations on reprivatization.[72]

Although federal funds were not available to the province, patients continued to be transferred to the residential units until 1972. At that time the Health Insurance Act of July 1972 provided that care in residential units was an insured service. However, on March 15, 1972, Dr. G. A. Ives, the director of the psychiatric services branch, wrote to the executive director of the mental health division: "As I have pointed out in a previous memorandum to you, in some places in the system many of the patients now placed in the residential units are people who are ill-selected for such a situation." Dr. Ives then recommended "phasing the program out."[73] A little later, the executive director wrote to the deputy minister about the residential unit program observing that it

> has many disadvantages. Because the individual has been discharged from the "hospital" he is liable for maintenance charges, although he remains within the institution and is cared for by the same staff. In effect, he has access to the same benefits, but is charged for this. In most institutions the distinction is artificial, and many patients in the hospital present the same requirements for care and treatment as those in the residential units. There is a tendency to neglect those in residential units. Many discharged to these units have been in an institution for many years and it is doubtful that they could maintain their level of function in another setting.[74]

Dr. Ives noted that the residential units had "served a useful purpose in the earlier times of their introduction. They freed up staff to concentrate on patients...and...played a definite role in allowing many of our staff to start off a most desirable reduction in patient numbers by focusing on a number of priority program areas." Here Dr. Ives was referring to an earlier suggestion that staff not needed for the residential units could be used more profitably to care for acute patients. But, in a phrase of unconscious irony, Dr. Ives observed that "the concept of the residential unit patient has really not in recent times been accepted by therapeutic staff who have treated them vigorously, and in many cases, altered the patient's status frequently to full return to the community." Translated this means that the original idea behind the residential units was to provide minimal care for chronic patients for whom active treatment would not provide further benefit. However, some staff ignored the policy and worked with residents to the point where they could return to the community. Dr. Ives admitted that: "The publicity (and perhaps political) feedback may be undesirable along the lines of 'why did you originally do something which you are now undoing.' In my opinion this can be reasonably dealt with by the statements made in my paragraph above."

In financial terms, the residential unit program had been a success. From September 1964 to February 1973, a total of 11,500 people, most of them over 65 years of age, had been transferred from residential units to the homes for special care. It is likely that more than half of this number was comprised of psychiatric patients. According to Richard T. Potter, the Minister of Health in 1973, the total revenue obtained from maintenance charges from the residents over the period 1967 to 1972 was $4.14 million.[75]

The abandonment of the residential unit program did not solve the continuing problem of residential care for chronic and elderly mentally ill and mentally retarded people. After 1964, the Homes for Special Care Program was constantly under attack from the opposition parties, the press, and pressure groups. A 1984 study of the program commissioned by the Ministry of Health for the mental health division noted that from 1964 to 1984,

> the administrative responsibility for the Program has changed on six different occasions... These frequent changes and lack of consistent management have resulted in a program with a wide range of resident types and an unclear role in the continuum of mental health services in the province.[76]

The list of weaknesses echoed past complaints about Ministry of Health policy. "There is no planning for future homes...the Program is more reactive than proactive...the management information system is fragmented and inaccurate...program expenditures are not monitored," services and programs provided to residents were uneven across regions and the per diem rate paid to the privately owned nursing homes was not based "on actual costs incurred or analysis of any historical cost data" but resulted from "annual nursing home negotiations."[77]

The residential unit system was established because the Department of Health hoped to obtain federal government funding by separating chronic mentally ill patients from those who were still, ostensibly, under active treatment. This was part of a general movement in North America to reduce overcrowding by transferring to nursing homes or homes for special care those patients, mainly elderly, who were no longer benefiting from active care. In Ontario, this policy was implemented in two stages. First, the residential units were established in the provincial mental hospitals, and second, existing nursing homes were authorized to become homes for special care and to receive residents transferred from the residential units. Since the residential units were located in the provincial hospitals, and since nothing changed in the way the individual resident was treated except that s/he was reclassified from patient to resident, there can be no question that the move was prompted by the expectation of federal funding for the residential units. Moreover, if there were therapeutic reasons behind the creation of the residential units, it was curious that equivalent units were not established for the chronically ill in general hospitals. After all, the Department of Health claimed that segregating chronic patients would allow staff to devote more time to the acutely ill. But the reason why residential units were not established in general hospitals was because chronically ill patients already qualified for federal cost-sharing funds whereas residents in the residential units in the provincial mental institutions did not.[78] Andrew Scull has suggested that: "Particularly in America, an effort is under way to transform 'social junk' into a commodity from which various 'professionals' and entrepreneurs can extract a profit."[79] Although Scull argues that there was a deliberate and conscious attempt by American mental health planners to help private entrepreneurs make a profit at the expense of discharged patients, there is no evidence that the Progressive Conservative government was overwhelmingly motivated by a desire to help the private sector profit from transinstitutionalization. Rather, policy evolved in the incremental, ad hoc way it always had. The government would have been quite happy to use public funds, as long as they were federal funds, to maintain elderly people in the provincial institutions. They would have been equally happy to house them in publicly supported municipal institutions—if federal cost-sharing funds were made available. But when it became clear federal funds were not available, the province turned to the private nursing home sector, not because it was eager to line the pockets of private entrepreneurs, but simply because the nursing homes were already in place, and because they could relieve the province of some of the administrative and financial burden of the residential units.[80]

Notes

1 Interview, Dr. M. Dymond.

2 "The blueprint which I submitted to the House in 1959 was really handed to me as a finished document, essentially, and then they gave me a crash course from Christmas 1958 until February." Interview, Dr. M. Dymond.

3 "He [Dr. Dymond] regretted that the program was announced without prior consultation, but this was unavoidable." AO, RG 10, B. 165, HS S–6, March 6, 1959, Minutes of Superintendents' Conference. Perhaps the lack of consultation was an indication that Dr. Dymond did not want to give the superintendents time to mount a campaign against reducing the size and role of the large institutions, or it might have been a deliberate move to show them who was boss.

4 *Debates*, February 11, 1959, p. 286. Dr. Dymond altered the language of the "Proposed Revision" document when presenting it to the legislature: "I only dressed it up more from the standpoint of presenting it." Interview, Dr. M. Dymond. In the document this passage read: "If we could start afresh, our organization of Mental Health Services would start at the community level. Up to the present, we have been working backward trying to bring the mental hospital closer to the community and this is the course that, by force of circumstance, we will have to continue, though hopefully at an increased rate."

5 The "Proposed Revision" stated: "There has never been a thorough-going renovation of the old pattern." The large hospitals were "usually overcrowded," and some centres

had only a "token psychiatric service." Department of Health, "Proposed Revision of Mental Health Program in Ontario," p. 2.

6 *Debates*, March 24, 1959, p. 1610.

7 AO, RG 10, Series 5, January 16, 1959, McNeel to Dymond.

8 *The Globe and Mail* 3 March 1959.

9 AO, RG 10, HS S–6, November 19–20, 1959, Superintendents' Conference.

10 *Debates*, December 14, 1961, p. 467.

11 Interview, Dr. M. Dymond.

12 *Debates*, March 26, 1962, p. 1512.

13 *Debates*, February 25, 1964, p. 907.

14 *Debates*, June 15, 1965, p. 4172. A study published in 1964 showed that the resident population of Ontario's mental hospitals, excluding patients in mental retardation facilities, began to decline in 1958, while resident rates per 100,000 population began to decline in 1951. K. M. McGregor, M.D., "Trends in Mental Hospitals," *Canadian Psychiatric Association Journal,* 9 (1964): 331. McGregor seems to have accepted official statistics which excluded patients in residential units from the total mental hospital population. However, these patients actually remained in hospital although they were formally discharged as patients and readmitted as "residents." If one includes patients in the residential units in the residential totals, then the decline did not begin until 1965. See Table 6–1.

15 Liberal James Trotter attacked the government for announcing the construction of a new, 1,000 bed hospital in Toronto: "Why would they announce a 1,000 bed hospital when they are told that the proper way to build a hospital is for the maximum of 500 people?" *Debates*, February 12, 1960, p. 357.

16 *Debates*, February 12, 1960, p. 360.

17 *Debates*, February 11, 1965, pp. 465–471.

18 *Debates*, June 15, 1965, pp. 4170–71.

19 AO, RG 10, HS S–6, June 13, 1958, Superintendents' Conference.

20 This was the story told to the author by Betty and Jerry Anglin concerning the plans used to build the Smith's Falls institution for mentally retarded people.

21 *More for the Mind* 42.

22 *Debates*, June 7, 1966, p. 4385.

23 *Debates*, May 1, 1967, p. 2819. "This is in keeping with a long-enunciated philosophy—and a philosophy on which all three parties in this House have been in agreement—that boards at the local level should operate many of these facilities."

24 *Debates*, February 23, 1962, p. 587.

25 *Debates*, June 15, 1965, p. 4159.

[26] *Debates*, June 9, 1965, pp. 3921–23. The first study of psychiatric manpower was done by the Ontario Committee on the Healing Arts in 1967. For a list of surveys see N. El-Guebaly and P. Leichner, "Psychiatric Manpower in Canada—The 1980 Surveys, Part I: National and Interprovincial Comparisons," *Canadian Journal of Psychology*, 27 (1982).

[27] *Debates*, Feb. 16, 1950, p. B–18.

[28] "I feel that every hon. member of this House will agree with me that the answer to our mental health problem today is not going ahead and building bigger and better mental hospitals." Mackinnon Phillips, Minister of Health, *Debates*, March 27, 1952, BB–5.

[29] Interview, Anonymous. In the event, the mental health bureaucracy convinced Dymond that building large institutions was not in keeping with current thinking, and, after a long battle within the Ministry of Health, he reduced their size to 300 beds.

[30] *Debates*, November 27, 1969, p. 9006.

[31] *Debates*, Oct. 20, 1970 S–156 and November 3, 1970, p. 5954.

[32] Interview, Anonymous.

[33] *Debates*, March 20, 1976, p. 223.

[34] AO, RG 10, Series 108, B. 12, March 1966, "Report of the Interdepartmental Committee on Emotionally Disturbed Children," p. 5.

[35] Interview, Anonymous.

[36] *Debates*, February 11, 1959, p. 290.

[37] *Debates*, February 11, 1959, p. 290.

[38] *Debates* February 11, 1959, p. 290.

[39] AO, RG 10, B. 50, HS 1–2, May 26, 1944, Dr. T. D. Cumberland, Superintendent, Ontario Hospital, New Toronto, to McGhie.

[40] Mental Hospital Survey Committee *Report* 9.

[41] Canada, House of Commons Special Committee on Social Security, *Minutes of Proceedings and Evidence*, Tuesday, May 18, 1943, p. 321.

[42] AO, RG 10, B. 50, HS 1–2, May 8, 1944, Memorandum on mental health services from B.T. McGhie to "All Superintendents."

[43] AO, RG 10, B. 50, HS 1–2, May 12, 1944, Fletcher to McGhie.

[44] AO, RG 10–20-A–1, June 28–29, 1944, Superintendents' Conference.

[45] AO, RG 10, B. 52, HS 2–1, January 31, 1947, "The Further Development of Mental Hospitals and Community Psychiatric Work in Canada," Address to Ontario Neuropsychiatric Association.

[46] AO, RG 10, B. 50, H 1–2, October 14, 1949, Superintendents' Conference.

[47] *Debates*, March 30, 1949, DD–10.

[48] *Debates*, March 23, 1955, p. 1140.

[49] *Debates*, March 23, 1955, p. 1141.

[50] "Proposed Revision" 7.

[51] *Debates*, February 11, 1959.

[52] AO, RG 10–37, December 15, 1960, Residential Units Correspondence, unsigned mimeo describing meeting.

[53] AO, RG 10, Series 6, January 4, 1961, Dr. W.G. Brown, to Dr. M. R. Elliott, deputy minister of Health, Manitoba. The Manitoba Department of Health and Public Welfare had got wind of what Dymond was attempting in Ontario, and wrote for further details. Brown then replied outlining the Ontario plan.

[54] One participant at a meeting between Dr. Dymond and the superintendents remembers Dr. Dymond lecturing a reluctant Dr. C. H. Moorhouse, superintendent of the New Toronto institution, on the need to establish a residential unit: "Moorhouse really felt responsible for his patients and he didn't like the idea of the units." Interview, Cyril Greenland.

[55] AO, RG 10–37, 1962, "Rehabilitation or Residential Units."

[56] AO, RG 10, B. 50, HS 1–2, March 1972, H. W. Henderson, "Community Placements."

[57] G. C. Cormack and S. A. Hollings, "Homes for Special Care Program, Province of Ontario," *Canadian Journal of Public Health*, 56 (1965): 472. Cormack was in 1966 the director of the mental hospitals branch of the mental health division and Hollings was the administrator of the homes for special care program. On the Homes for Special Care Program and mental retardation policy see Simmons, *Asylum to Welfare* 176–77 and 186–188.

[58] *Debates*, Oct. 19, 1970.

[59] AO, RG 10–108, B. 7, July 9, 1973, Dr. G. A. Ives, Director, Psychiatric Hospitals Branch to Mr. G. J. Chatfield, General Manager, Direct Services Division. On the Homes for Special Care Program, See Sherill Maud Carden, "All Dressed Up and Nowhere to Go," diss., York University, 1985.

[60] C. A. Roberts, "A Report on Ontario Mental Health Services", 1963, p. 82.

[61] AO, RG 10, Series 6, September 30, 1962, Deputy Minister's Files: Residential Units, "Per Capita cost statements, April 1, 1962-September 30, 1962."

[62] AO, RG 10–37, 1963, Unsigned memo to the Honourable M. B. Dymond, M.D.

[63] AO, RG 10–06, January 9, 1976, Estimates, Meeting with Treasury, Memo to C. E. Brannan, Secretary Treasury Board, re: Department of Health proposed reductions in estimates for 1967/68 and Anticipated Revenue from CAP from K. Charron, Deputy Minister.

[64] AO, RG 10, B. 29, File 6, January 1970, Dr. H. W. Henderson, "Progress Report and Review of MH Program."

[65] AO, RG 10–06, January 9, 1967, Estimates, Meeting with Treasurer.

[66] *Debates*, April 24, 1968, p. 2075.

[67] *Debates*, May 6, 1968, 2527.

[68] Roberts, "A Report on Ontario Mental Health Services," p. C-R 83.

[69] AO, RG 10–108, B. 18, July 18, 1972, Department of Health, Submission to Cabinet, "Revised Mental Health Program (Project '77). The submission states that "lower cost nursing and residential homes" for the 2,000 mental patients would provide space for the "temporary reallocation of retardates in provincial hospitals while making potential cost savings." Transferring mentally retarded people to vacant beds in the mental hospital would meet the criticisms of parents, the Ontario Association for the Mentally Retarded and others regarding the overcrowding in the mental retardation institutions. The submission also recommended the establishment of five community "residential care and assessment centers" of 695 beds for mentally retarded people. Apparently most of the proposed $6.8 million expenditure would go toward these five centers, an increase in the number of children's mental health centres as well as toward additional children's beds in the Ontario Hospitals.

[70] Simmons 187ff.

[71] *Debates*, Supply Committee, October 19, 1970.

[72] *Debates*, Supply Committee, October 19, 1970.

[73] AO, RG 10–37, March 15, 1972. Memo from Dr. G. A. Ives, Director Psychiatric Services Branch to Dr. H. W. Henderson, Executive Director.

[74] AO, RG 10–108, B7 March 15, 1972. Memo from Dr. H. W. Henderson, Executive Director, Mental Health Division to Dr. K. C. Charron, Deputy Minister, Department of Health re: Residential Beds.

[75] AO, RG 10–37, February 1973, "Submission to Cabinet: Health Insurance Benefit Coverage, Residential Units in Provincial Psychiatric Hospitals," Richard T. Potter, M.D., Minister of Health.

[76] Touche Ross and Partners, April 1984, "A Review of the Homes for Special Care Program for the Mental Health Division, Ontario Ministry of Health," Touche Ross and Partners, p. 1.

[77] Touche Ross 13.

[78] C. A. Roberts 11.

[79] Scull, *Decarceration* 150.

[80] Herein lies one difference between the Progressive Conservative ideology, such as it is, and a free enterprise, capitalist-oriented political ideology such as characterized the Conservative Party under Margaret Thatcher. In the latter case, the Thatcher government was not only eager, it was ideologically impelled to search for some means to help private enterprise play a role in the health and social services. The Progressive Conservatives, however, were willing to turn over responsibility for social or health services to the private sector if it was politically feasible to do so, but they did not feel it as an ideological or political obligation.

7

The System Under Scrutiny

"Roberts and Hanly reports? Never heard of them."

Former Minister of Health, 1970s

The Roberts Report

The 1960s were a time of ferment in the health services. In 1964 and 1965, two volumes of the Royal Commission on Health Services (the Hall Commission) were published. During the summer of 1965 the provinces and the federal government met in Ottawa to discuss a nationwide health insurance plan, while in June 1965, the Ontario legislature passed the Ontario Medical Services Insurance Act. At the same time, despite protests and appeals from the provinces, the federal government refused to include mental hospitals in the hospital insurance program.

This was also a time of reorganization within the Department of Health. In April 1966, mental health was upgraded from branch to division status and its four branches were given responsibility for all aspects of mental health care including the operation of the provincial hospitals for mentally ill and mentally retarded people. According to the Minister of Health "mental health is the most important single health problem in Canada and likewise in the province of Ontario."[1]

The decade 1960–1970 also saw the publication of major reports on Ontario's mental health care system. In 1963, Dr. C. A. Roberts, medical superintendent of the Verdun Protestant Hospital, assistant professor of psychiatry at McGill and ex-chief of the mental health division of the federal Department of Health and Welfare, was asked to do a report on the Ontario mental health system. Perhaps because it was the most comprehensive, and critical report of its kind, it was neither published nor publicized, nor were its conclusions known outside the confines of the Department of Health.[2]

In June 1967, the newly established Committee on the Healing Arts commissioned Professor Charles Hanly of the University of Toronto to conduct a study of mental health professions and services in Ontario. His report was submitted in 1968. Hanly also criticized the existing state of mental health services, sharply attacked the medical model of care, proposed a diminution in the power of psychiatrists and suggested a model of mental health care emphasizing psychotherapy and the establishment of community mental health centres. His report as well was almost totally ignored. Yet, together, the Roberts and Hanly reports provide a unique insight into the state of Ontario's mental health services in the 1960s.

Although he recognized the "considerable progress" that had been made in Ontario in "protecting the community from the effects of psychiatric illness" and in providing "humane care for...patients in a protective environment," Roberts was deeply critical of a program philosophy which was "rooted in another era." Roberts found a system that was uncoordinated, funded in a haphazard manner and based on priorities unrelated to the needs of psychiatric patients.

The problems began at the top, where, despite the existence of organizations specifically endowed with formal responsibility for mental health care, priorities were set without paying much attention to the mental health care bureaucracy. "The Chief of the Branch, while appearing to have responsibility for the program as a whole, does not appear to play the role of Advisor to the Government on all matters related to mental health."[3] The director of hospitals had little to do with the actual operation of the hospitals but rather had responsibility for the personnel of the mental health branch.[4] At the same time, the director of community mental health "is increasingly involved in the organization and provision of all services other than those provided by the inpatient services of the Ontario Hospitals." The problem was that "[t]he roles of the other professional personnel are not at all clear." Roberts also found that the superintendents had little influence on policy, while neither the superintendents' conferences, the meetings of the directors of the mental health clinics, nor "the reports of the special committees play any effective part in the development of program or the establishment of policy."

Roberts was equally critical of the large provincial hospitals. Despite the efforts of professional staff, he noted "adequate psychological and social treatment cannot and is not being provided by the staff available."[5] Industrial therapy was "very spotty", and yet, at the same time the provincial hospitals were being equipped with diagnostic services more appropriate for general hospitals. Dr. John Pratten, formerly superintendent of the Kingston psychiatric hospital remembers that,

> there were rooms full of hundreds of thousands of dollars of equipment just sitting unused, just stored, most of it rusted and rotting. They bought chemical analyzers and a whole set of pathology equipment because pathology and mental hospitals were a big thing in the 1850s so they bought all the equipment to do it in the 1960s when no one had the slightest interest in doing pathology in the 1960s.[6]

Roberts also found that there was no relation between the needs of mentally ill people and the location of new hospitals or the number of beds provided. "The present large scale renovation and building program in Ontario Hospitals does not seem to be based on a set of principles clearly stated and clearly understood by those responsible for construction and those responsible for the provision of patient care." New construction was taking place in old hospitals without reference to any overall plan, old buildings were scheduled for demolition when they could be renovated, and in some cases, "major expenditures are being made on buildings which have been earmarked for demolition during the next few years."[7] Roberts noted that it was "impossible to determine the basis on which decisions are made regarding capital expenditures." In some areas of high need there were no facilities, while in areas of low need unnecessary facilities were being constructed. In addition, the architecture and capacity of buildings seemed unrelated to accepted standards or needs. Nursing units of over 50 beds were being constructed when it "had been held for many years that nursing units of over 40–50 beds are unsatisfactory." There was a "marked shortage of space for day and recreational activities." Thus, Roberts observed: "It is...apparent that the Ontario service and the Public Works Department either have no philosophy about hospital construction, or...they reject many presently held principles about hospital construction without enunciating their reasons for doing so."[8] In an interview in 1986, Dr. Roberts said:

> Right across this country, the location of mental hospitals was based on patronage. Palmerston, Goderich, Owen Sound were all built after we said to the government: "For Heaven's sake, you don't need a 300 bed hospital outside Timmins." I really can't see any explanation except that it was decided that some district had to get something so it was decided to build a mental hospital. Brockville Psychiatric Hospital has always been maintained at an unrealistic level because Brockville had a very influential Minister. If you look at the development of general hospitals across the province it bears no relationship to planning. You have all of the studies and suddenly a political announcement is made. It can't be changed. No decision seems to be made on the basis of data, except the data about how to get elected.[9]

The key ministry was Public Works which injected funds into local economies as a means of winning political support for the government. Or, as Roberts delicately put it, "one cannot fail to be impressed by the apparent absence of a common philosophy or set of principles underlying the development of services and the operation of existing facilities."[10]

With regard to the residential units, Roberts pointed out one of the principal ambiguities of the program. The declared intention of the policy was to identify patients who could be discharged to the community or to community care facilities if such facilities were available. However, these patients were kept in locked residential units. "In our society," Roberts said, "one generally thinks of locked facilities as being present in either penal institutions or mental hospitals... It hardly seems reasonable to decertify a patient, which presumably indicates that the patient should have all of his civil rights returned to him, and then to lock him in a ward and deny him his freedom."[11] Moreover, it was impossible to tell from staffing patterns what the difference was between the residential units and the rest of the hospital wards.

Finally, Roberts noted that the Department of Health tended to lump under the heading of community services a disparate array of services such as mental health clinics, travelling clinics, and the psychiatric units in the general hospitals. "This does not appear to be the best way of organizing or designating psychiatric services..." Rather, Roberts suggested that psychiatric treatment services be organized so as to provide "professional treatment for patients and to recognize that there are other needs of patients in the area of financial and social support which should be the responsibility of community services which are not responsible for the provision of psychiatric treatment as such."[12] Roberts was suggesting a division of responsibility, with community services fulfilling mainly a social welfare function, and psychiatric services providing treatment services. The difficulty was that, in 1963, social services were provided through the Ministry of Public Welfare and there were no community mental health services except for the boarding-out program which placed hospital patients in private homes. Moreover, as Roberts pointed out, "present arrangements for the rehabilitation of patients in the mental hospitals are in a state of development." Since, within the hospitals, it was sometimes the rehabilitation branch of Health that assumed responsibility for social welfare functions, or at other times the Department of Welfare, there was a continuing lack of coordination between ministries.

But what was the reason for this pattern of services? Roberts explained it in terms of the differing historical development of mental health services in Canada, Great Britain and the United States. In Great Britain, he noted, the hospitals were generally under the control of a variety of local bodies. When the National Health Service was established in 1948, the hospitals were placed under regional boards centred around university medical schools and these boards, in turn, established management committees which administered a small group of hospitals.[13] Thus, even after the passage of the National Health Service Act, there were two semi-independent authorities located between the central government and the hospital. Roberts compared the highly centralized Ontario system unfavourably with the English system where,

> one...gets the impression that...the system may indeed be more flexible than are the administrative arrangements with which we are familiar on this continent. It is quite likely that this is because of the British attitude towards administration—a minimum of central direction with a maximum of confidence that the individual will do the right thing in any given situation.[14]

Roberts contrasted community indifference toward mental hospitals in Ontario with England where there was a feeling that "this is our mental hospital." Roberts attributed this difference to the fact that the local management committees of the English hospitals had a degree of administrative and budgetary independence of central government that did not exist in Ontario.[15]

In the United States, the organization of the mental hospital system varied from one state to another, but, generally, the state hospitals were run by boards of trustees which then reported to a state mental hygiene or state mental health authority. In Ontario, however, the government was responsible for the entire operation of the mental hospital system including funding, management, construction, planning and research. The inevitable consequence was that the mental hospital system was used by government as a means to achieve a wide variety of goals, many of which had no relation to the mental health needs of the patients. "These governmental practices," Roberts wrote, "were not, in the first place, established to meet patient care needs, but were designed to meet the needs of other governmental services not intimately concerned with the day-to-day needs of sick and dependent people." Roberts drew a comparison between the provincial psychiatric hospitals and the tuberculosis sanitoria which, though financed from provincial funds, were run by independent boards. "It does not seem unreasonable to state that the standards of care provided came closer to meeting the needs of the patients with tuberculosis than the program operated directly by the Government has come to meeting the needs of psychiatric patients."[16]

For Roberts, one way to improve the mental health system was to decentralize control and to ensure that priorities were determined with a view toward improving mental health services, rather than fostering other governmental objectives. Toward this end, Roberts suggested putting the mental hospitals under the Public Hospitals Act as were the general hospitals, so that they would be operated by local boards of management and their budgets formulated in the same way as the general hospitals. If the mental hospitals were turned over to management boards with local representation, there would be demands for increased funds, but the community might take more interest in institutions which traditionally were isolated from the community and were often an object of suspicion or hostility. In line with British practice, Roberts recommended a block system of financing whereby the Ontario Hospital Services Commission would give the mental hospitals lump sum grants to be used as the management committee saw fit. Ulti mately, Roberts argued, divesting government of "direct responsibility for the construction, reconstruction, maintenance and operation" of the mental hospitals would lead to a greater sense of initiative and responsibility. But if control over the individual mental hospitals was relaxed, then there would also have to be a change in the organization of central authorities. Thus, Roberts proposed that the mental health branch of the Department of Health be divested of its responsibility for the day-to-day operation of the psychiatric services, and that it play a policy advising, formulating, monitoring, and coordination role. This would allow the individual hospitals to deal directly with government service agencies. In order to establish links between the government and the community, Roberts recommended the establishment of a "consultative committee on mental health." This would consist of representatives from the medical schools, professional interest groups and government, as well as two lay representatives. Its role would be to advise the government on "the development and coordination of all psychiatric services in the province."[17]

In his report, Roberts did find something positive to say about Ontario's mental health system. He endorsed the policy of establishing psychiatric units in the general hospitals and he proposed an extension of the provincial boarding-out program. However, he also touched on one of the major problems in Ontario's mental health care system, the continuing short-fall in the number of psychiatrists employed in the provincial psychiatric hospitals. The problem was that hospital psychiatrists were paid on a salaried basis while their colleagues in the general hospitals and in private practice were reimbursed on a fee-for-service basis. Here again, Roberts drew an unfavourable comparison with Great Britain where, because of the National Health Service, "[h]ospital work, community practice, teaching and research—job for job—bring the same rewards."[18] Roberts argued that "one should strive to ensure that psychiatric work brings the same reward as any other field of medicine."

With regard to legislation, Roberts suggested that the law be amended so that mental hospitals would no longer enjoy a special status in law but would be brought under the same laws as the general hospitals. In this way, the special status of mental patients would end and, except for "special legislation for the few patients who need it," they would no longer have to suffer the loss of civil rights and be subjected to special legal requirements.

Finally, Roberts endorsed the recommendation of the Canadian Psychiatric Association to the Royal Commission on Health Services (which was then conducting hearings) that the federal government include mental hospital patients in the Hospital Insurance and Diagnostic Services Act of 1957.[19] The question of including mental hospital patients had been a bone of contention between the federal government, the provinces and the CMHA ever since the proposal had been raised in 1943. At that time, the provinces were reluctant to accept the federal proposal because their calculations showed that they would lose more federal funds than they would gain through funds recovered from patients. In 1956, when the Hospital Insurance and Diagnostic Services Act was being discussed, the Minister of National Health and Welfare stated that the costs of patients in provincial mental and tubercular hospitals would be excluded since these were already covered by provincial general revenues while the federal plan was intended to assist insurance schemes.[20] Twenty years later, in discussing the background to the Tyhurst Report, Dr. Roberts mentioned that Dr. D. G. McKerracher, formerly of the mental health services in Saskatchewan and one of the co-authors of the report of the Royal Commission on Health Services, had opposed including mental hospitals under the federal plan in order to force the provinces to redirect funds away from the provincial mental hospitals and toward psychiatric units in general hospitals.[21] Services in the latter were covered under the federal plan.[22]

The Roberts report came four years after Dr. Matthew Dymond had been appointed Minister of Health and three years after his speech to the legislature promising major changes in Ontario's mental health policy. Few of Roberts' recommendations were accepted by the Department of Health. Like every previous report on Ontario's mental health services, the Roberts report soon began to gather dust on the Department's shelves.

The Hanly Report 1968

The Hanly report is as interesting as the Roberts report although for different reasons. Roberts approached the question from a medical point of view. Hanly, on the other hand, was a member of the University of Toronto's Philosophy Department and at that point, training as a psychoanalyst. It is not surprising, therefore, that Hanly was highly critical of the medical model of care and suggested an alternative model based on community services with a heavy emphasis on psychotherapeutic treatment.

As had been the case with every previous study, Hanly's was a tale of insufficient resources, lack of trained personnel and of misplaced priorities.[23]

The "basic problem" was the lack of trained professionals and subprofessionals, such as child care workers, psychiatric nurses, and social workers.[24] Almost all the facilities queried by Hanly's researchers mentioned staffing problems. Public institutions affiliated with medical schools or university departments of medicine or psychiatry had little trouble in recruiting psychiatrists and medical doctors, but encountered problems in recruiting psychologists and social workers. On the other hand, small private institutions or institutions unaffiliated with universities had difficulty in recruiting professionals and depended on social workers for staff. The "most general shortage is child care workers."[25]

On this point Hanly departed sharply from the medical-psychiatric orientation which characterized previous studies of Ontario's mental health system. Hanly noted that there was really little need for medical attention or treatment for emotionally disturbed children because most of them suffered from psychological rather than organic problems. Yet, it "is generally the case that a psychiatrist is the chief of the services in a residential treatment centre, and acts as the head of a treatment team when the professional services are organized on the team principle."[26] Hanly suggested that the explanation for the dominance of the psychiatrists had less to do with the specific needs of their clients and more to do with the "accident of the traditions of mental health services in Ontario, and of the traditions of education and training in clinical psychology and psychiatric social work in Ontario."[27] In other words, because medical doctors and psychiatrists had traditionally staffed both the federal and provincial mental health systems they had ensured that the medical model of care was the accepted treatment paradigm and that medical doctors and psychiatrists were the key interpreters and guardians of that paradigm. Moreover, because of their dominance, it had been very difficult to get the universities and government to accept the possibility that trained clinical psychologists might have a role to play in the mental health system equal to that of the psychiatrists. Hanly condemned not only the medical and psychiatric professions but also the Department of Health for the shortage of clinical psychologists and for the barriers raised against them in the mental health system. "Medicine and psychology are in a state of cold war in the field of mental health."[28]

Hanly also swam against the current of mental health policy in Ontario by recommending the establishment of "many more well-staffed *local* [his italics] mental health centres... Mental health personnel, in both public and private hospitals, as well as those working in community clinics were practically unanimous that the lack of these facilities is a major gap in the province's mental health services." Ironically, by this time, the Department of Health had already taken the decision to abandon local mental health clinics and to turn over their functions to the provincial psychiatric hospitals or to the psychiatric units. With regard to the provincial hospital system, Hanly also noted that nothing had been done to replace the provincial mental hospitals or to reduce their size. In fact, this was not completely accurate. The number of residents in mental hospitals in Ontario had begun to decline in the mid–1960s. If, however, Hanly meant to imply that there was no deliberate, explicit program of deinstitutionalization of mentally ill people, then he was correct. What happened in Ontario was that, due to a number of reasons including the increasing effectiveness of psychotropic drugs, there had been a secular decline in the mental hospital population. But rather than confronting this fact head-on and trying to lay down some kind of coherent long-range policy for mental health services, the Department of Health was reacting in its usual ad hoc fashion.

In his critique, Hanly discussed the question of recruiting sufficient staff to man and to run the psychiatric hospitals. The problem was the perennial one of trying to find staff willing to work in remote, often isolated hospitals, far from centres of population and without any links to hospital or university communities. Although Hanly noted that it would be hypothetically possible to improve the Ontario Hospital system by recruiting additional professional staff and by improving rehabilitation programs, he concluded that: "The Ontario Hospitals could gradually wither away. No one would mourn their passing."[29]

Not only was Hanly critical and, ultimately, condemnatory of the psychiatric hospitals, he was equally critical of the policy of establishing psychiatric units in the general hospitals. Noting that the Royal Commission on Health Services had recommended in 1964 that there be an increase in the number of psychiatric units, Hanly pointed to its "inherent limitations...general hospitals are reluctant to admit to their psychiatric units children, adolescents, patients with behaviour disorders, geriatric patients or patients suffering from acute psychiatric disorders requiring long-term treatment."[30] Hanly also quoted from the 1953 World Health Organization report which criticized psychiatric units. Citing provincial statistics showing that the turnover of patients in the psychiatric units was two-thirds more than that of the psychiatric hospitals, Hanly argued that the psychiatric units were deliberately selecting for treatment those patients who were easy to treat and sending the difficult patients to the Ontario Hospitals. However, in 1966, a year before Hanly began his study, the director of community mental health services said: "There is very little selection practised today, and the units have clearly demonstrated that the general hospital can look after most patients in need of diagnostic assessment and short-term intensive treatment."[31] On the other hand, Hanly referred to "[o]ur field work" which suggested that "the Ontario Hospitals are used by the general hospitals as repositories for the most severe and chronic cases."[32] And he suggested that "psychiatric units of general hospitals could be converted to other medical uses as the population increases without loss to the taxpayer."[33] As an alternative to the psychiatric units, Hanly proposed the establishment of "comprehensive community mental health centres that can provide high quality services for the entire spectrum from the care of geriatric, senile patients, to the treatment of emotionally disturbed children, to family therapy in an outpatient clinic."[34] These CMHCs would be distributed throughout the province on a catchment area basis and would be "deeply rooted in the community." Noting that the Ontario Committee on Taxation had proposed a system of regional government for the province, Hanly suggested that these regions form the basis for the CMHC catchment areas.[35] Because they would provide services for a variety of people such as the elderly, emotionally disturbed children, psychoneurotics, and psychotics, they would attract professionals with different skills. The heterogeneous composition of the staff would make the CMHCs attractive for professionals even if they were located in rural settings or far from hospitals or universities. The CMHCs could provide a valuable training center for local "professionals and subprofessionals." They would be better placed than large institutions to perform public education and planning functions in the community, and they could also provide diagnostic services to the courts, thus obviating the reliance on the Department of Reform Institutions.[36] They would also be particularly advantageous for emotionally disturbed children because they could treat the child in his/her community in close contact with family, school or other local institutions. Hanly predicted that integrating public mental health services in the CMHCs would eliminate fragmented service patterns, that is, situations where individuals in difficulty were confronted by a confusing array of government departments, institutions and professionals all trying in an unintegrated way to help resolve their problems. However, there would have to be links between the CMHCs and community health centers, necessitating coordination between the Departments of Education, Health, Reform Institutions, and Social and Family Services. Hanly proposed that the CMHCs vary in size from 40 to 100 beds and that they have a full professional staff. In this way, they could replace the psychiatric units in the general hospitals. As regards administration, Hanly suggested that the CMHCs could avoid the "undesirable trend towards bureaucratic centralization" if they were given a large degree of autonomy including the ability to determine the size and architecture of buildings. In this, they would be "confident in the realization that they could not do worse than has already been done."[37] Hanly criticized the Department of Public Works for their "order of priorities...which do not seem to relate to the needs of the hospitals."

On the other hand, Hanly noted that local communities were reluctant to assume any financial or administrative burden in the mental health system, and he suggested that the apathy of local government officials might be "itself derivative of psychopathology." This is, of course, exaggerated and reductionist. There are ideological and budgetary reasons why local governments in Ontario have been reluctant to assume the administrative and financial costs of social expenditures for mental health. Many local governments in Ontario are politically conservative and most are reluctant to add to their property tax burden by assuming additional expenditures for socially dependent and often stigmatized groups such as the mentally ill and mentally retarded. It is this, rather than any psychopathological reason which explains the negative attitude of local government officials in Ontario toward mental health expenditures.

Hanly also spent some time discussing the state of children's services in Ontario and he drew particular attention to the "major issue [of] the shortage of...facilities."[38] The lack of facilities for emotionally disturbed children was not a new problem.

Six months before Hanly and his researchers began work on his report, Minister of Health Matthew Dymond had tabled a White Paper in the legislature sketching the outlines of a new program for children "suffering from mental and emotional disorders."[39]

Better collaboration among departments dealing with children was promised, there would be improved facilities for the identification and assessment of children with emotional disorders and a series of regional children's centres would be established.

Finally, Hanly raised an issue of crucial importance to mental health policy: the question of numbers. Hanly referred to two studies which had had a major impact on mental health planning: *The Midtown Manhattan Study* and the Stirling County Study by D. C. Leighton.[40] These showed that approximately 20 percent of every population was disabled by a serious mental illness. Although Hanly did not call this figure into question he stated that "it would be unwise to use the 20–25 per cent prevalence figure as a definition of need against which to measure the mental health resources of the province; for it is unlikely that the mental health needs of such a large number of people can be met in the foreseeable future."[41] Rather, he recommended adoption of "the somewhat arbitrary objective" of establishing sufficient mental health resources to treat 10 percent of the population. In 1970, that meant around 700,000 people. Of course, adjusting the figure in this way could be extremely useful, for by Hanly's criterion a downward adjustment of one percent would eliminate the need for services for 70,000 people, while an increase to 11 percent would work in the opposite direction. Ironically, more than a decade after Hanly's report was published, Dr. G. F. Heseltine noted in his *Blueprint* report to the Ministry of Health that "there continue to be strong pressures to encompass an ever-broader range of states of mental distress and dissatisfaction within the mandate of the service system."[42]

Hanly's proposals were in radical opposition to three of the major assumptions of the provincial mental health system: that psychiatrists and medical doctors would play the dominant role in determining the shape and priorities of that system; that the provincial mental hospitals would continue as the major care providers and that "community services" would refer mainly to the psychiatric units in the general hospitals. By contrast, Hanly proposed giving a more important role to psychotherapists and to other professionals and nonprofessionals, he advocated the withering away of the psychiatric hospitals and the establishment of community mental health centres in place of the psychiatric units.

Hanly's report was released in 1970, but it did not get a receptive hearing either in the Department of Health or in the wider psychiatric community. As was the case with the Roberts report, its recommendations were completely ignored.

Notes

1 *Debates*, April 20, 1967.

2 Dr. C. A. Roberts, "A Report on Ontario Mental Health Services," Department of Health, February 1963. In an interview Dr. Roberts was surprised that the author had obtained a copy of the report since he assumed it had been kept confidential.

3 Roberts CR–2.

4 Roberts CR 2.

5 Roberts CR–11.

6 Interview, Dr. John Pratten.

7 Roberts CR–14.

8 Dr. Pratten recalls that in the 1960s "research was going on at Queen's University when they built this beautiful new wing at Kingston called Westwood. It was built in conjunction with Queen's including laboratories, lecture halls, and amphitheatres. But there had been no consultation, this was one of those terrible things where the government got into a fight over who would build it and how it would be built, so they gave it out to three separate architectural firms, kind of a patronage deal. When I got to Kingston in 1962 there wasn't one part of it that was being used for what the architects said it should be used for. It was built like a bastardized general hospital, neither as good as a general hospital and just as bad as a mental hospital. The admitting wings were the infirmaries like general hospital units, the chronic care wings became admitting units." Interview, Dr. John Pratten.

9 Interview, Dr. C. A. Roberts.

10 Roberts CR–20.

11 Roberts CR–82–83.

12 Roberts CR–85.

13 Kathleen Jones, *Mental Health and Social Policy, 1845–1959* (London: Routledge and Kegan Paul, 1960) 151.

14 Roberts CR–15.

[15] Roberts CR–16.

[16] Roberts CR–6.

[17] Roberts CR–7. In 1988 the Provincial Community Mental Health Committee recommended that the Ministry of Health establish a Provincial Advisory Committee which would report to the Ministry of Health and the Premier on mental health matters. See *Building Community Support for People: A Plan for Mental Health in Ontario* (Toronto: The Provincial Community Health Committee, 1988) 11.

[18] Roberts CR–17.

[19] Roberts CR–90. See also, "Editorial; The CPA Brief to the Royal Commission," *Canadian Psychiatric Journal*, 7 (1962): 109–111.

[20] See Eric J. Hansen, *The Public Finance Aspects of Health Services in Canada* (Ottawa: Royal Commission on Health Services, 1963) 35.

[21] C. A. Roberts, "'More for the Mind': Twenty Years Later," p. 9.

[22] See Department of National Health and Welfare, Information Services Division, *The Hospital Insurance and Diagnostic Services Program in Canada* (Ottawa, 1962) 38.

[23] Charles Hanly, *Mental Health in Ontario* (Toronto: Committee for the Healing Arts, 1970) 303–304.

[24] Hanly 313.

[25] Hanly 296.

[26] Hanly 298.

[27] Hanly 298.

[28] Hanly 231.

[29] Hanly 278.

[30] Hanly 262.

[31] H. W. Henderson, "Community Mental Health—Mental Health Administration, Implications," *Canadian Journal of Public Health* 57 (1966): 147.

[32] Hanly 265.

[33] Hanly 278.

[34] Hanly 276.

[35] Hanly 392.

[36] Hanly 394.

[37] Hanly 277.

[38] Hanly 288.

[39] Quoted in H. W. Henderson, "Original Concept," in Jalal Shamsie, editor, *Experience and Experiment* (Toronto: Leonard Crainford, 1977) 115.

[40] D. C. Leighton, et al, "Family Survey of Stirling County," in *The Character of Danger* (New York: Basic Books, 1963).

[41] Hanly 21.

[42] G. F. Heseltine, *Towards a Blueprint for Change: A Mental Health Policy and Program Perspective* (Toronto: Ministry of Health, December, 1983) 30.

PART III: 1970–1985

8

Internal Politics in the Ministry of Health

When the new broom comes in, especially when it doesn't know what it is doing, it comes in with a set of assumptions which are remarkably similar from one new broom to the next. The first is that the system is in a mess otherwise they wouldn't have appointed me, second, that if the system is in a mess it's because the people who are there are the ones who screwed it up, and based on that, the third assumption is that I'll do everything the opposite of the way the last guy did it. This leads to the conclusion that opposites are really not opposites, the thing and its opposite equal each other and the new broom winds up doing exactly the same as the old broom.

Former civil servant in Mental Health Division,
Ministry of Health

The Committee on Government Productivity and Mental Health

The 1970s ushered in a period of major change in the administration and structure of government. In 1969, Premier John Robarts appointed the blue-ribbon Committee on Government Productivity (COGP) to examine and make recommendations for a major reorganization of government structures.[1]

The committee quickly turned out interim reports on various aspects of government administration, with the Robarts government implementing the COGP recommendations as they were published. Two of the most important reforms were the creation of policy field ministers to oversee and coordinate the work of line ministries, and the internal reorganization of ministries along functional lines.

In order to broaden the narrow perspectives of line ministries like the Ministry of Health, the COGP recommended, and the government established, a series of policy ministers whose job was to develop broad-based, integrated policy cutting across ministerial boundaries. To ensure that the policy ministries had some power they, along with the chairman of the newly created Management Board (ex-Treasury Board), the Minister of Finance and Intergovernmental Affairs, (ex-Treasurer) and the Premier as Chairman comprised the Policy and Priorities Board of Cabinet. As the name implies, the Board was to vet all major policy proposals from the various ministries and to establish a hierarchy of priorities for spending. On January 5, 1972, Robert Welch was named Minister of Social

Development Policy. The Social Development Policy field included the Ministries of Colleges and Universities, Community and Social Services, Culture and Recreation, Education, and Health.

In the same year that Premier Robarts appointed the COGP, there were stirrings within the mental health division. The executive director praised the establishment of psychiatric units in the general hospitals but admitted that some provincial "facilities for the mentally ill and the retarded...offer very poor accommodation...limited numbers of staff make it difficult, if not impossible, to provide a satisfactory level of service." He noted that the shortfall in staff in the Ontario Hospital system was "comparable" to the 25 percent figure reported by the United States Department of Health, Education and Welfare.[2] On May 27, 1969, Dr. Henderson wrote to the deputy minister of health noting the "critical problems of limitations imposed by the shortage of professional staff in senior positions...[and] the difficulties imposed by inadequate physical accommodation and excessive overcrowding, particularly in the facilities for the retarded."[3] Dr. Henderson proposed internal administrative changes within the mental health division including implementation of a new cost accounting system, a new system of departmental organization, and changes affecting the organization of the medical staff and services for children and adolescents. In the fall of 1969, Henderson again wrote to deputy minister Charron, this time proposing that Mr. Justice Kelly be appointed by the government to conduct a study of the role of government in providing services to the mentally ill and mentally retarded.[4] Henderson implied that one reason for conducting a study was to defuse possible protests from staff over reorganization.

> It is my opinion that considerable advantage could be gained by reinforcing our position with the findings of such a study if it is the intention of government to adopt a vigorous course of action directed to the inadequacies. Because of the severe limitations which have been imposed on our program and the efforts that are being made to raise the standards of care in the provincial facilities, we should anticipate strong protest from our staff if these shortcomings are documented in the manner proposed and no corrective action taken. In order to counteract the possibility of an unfavourable response from the staff, it would helpful to discuss the proposal at the Senior Management Conference...[5]

However, neither Mr. Justice Kelly nor anyone else was appointed at that time to investigate the mental health or mental retardation system. It is true that Walter Williston, Q.C., was appointed in 1971 specifically to review mental retardation policy, but Williston's appointment was in response to a quite different set of circumstances, and he was limited to a study of mental retardation policy.

Reorganizing Mental Health

Rather than make major changes in the mental health system, the Department made minor changes in the organization of the mental health bureaucracy. Despite the establishment of a Policy Secretary for Social Development, no attempt was made to integrate the delivery of mental health and social welfare services.

At the end of the 1960s there was a series of reorganizations in the mental health division. From an office headed by the chief of the mental health branch and a few officials, by 1970 the mental health division was staffed by close to 90 people distributed among five branches: professional services, hospital management services, psychiatric services, mental retardation services and children's services. Prior to the passage of the 1967 Mental Health Act, responsibility for various aspects of mental health policy had been scattered throughout the various social service ministries; however, the 1967 Act centralized responsibility for mental health policy in the hands of the Department of Health, and specifically in the hands of the mental health division. In the late 1960s as well, the Department of Health also modernized its administrative and accounting system so as to better monitor and control expenditures and management procedures throughout the province.

The Department of Health had begun to move toward a functional administrative system in early 1966, organizing the various branches within the mental division on the basis of specific functions, such as hospital management or personnel, rather than on the basis of client groups such as mentally ill or mentally retarded people. By the 1970s, the system whereby provincial mental hospitals were headed by medical doctors had been altered, with trained non-medical administrators taking over the direction of the hospitals, assisted by a medical director. When the COGP proposals were implemented, the functional approach was extended to within the Ministry of Health itself. Whereas previously the Ministry of Health had been organized around program areas (health promotion and disease prevention, treatment and rehabilitation and psychiatric and retardation services), in August 1972 the Ministry was reorganized along functional lines (development of standards, health care delivery services and ministry administration).[6] This meant that the mental health division was disbanded and its personnel assigned to various posts within the new functional organization of the Ministry, most of them being assigned either to the health standards or health services divisions.

It was the COGP which initiated the gradual replacement of doctors by professional administrators in Health partly because of the committee's stated goal of improving what the authors called the "corporate" allegiance of bureaucrats.[7] One of the problems with the bureaucracy, as COGP saw it, was that individual ministries tended to become parochial and to lose sight of the overall objectives of the government as a whole.[8] This led the COGP to recommend the creation of policy secretariats, Management Board and the Policy and Priorities Board. These bodies would provide a forum where separate program ministers would exchange information, get an overview of developments within policy fields and coordinate their actions and establish priorities amongst policies. The decision to employ generalists who would take a corporate view within ministries led to a search for bureaucrats with management or administrative training. This spelled the end of medical dominance of the mental health bureaucracy. As Graham Scott, ex-deputy minister of health, put it: "The kind of administrative talents you require amongst doctors are usually mixed up with a desire to be involved with the action as opposed to the policy."[9] Another ex-deputy minister of health stated that "I was told when I went to the Ministry of Health that there was a lack of competent medical people in the Ministry."[10] Whatever the reasons, as long as medical doctors and psychiatrists dominated the mental health division of the Ministry of Health it was inevitable that policy would follow a medical model of mental health care. But as psychiatrists gave way to professional managers or (as in the case of David Corder, a former nurse who was to become assistant deputy minister of mental health in 1985) to people trained in associated professional fields, the mental health bureaucracy began to take a greater interest in patients' rights, community services as opposed to hospital care, and to impose tougher accounting and financial controls on the large institutions than had been previously been the case.[11]

Over the next few years there were a bewildering variety of changes as divisions and branches were created, reorganized or disbanded. In 1974, responsibility for mental retardation policy and the provincial institutions for mentally retarded people was removed from the Ministry of Health and given to the Ministry of Community and Social Services. Despite, or perhaps, because of these frequent reorganizations and because of problems caused by the functional organization of the Ministry, a report from the Ontario Council of Health in 1979 noted that "everyone was responsible for mental health services and...no one is responsible for them."[12]

The Task Force on Health Care Costs

By the late 1960s and early 1970s the glaring inadequacies of the mental health system prompted reform proposals from professional organizations and from within the mental health bureaucracy itself. In the end, these proposals failed, but they demonstrate that even mental health bureaucrats were willing to put forward radical suggestions for change.

In the summer of 1969, the Minister of Health appointed a committee on health care costs to parallel the recently completed work of a federal committee on health costs. In turn, the deputy minister of health, K. C. Charron, appointed a series of subcommittees, including a mental health subcommittee on health care costs, (sometimes referred to as the task force on mental health care costs). The task force consisted of representatives from the major pressure and professional groups in the field—the Ontario Mental Health Association, Ontario Psychiatric Association, Ontario Psychological Association, Ontario Welfare Council, Ontario Mental Health Foundation, and the Ontario Hospital Association. It was chaired by Lawrence G. Macpherson, the vice-principal for finance at Queen's University, and assisted by Dr. H. W. Henderson, the executive director of the mental health division, and Henderson's executive assistant.

We have seen how, in 1967, the deputy minister suggested to Treasury Board that the provincial government reduce its contribution to chronic care, to services for emotionally disturbed children and to mental hospitals, pick up additional revenues from the Canada Assistance Plan revenue and patient charges, and in the process make a small profit.[13] But the task force on mental health care costs had no such solutions to offer. The committee recommended the establishment of "public advisory boards or...boards of governors" for provincial mental hospitals, a study of methods whereby the mental hospitals would be funded in the same way as the general hospitals, and a freeze on new beds for "psychiatric care" until a study had been completed concerning the development of additional community services.

Ironically, each of these recommendations struck at the very heart of mental health policy since they would have increased rather than decreased costs, as well as undermining government hegemony over mental health policy. The difference between establishing advisory boards or boards of governors was crucial since advisory boards were exactly what the name implied, while boards of governors implied putting the psychiatric hospitals on the same administrative and financial basis as the general hospitals. This certainly would have led to a call for increased expenditure.

The committee also recommended changes in the method by which mental hospitals were financed in Ontario. Since the inception of the provincially funded hospital insurance program, premiums collected by the government were used to fund the general hospitals. This was not the case with the mental hospitals whose funding came directly from general revenues. The general hospitals argued that revenues derived from premiums should be devoted to health care, and the totals used as a benchmark against which to measure the sufficiency of funds the province put into the hospital system. But there was no equivalent benchmark in the case of the mental hospitals. According to the committee "[t]his system invites a number of consequences, mostly, it seems, unfavourable to the development and maintenance of a quality of care comparable to that of the general hospitals."[14] But the committee could do no more than suggest that a study of new financial arrangements be undertaken. The last recommendation was for a freeze on the provision of additional psychiatric beds until there had been further study "of the prospects for the development of ambulatory, day care, and community services..." Although no additional psychiatric beds were being added to the provincial hospitals, beds continued to be provided in the psychiatric units in the general hospitals and the province continued its program of reconstruction and renovation of existing mental hospitals. Moreover, the apparent paradox of a province spending millions of dollars to renovate the large institution at 999 Queen St. while at the same time appealing for restraint in public expenditures is easily resolved. As has been shown above, the Ministry of Health was very careful to explore every possible road to economy, especially those which led to federal government cost-sharing. But given the long tradition of using mental hospital expenditures as a method of currying political support or boosting local economies, the government was loath to reduce expenditures on 999 Queen Street thus provoking the inevitable reaction from the City of Toronto.

In the end, the work of the task force on mental health costs was in vain. According to its chairman, the task force was hamstrung from the start by the apparent unwillingness of the executive director of mental health to provide it with statistical information about the mental hospitals.[15] According to another member, the executive director of the mental health division was extremely reluctant to give the task force room to maneuver and was highly protective of the mental health bureaucracy.[16] The result was that while the task force was under considerable pressure to produce a report, its work terminated prematurely due to lack of information and cooperation. In January 1970, James G. Wilson, the administrator of the Brockville general hospital and the representative of the Ontario Hospital Association on the committee wrote to Lawrence G. Macpherson, the committee chairman: "I must say that I have a feeling of frustration and some disappointment that there has been no apparent progress with the plan of study," and he observed that no information had been provided regarding the number of people employed in the Department of Health, in the mental health branch or the psychiatric hospitals."[17] Wilson then went on to express "surprise" at the fact that "when various levels of government are urging restraint for our economy" the Minister of Health announced plans to spend $24 million to replace the old mental hospital at 999 Queen Street West. "It is even more surprising," Wilson wrote, "when all of the expert opinion which I can read has condemned the large mental hospital." Wilson also referred to "a report prepared some time ago by Dr. C. A. Roberts...which is probably quite interesting." Whether Wilson ever obtained the report is not clear, but if he had he might have been surprised to see how similar the criticisms were and how little things had changed in the intervening seventeen years. Because of the apparent lack of cooperation from the mental health division and the lack of data, the Committee disbanded in 1970. It never produced a final report.

The Mental Health Bureaucracy and Reform

In the early 1970s, there was a massive expansion of the Department of Health.[18] In 1972, it took over the administration of the Ontario Health Insurance Plan (OHIP), and in 1972/73 the budget of the Ontario Hospital Services Commission was included in the budget of the Department of Health. The result was that by the mid–1970s the Health budget was larger than the budgets of any of the other ministries, including the Ministry of Education, previously the top-spending ministry in the Ontario government.[19] These developments did little to improve coordination and planning within the Department. In his 1970 report for the Committee on the Healing Arts, Charles Hanly noted that the mental health delivery system had "developed without any overall plan in response to both changing demands in various sectors of society and changing therapeutic capabilities in psychiatry and psychology."[20] Two years later, in 1972, there was still concern about the "fragmented, uncoordinated, and poorly planned system over which the Minister presides."[21]

A dramatic illustration of discontent about the state of mental health administration and services comes from an April 1971 confidential memo from Dr. R. A. Farmer, the director of the hospital management services branch, to his superior, Dr. H. W. Henderson, the executive director of the mental health division.[22]

> A tremendous disparity currently exists between the resources applied to the care of the mentally ill and retarded in Ontario when compared to the resources applied to the operation of general hospital facilities. This has always been the case and will, undoubtedly, continue for some time in the future. In many instances, the physical facilities leave much to be desired, the quantity and quality of staff does not compare favourably with that found in other hospital systems, the number of patients under care exceeds the numbers of beds available, the facilities operate in virtual isolation with little direct community involvement, and the net result clearly indicates that one department of government, namely Health, has established a double standard in the care and treatment of the same general population at large.

Farmer further argued that the reason for the dramatic difference in levels of quality between the mental health and mental retardation system, and the medical hospital system was because the mental hospitals were run as direct services by the Ministry of Health, while the general hospitals were owned, operated and directed by community-based boards, with the government exercising indirect control through financing policies. The solution was to "begin placing full operational control and ownership at the community level through the establishment of Boards of Directors, incorporation, and the sale by government of the physical assets to the new corporation."

Dr. Farmer suggested that up to 1,800 patients in provincial mental hospitals and up to 1,300 patients in mental retardation facilities might be transferred to the Homes for Special Care Program, thereby saving the province "millions of dollars in both capital and operating costs." Farmer also advocated increased involvement in mental health services by the community and specifically by the local public health services. "For some reason or another, we are reluctant to engage the services of local public health authorities and fire inspectional authorities, and have attempted wherever possible to provide a completely 'inward looking' self-sustaining system in isolation when compared to all other health services in various regions throughout the province." To improve relations with the community Farmer advocated,

> that we do everything possible and within our power to clearly identify with the community and not central government. For example, I see no reason why in all our facilities the local medical officer of health should not be appointed to the consulting medical staff, attend medical and professional advisory board meetings and play a vital and meaningful role in our day to day operations... Two levels of care and two systems of care cannot continue in future. Close integration between the Mental Health Division and the Ontario Hospital Service Corporation is essential, sharing of services wherever feasible and justified should

> be mandatory, the financing of mental health care as well as general health care should be consistent and based on the same insurance principle...and the organization and operation of facilities in both systems should be similar, under the authority of a Board of Directors with control vested in the Department through legislation and fiscal authority. I cannot believe that the double standard of care in this province will ever be completely rectified through the slow process of mental health attempting to "catch up" through improving the administration and technology at divisional and local level. There must be a clear understanding that the integration of these two systems of health care is essential and straightforward methods should be proclaimed to bring the desired result about... Until this happens, I cannot foresee a major improvement in the overall standard of care provided and, if anything, the gap between the general system of health care and our system of health care may widen further.

Although these proposals would have led to a radical re-shaping of the mental health system, they were not completely arbitrary. Not only did they reflect the thinking of a senior mental health bureaucrat, they were in line with the overall direction of the COGP Report. According to the deputy minister of health, the COGP had stipulated that the Ministry should adopt a policy of decentralization: "The policy of decentralization is firmly established," the report notes, "and has been accepted as the direction we will take in the future as we approach our assignments."

In the late 1960s, student rebellions swept European and American campuses, urban riots occurred in major American cities, while in Canada student radicals set fire to computers at Sir George Williams University in Montreal. The New Left had popularized ideas on participatory democracy and community involvement in political decision making as correctives to the perceived deficiencies of big bureaucracy. Thus, all levels of government, some in response to actual events, others fearing future disruptions, were casting about for ways to give more participation to service consumers and to lighten the burden of centralized government. In this climate, it is not surprising that the COGP report noted that "terms [such as] 'citizen involvement' and 'citizen participation' are frequently heard expressions of a public concern."[23]

Support for this point of view can also be found in a task force appointed in 1972 in line with COGP recommendations that individual ministries examine their administrative structures and make recommendations for reorganization.[24] In 1972, a coordinating committee was established for the reorganization of the Department of Health, including a task force and various subcommittees on different aspects of psychiatric and retardation services.[25]

On key issues, the task force and its subcommittees demonstrated enormous disillusionment with the existing state of mental health services and a desire to embark on a program of decentralization, divestment, and a merging of health and social service delivery that went far beyond anything previously proposed.

The adult psychiatric services subcommittee proposed that the Ministry of Health get out of the business of direct delivery of adult mental health services and establish "local Management Boards" for the provincial psychiatric hospitals. These boards would be composed of members appointed by Health and of members elected in the community. The Ministry's role would be confined to providing funding and "these funding responsibilities should relate to the Boards..."[26] A second recommendation was that Human Resource Centres be established performing an ombudsman service helping patients and clients to locate appropriate services and ensuring that such services met their needs. "They should be responsible for fixing accountability for care in unambiguous terms." In addition, the subcommittee recommended that rehabilitation be "emphasized for the treatment of the mentally ill" and that the local management boards would receive funds through Health in order to "coordinate all appropriate agencies and facilities within their particular area" for the purposes of rehabilitation.

In an interim report, the subcommittee on regional and local service delivery unanimously recommended that the primary obligation for the delivery of service be placed at the community level.[27] But the subcommittee went even farther, recommending not only the decentralization of mental health services, but of social development programs as well. Central government would "transfer all operating authority and responsibility of social development programs (including all health and mental health programs) to local community levels thereby ensuring by whatever means necessary that a clear direct obligation exists at community level for the provision of such services and programs." Community boards would be established for all psychiatric, mental retardation and children's facilities, and they would have direct responsibility for service delivery. All this would be organized in a three tier system along district, regional and central lines. There would be district and regional social development councils with planning and coordination responsibilities and they would even be given some financial authority by the Ministry. At the provincial level a separate organization would be established reporting to the Provincial Secretary of Social Development and overseeing the work of the regional and district councils. In addition, the subcommittee emphasized that it "*strongly supports the recommendation that at the very least government define standardized and uniform boundaries for regions within the social development policy field* [their italics]." In its conclusion the subcommittee argued that "the coordination of all social development programs including health and mental health...should...result in improved social development services to the population at large, and will overcome the existing fragmentation of the system with the development of individualized vested interests at various levels."[28] The final report of the subcommittee added that "consideration be given to the complete integration of mental health care within the program of general health care with a view to *eliminating all inappropriate differences between the two systems in future* [their italics]."

Needless to say, this radical proposal for an integration of the mental health and social service fields was ignored, although two years before, in 1970/1971, Quebec had combined the Ministries of Health and Family and Social Services in a new Ministry of Social Affairs. Thus, Quebec embarked on a completely different road toward the delivery of health and social services.[29]

At this time, other branches in the Department of Health were also thinking about the advantages of divesting government of responsibility for the provincial psychiatric hospitals and of decentralization of authority. When the coordinating committee requested information from the research and planning branch of the Ministry, it was sent a paper entitled "Trends and Developments for Health Services" which stated that the Ministry of Health would "over time, progressively divest itself of responsibility for the direct delivery of health services and would decentralize the responsibility for planning, organizing and coordinating delivery of services to authorities in designated geographic areas."[30]

But not everyone agreed with these proposals. One month before the final reports were submitted to the full committee, Dr. Farmer wrote to Dr. H. W. Henderson, the chairman of the full committee, concerning changes in the draft of the final report.

> I cannot help but note that the Ministry of Health will continue to be the primary authority in the area of planning, development, funding, standard setting and provision of consultation and other supporting services. It would appear that this general statement which relates to organization is perhaps in conflict with the recommendations of the subcommittee on Regional and Local Service Delivery.[31]

Dr. Farmer admitted that his subcommittee's recommendations "will indeed be contentious" and he noted differences between Henderson's draft and the subcommittee's recommendations. But, in the end, the recommendations of the various task forces went for naught, and the final report of the psychiatric and retardation services task force was a bland distillation of the reports of the various subcommittees. Whereas the subcommittees had all recommended that local or regional bodies be established with a high degree of administrative and operating responsibility, the task force report merely referred to,

> two essential requirements: 1) A suitable means of planning programs which pertain to mental illness and mental retardation with the close collaboration of all Ministries within the Social Development Policy Field...2) The delivery of services in a manner that will meet the needs of the individual and his family for assistance.

The final report also proposed that "local and regional services should be provided by agencies under Management Boards."

Why were none of the recommendations concerning mental health policy implemented?

Dr. Farmer says he does not understand why they were rejected although he thinks that the possibility of increased costs deriving from divestment and decentralization might have posed an obstacle to reform.[32] Another major obstacle was the immense administrative upheaval entailed in the proposal for social development councils. It was perhaps naive to expect that the Ministries of Health and Community and Social Services would collaborate in handing over to the Provincial Secretary for Social Development responsibility for an entirely new administrative structure. It is also unclear whether these proposals enjoyed any support within the Ministry of Health—or even if they got beyond the deputy minister level. The evidence does indicate that Dr. Henderson was unwilling to accept the recommendations of the subcommittees, but whether this reflected his own feelings or those of the Minister of Health is unclear.[33]

The fact that the recommendations of the various subcommittees, staffed by senior mental health bureaucrats, went completely unheeded demonstrates that, in the case of mental health policy, civil servants cannot make major policy changes on their own. Certainly bureaucrats can formulate policies, and they may even formulate radical and innovative policies, but they cannot implement them without support from their political masters or without outside pressure. The proposals failed because there was neither public pressure forcing government to implement them nor powerful allies at the top of the political structure to support them. Lacking such support the task force reports disappeared into obscurity.

The Divestment Controversy

This was not the first, nor was it to be the last time that arguments were unsuccessfully put forward suggesting that only when government divested itself of control over the mental hospitals and gave the community a much bigger role to play in their operations could any real improvements in the system take place. However, aside from the establishment of community advisory boards which, as the name implies, had only very limited advisory powers and the establishment of district health councils, also with limited advisory powers, the government refused to countenance turning the mental hospitals over to the community, integrating the mental health system with the general medical system, or of integrating health with social services.[34]

There were a number of reasons why the Ministry and government were reluctant to act. Giving the public a greater voice in the administration of the system would inevitably have led to demands for increased funding. Divestment would have led to increased participation in decision making and to increased difficulties in reaching a decision. Few bureaucrats favour changes which will make their own lives more difficult. As the COGP report put it: "It can be claimed that the more citizens are able to contribute, the slower the decision-making process becomes, since many opinions and pressures must be considered. No government can please all of the people all of the time."[35] Divestment would have prevented or at least made it more difficult for governments to use mental hospital policy as a means to achieve other ends such as providing employment in politically or economically necessitous regions. After all, as a former assistant deputy minister pointed out, independent boards would have taken one look at the mental hospitals and demanded an increase in funds.[36] Given that maintenance costs at the mental hospitals were much lower than at the general hospitals (at that time the per diem rate for the mental hospitals was $13.00 to

$14.00 as compared with a rate of $50.00 for the general hospitals, and $9.50 for homes for special care) one member of the committee pointed out that turning the mental hospitals over to a board of governors would lead to increased expenditures.[37]

Divestment of the mental hospitals would have led to conflict with the trade unions whose members would no longer enjoy the comparative salary advantage that came from being employed by the Department of Health as well as sharply curtailing the ability of Health to determine policy at the local level.[38] It was pointed out in the legislature on October 22, 1973 that at the Toronto general hospital, workers' salaries were on average about $17.00 below the rate for comparative positions at the provincial mental hospitals. Moreover, employees in the provincial hospitals earned the same wage regardless of where the hospital was located, whereas the wages of general hospital workers varied from one hospital to another. Although in principle divestment might have reduced the wages paid to mental hospital workers, in fact the government knew it would provoke an enormous fight with the trade union movement. According to Tom Campbell, former deputy minister of health from 1979 to 1981, the question of divestment was discussed but there were two main objections. First, unlike the general hospitals which had no difficulty in attracting loyal and energetic board members, it was thought that most provincial psychiatric hospitals would have difficulty in attracting people to their boards.

> After all, the patient population of general hospitals is usually made up of people who live in the area, they see it as their hospital. But people in the psychiatric hospitals often come from far away. So it is easy to attract people to serve on the boards of the general hospitals, but we thought it might be difficult to get people to serve on the boards of the psychiatric hospitals.

Second, once the psychiatric hospitals had been divested, it would have been extremely difficult to limit their size or, if necessary to close them down. According to Campbell, "it is nearly impossible to close down a general hospital, no matter how good or bad it is, and the same obstacles would have confronted us in the case of psychiatric hospitals." According to this reasoning, divestment was opposed because government had to retain firm control over the psychiatric hospital system if deinstitutionalization was to proceed and hospitals were to be closed. Finally, many ex-civil servants who worked in the Ministry of Health or in the mental health division during this time remarked that they were proud of the mental health system in Ontario, and they believed that the centralized bureaucracy had played a positive role in bring that system about. Moreover, as one deputy minister put it, one of the major problems in the mental health system was the tendency of some mental hospitals to "dump on each other," that is to fob off their most difficult patients onto other hospitals. His argument was that such fobbing-off was more difficult in a centralized than in a decentralized system, and he suggested that if the mental hospitals were divested to community boards, in the absence of central control, they might find it easier to get rid of the difficult patients.[39]

The reluctance of the Ministry of Health to decentralize was not a peculiarly Ontario phenomenon but was characteristic of mental health authorities across Canada. On September 24, 1974, the provincial directors of mental health met in Toronto, and, among other things, discussed decentralization, and the integration of the mental health services with general health services and social services. In principle, the provincial mental health directors were in favour of decentralization and regionalization—but only of mental health services. "There is less agreement," they noted, "on the desirability of decentralizing and regionalizing *administrative* functions. [their italics] Whether the electorate loses or gains control by decentralization is debatable. In any event, it seems unlikely that the provinces, as the taxing authorities, will ever be prepared to give up final fiscal control to regions."[40] With regard to integration of mental health services, the provincial directors noted a clear trend toward greater "*co-ordination* [their italics]" of mental health services with general health and social services, although they also observed that integration was very difficult to achieve. Moreover, the provincial mental health directors argued that "[i]ntegration should not mean absorption of mental health services into other services. Experience has shown that, both from an administrative and service point of view, they should be kept separate." They emphasized that having a group of mental health experts organized separately was very important for setting priorities, distributing resources, and for providing psychiatric services.

During the late 1960s and 1970s, reform-minded bureaucrats and committees failed to make a dent in Ontario's mental health system. Unlike Quebec in the 1960s and 1970s, where a series of major scandals concerning the French psychiatric hospitals led to major reforms in the health system, the Ontario mental health system continued to run smoothly along policy rails laid down in the distant past. But a political time bomb was ticking away and it was to go off at the end of the decade.

Notes

1 On the background to the establishment of the committee see James D. Fleck, "Restructuring the Ontario Government," *Canadian Public Administration* 16 (1973): 55–66. According to Professor George Szablowski of York University one of the reasons for government reorganization was to keep up with Ottawa which had already completed a similar reorganization. However, the policy fields began to fall into desuetude during the latter part of Premier Davis's tenure, and were finally abandoned when the Liberal Government took power in 1985. Interview, George Szablowski.

2 H. W. Henderson, "Mental Health Services: A Review of Programs and Expenditures in Ontario," Ministry of Health, May 8, 1969, p. 13.

3 AO, RG 10–108, May 27, 1969, Dr. H. W. Henderson, Executive Director, Mental Health Division to Dr. K. C. Charron, Deputy Minister.

[4] AO, RG 10–108, B. 12, September 8, 1969, Dr. H. W. Henderson Executive Director, Mental Health Division to Dr. K. C. Charron, Deputy Minister.

[5] AO, RG 10–108, B. 12, September 8, 1969, Henderson to Charron.

[6] AO, RG 10–108, B. 12, September 8, 1969, Henderson to Charron.

[7] Committee on Government Productivity, *Interim Report Number Six*, (Toronto: Committee on Government Productivity, 1972) 5.

[8] In a March 1981 article in *The Globe and Mail*, Professor Cyril Greenland of the School of Social Work at McMaster University tried to explain why mental health policy had gone wrong. The large mental hospitals discharged patients to the community without ensuring adequate supports while the psychiatric units ignored chronic patients in favour of the less seriously ill, "well-behaved, middle-class patients with good prognoses." Equally important was the fact that the psychiatrists who traditionally staffed the upper reaches of the mental health bureaucracy in Health had been replaced by a "nomadic band of bureaucrats, mostly administrators and managers. Lacking psychiatric experience and exhausted by managing 10 psychiatric hospitals...these civil servants have little time to consult mental health specialists."

[9] Interview, Graham Scott.

[10] Interview, Anonymous.

[11] "Studies of those fields of public policy where knowledge, expertise and information tend to be restricted to certain groups of participants illustrate the importance of the dominant paradigm. In these instances the monopolistic tendencies and practices of bureaucratic, professional and technological organizations result in policymaking arenas where change can often be effected only if revolutions—major or minor—occur in regard to the dominant assumptions and modes of thought that constitute the prevailing paradigm. Such revolutions, in other words, are a necessary, although not always a sufficient, condition for changes in public policy." Peter Aucoin, "Public-Policy Theory and Analysis," in *Public Policy in Canada*, edited by G. Bruce Doern and Peter Aucoin, (Toronto: Macmillan Company of Canada, 1979) 16. It must also be remembered that the government had entered a period of tight budgets and fiscal restraint in the 1970s, which gave added impetus to the search for administrators with the necessary skills to get the most out institutional budgets.

[12] Ontario Council of Health, Committee on Mental Health Services in Ontario, *Agenda for Action*, 1979, p. 147.

[13] AO, RG 10–06, January 9, 1967, Estimates, Meeting with Treasurer.

[14] AO, RG 10–108, B. 17, January 15, 1970, Task force on Mental Health Care Costs, Interim Report No. 1.

[15] Telephone interview, Lawrence G. Macpherson.

[16] Interview, Dr. R. Ian Hector.

[17] AO, RG 10–108, B. 17, January 7, 1970, Wilson to Macpherson.

[18] On April 7, 1972, the Government Reorganization Act changed Department of Health to Ministry of Health.

[19] See D. K. Foot, *Provincial Public Finance in Ontario: An Empirical Analysis of the Last Twenty-Five Years* (Toronto: Ontario Economic Council Toronto, 1977) 78 *et passim.*

[20] Hanly 390.

[21] AO, RG 10, January 17, 1972, E. V. Margetts, Program Analysis Coordinator, Policy and Executive Secretary, Coordinating Committee for the Organization of the Department of Health, "Centralization and Decentralization," January 27, 1972.

[22] AO, RG 10–108, B.12, April 6, 1971, Dr. R. A. Farmer, Director Hospital Management Services Branch to Dr. H. W. Henderson, Executive Director MH Division.

[23] Committee on Government Productivity, *Interim Report Number Three*, December 1971, p. 52.

[24] At a meeting of the coordinating committee which organized the various subcommittees, Dr. Henderson had expressed reservations about including representatives from "voluntary organizations" on the subcommittees. But on this he was overruled by deputy minister K. C. Charron, chairman of the committee. Thus, Dr. Farmer included on his committee representatives of the major pressure groups in the field including Dr. J. D. Griffin of Mental Health Canada, Mora Skelton of the Ontario Association for the Mentally Retarded, as well as private individuals and pressure group representatives. AO, RG 10–108, B.3, January 7, 1972, Coordinating Committee for the Organization of the Department of Health, 1st Meeting.

[25] When the Ministry established a coordinating committee for the organization of the Department of Health, it claimed that it was "in advance of the COGP and therefore no outside push has been necessary." Coordinating Committee for the Organization of the Department of Health, January 7, 1972. At a January 7, 1972 meeting of the Coordinating Committee, W. J. Lane of the Treasury Board Secretariat noted that: "The Management Policy Branch of the Treasury Board Secretariat will be watching the organization of this Department with great interest as we are well advanced in our planning and are considered as a 'prototype'." AO, RG 10–108, B. 1.

[26] AO, RG 10–108, B. 3, February 19, 1972, Task Force Subcommittee report, Sub-committee on Adult Psychiatric Services, pp. 2–3.

[27] AO, RG 10–108, B.3, February 29, 1972, Report of the Subcommittee on Regional and Local Service Delivery, p. 3.

[28] Although Ontario never adopted a policy of combining social service and health delivery within the same structures, just two years before, in December 1970, the government of Quebec had passed a law establishing a network of local and regional health and social service centres. See Françoise Boudreau, *De l'Asile à la Santé Mentale* (Montreal: Editions Saint-Martin, 1984) 159.

[29] Boudreau 153–165.

[30] AO, RG 10–108, February 16, 1972, Margetts to Henderson, Re: Trends and Developments for Health Services.

[31] AO, RG 10–108, B.3, January 28, 1972, Farmer to Henderson.

[32] Interview, Dr. R. A. Farmer.

[33] In an interview Dr. Farmer suggested that Dr. Henderson may have been reflecting the views of the Minister rather than his own views on the matter.

[34] At the same time the Ministry declared its support for the establishment of district health councils whose job would be to "identify the needs, establish priorities and plan and coordinate a comprehensive health care program within policies established by the Ministry of Health." Executive Director's Column, *Canadian Journal of Public Health* 62 (1972): 465–469.

[35] COGP, *Interim Report Number Three*, p. 53.

[36] Interview, Dr. Boyd Suttie.

[37] AO, RG–108, B.17, July 25, 1969, Robert E. Bunn, Ontario Mental Health Association in Minutes, Mental Health Sub-Committee on Health Care Costs.

[38] Many of those interviewed expressed this view, including one senior bureaucrat appointed in the 1980s. He prefers to remain anonymous.

[39] Interview, Graham Scott.

[40] AO, RG 10–20-A–5, October 16, 1974, Memo from J. K. Maynard, Director Psychiatric Hospitals Branch, to S. W. Martin, Deputy Minister, MOH, re: Report and recommendations from the Provincial Directors of Mental Health to the Conference of Deputy Ministers.

9

Deinstitutionalization in a Vacuum

> There was the assumption that it would be cheaper to get people into the community rather than keep them in the mental hospital.
>
> Former Director Mental Health Services

Deinstitutionalization Defined

The question of deinstitutionalization is wracked with controversy—even the definition of the term causes problems.[1] Deinstitutionalization can be defined narrowly in terms of releasing large numbers of people from psychiatric hospitals, or broadly as referring to a decline in the number of mental hospital beds due to a rising rate of discharge. An even broader definition would stipulate that deinstitutionalization does not occur unless community support systems are in place for ex-patients. Whatever definition one chooses, however, the term has ideological implications.

The humanitarian argument holds that the introduction of the neuroleptic drugs as well as more positive attitudes toward the mentally ill were contributing factors to deinstitutionalization. The economic argument holds that the decline in the number of patients in large mental hospitals was a direct result of fiscal pressures on state and provincial governments unwilling to bear the continued and rising costs of mental health care. The first argument assumes that deinstitutionalization was prompted by the best of motives—the desire to remove mentally ill people from large institutions and to reintegrate them into the community. It explains the lack of community services and the consequent crisis of deinstitutionalization as an accident or an oversight on the part of mental health bureaucrats, psychiatrists and pressure group representatives who did not weigh the consequences of deinstitutionalization. The second argument assumes that deinstitutionalization was prompted by the fiscal crisis of the state in the 1960s. Falling revenues forced governments to look for areas in which to economize. The mental health system was one such area, and mental health bureaucrats cynically decided to discharge large numbers of mentally ill people from hospitals knowing full well there were no community services to receive them. Andrew Scull contends that "the attempt to manage an increasing proportion of the 'deviant' within the community...will be seen to be a response to the changing exigencies of domestic pacification and control under welfare capitalism."[2] For

Table 9.1
Number of Patients in Hospital and Residential Units

Year	*In Hospital*	*In Residential Units*	*Total*
1961	14,368	1,234	15,602
1962	12,513	3,466	15,979
1963	12,470	4,133	16,603
1964	12,528	4,209	16,737
1965	11,441	3,732	15,173
1966	11,002	3,217	14,219
1967	9,517	3,332	12,849

[Source: Ministry of Health, *Annual Reports*]

Scull, deinstitutionalization was not aimed at improving the situation of the mentally ill, retarded and elderly but rather at the social control of deviant populations and by a desire to give the private sector an opportunity to profit from providing institutional care for deviant populations. A third position is that deinstitutionalization resulted from a fortuitous linkage between the forces of fiscal conservatism anxious to save money by closing large mental hospitals and returning patients to the community, and pressure groups and other humanitarian forces which saw the large mental hospital as the symbol of everything that was wrong with mental health policy.[3]

Part of the problem is that the term deinstitutionalization sometimes refers to the *process* whereby large numbers of mental patients left hospital beginning in the late 1960s and 1970s, while at other times it refers to a *policy* whereby authorities deliberately set out to reduce the size of mental hospitals by discharging people to a network of services which had been prepared to help their reintegration into the community. However, if we define deinstitutionalization as referring simply to the discharge of mental patients from hospital then it is easy enough to discuss deinstitutionalization in terms of the rate of discharge and falling patient populations.

From the very beginning, a certain proportion of patients was always discharged from the psychiatric hospital. The number of discharges was inversely correlated to the length of stay, that is, the longer a person was in the mental hospital the less likely he/she was to be discharged. But, as chronic patients accumulated in the back wards, total patient population grew. The high point was reached in 1960 when there were 25,630 patients in Ontario institutions for the mentally ill and mentally retarded (this figure includes patients in the psychiatric and mental retardation hospitals, in approved homes, on probation and "on escape but not discharged").[4] A close look at the statistics shows that the apparent decline in the psychiatric hospital population which began in 1960 was due almost exclusively to the inception of the residential unit program, and not to a

Table 9.2
Rate of Mentally Ill in Psychiatric Hospitals

Year	*per 100,000*
1937	278
1942	275
1946	270
1951	268*
1956	252
1961	203

* The neuroleptic drugs were first introduced to Ontario Psychiatric Hospitals in 1953.
[Source: Department of Health, *Annual Reports*]

policy of deinstitutionalization.[5] Statistics for Ontario mental hospitals (excluding provincial institutions for mentally retarded people) show that in 1959, there were 15,739 patients "in hospital" for that year. That number excludes all patients in approved homes, on probation, and "on escape." The following year the figure dropped slightly to 15,507 and in 1961 to 14,368. On the surface this looks like the beginning of a secular decline in the mental hospital population. But in 1961, 1,234 people were discharged from hospital and transferred to residential units. Since these residential units were in the mental hospital and, to all intents and purposes, hardly differed from the rest of the hospital, the patients in the residential units were hardly "deinstitutionalized" in any sense of the word. Thus, if the numbers of patients in the residential units are added to the "in hospital" totals, then the total in 1961 was 15,602.

From a different perspective, although the absolute numbers of patients in Ontario's psychiatric hospitals continued to rise until the mid–1960s, in 1938, the rate of patients in residence in psychiatric hospitals per 100,000 population began to decline.

In 1959, the number of days of care provided by the provincial psychiatric hospitals peaked at 6,260,000 and then began to decline. In that same year, psychiatric units provided 109,990 days of care. By 1970, the provincial mental hospitals provided 2,993,692 days of care, and the psychiatric units, 434,643. Whereas in 1959, the psychiatric unit provided 1.7 percent of the days of care, by 1970 they were providing 14.5 percent. In addition, approximately 40,000 people attended 68 outpatient departments and mental health clinics, and of these about 38 percent were children 16 years of age and under.[6] Although staffing levels were higher than ever before, there were still shortages. In 1972, there were 154 physicians in provincial mental hospitals—a short-fall of 20. Total staff in 1970 numbered 10,630, with an official shortage of 192.

By the 1970s, the full effects of deinstitutionalization were finally making themselves felt. But what did deinstitutionalization mean in the Ontario context?

If by deinstitutionalization we mean a clearcut policy directed toward reducing the population of provincial psychiatric hospitals and establishing community services to receive discharged patients, then no such policy ever existed in Ontario. However, if by deinstitutionalization we mean a deliberate policy of reducing the long-stay population of the large mental hospitals regardless of what happened to the patients afterward, then deinstitutionalization began in 1965. The ex-medical superintendent of the Queen Street Mental Health Centre recalls that, by the early 1970s, there were,

> pretty explicit messages that were associated with budget cuts, close units, lock the door, and don't use them. That meant you could move the staff that was operating a unit and consolidate. I think I can remember reading pretty specific directives that this was what the government wanted to see happen...[7]

Thus, the initial decline in the rate and ultimately in the number of people resident in Ontario institutions was not due to a carefully planned and executed policy of releasing people from the institution to a network of community support services. At first it was due to the fortuitous inception of the neuroleptic drugs in the 1950s and to the discharge of patients to residential units and then re-labelling them residents. Later, there were deliberate attempts to discharge patients to the community. Like almost everything else in the Ontario mental health system, deinstitutionalization came about slowly and in an ad hoc fashion.

In this sense, the process of deinstitutionalization in Ontario hardly differed from what took place in Great Britain or the United States where deinstitutionalization was, at first, a trend rather than a policy. "In the beginning," writes Douglas Bennett, "the 'deinstitutionalization' of the early 1960s was little more than the recognition by psychiatrists and by planners that the population of the mental hospitals was diminishing in spite of rising admission rates. True, there was a vague appreciation of changes in the relations of patients to staff and others. But it was not a policy." Bennett goes on to point out that both the 1957 British Royal Commission on the Law Relating to Mental Illness and Mental Deficiency and the U.S. Joint Commission on Mental Illness and Health were vague about what community living meant and about how mentally ill people would be received in the community.[8]

One psychiatrist put it this way.

> Deinstitutionalization was an incredible thing, and when I talk about it in retrospect I can't believe what I am saying, but there I was honestly saying that all you had to do was to load them with neuroleptic drugs and send them out into the community.[9] We began reading Erving Goffman and Ernest Gruenberg from New York State and how hospital screws people up. So we took tens of thousands of patients and threw them out of the hospital without any support system. We said there was going to be follow-up, but the fact of the matter is that nobody really understood, so the bureaucrats were delighted to get them out of hospital...and only in 1975 and later did we say, "Hey, this is crazy, what about housing, what about recreation?"[10]

Yet according to a senior civil servant, in the 1970s the feeling was,

> "what the hell do they want from us? Once they are out of the hospital they're on their own, they're just normal citizens, we won't interfere with that. It's not our job to provide services for these people, they are private citizens, somebody else can do it." I mean people aren't wrong in assuming that the government was being insensitive. I was appalled...I thought we could do better.[11]

Another psychiatrist observed:

> we were beginning to be concerned about where these people went, but we had the attitude that it was the community's responsibility and not the hospital's responsibility once they were discharged. We believed that the worst possible place a person could be was in the big institution, that if we could get them out they would be better off. But we didn't realize we weren't sending them out to a nice boarding home with Ma and Pa looking after them but to God knows what. But that wasn't our responsibility at that time. And so the hospital's concern for what happened to these people didn't really begin until the 1970s because we were getting the police bringing some of these people back, we were getting the coroner phoning because he found some guy dead under the bridge recently discharged from our place.[12]

By 1975, Minister of Health Frank Miller responded to accusations that deinstitutionalization was motivated primarily by the desire to save money. In the summer of 1975, he told the legislature:

> Regarding halfway houses, we have all kinds of halfway houses to talk about...but as we go back to more and more community support for the treatment of mentally ill persons, getting them back into the community faster and faster—and we are, not for dollars and cents, I say quickly; not for dollars and cents—it has been accepted that those people should be back in the community for their own sake.[13]

Aftercare

Until the 1930s, there was no organized aftercare program for patients discharged from the provincial mental hospitals. Some hospitals had hired social workers to keep track of and advise ex-patients, but social work programs were left to the hospital superintendents. When the mental health clinics were established in 1930, one of their responsibilities was to provide some form of aftercare for discharged patients. This was understood by the clinic teams to mean informing local physicians about the presence of a discharged patient in the community.[14] The clinics could not do much more because they were continually on the move and were swamped with work. By 1945, most of the provincial mental hospitals had implemented an aftercare program, but they lacked the personnel and the resources to do an effective job. Some people, even those who thought in terms of "community care," had only a vague idea of what aftercare meant. In a paper delivered in November 1949, the director of the aftercare department of the provincial institution at London advocated "citizen participation" in the development of aftercare organization, and then went on to suggest that families, friends, employers, government, hospital staff, charitable organizations, and a myriad of community organizations might play a role in the "re-establishment" of the patient.[15] The difficulty with this and similar proposals was the assumption that the community was interested in the problems of ex-patients and that almost every voluntary or professional organization in the community would want to get involved in an aftercare program. Both assumptions proved false. Interest in the problems of discharged patients waxed and waned over the years, but except for local branches of the CMHA, very few community organizations got involved. Even a report on the community mental hospital from the World Health Organization in 1953 had little specific to say about aftercare except to advocate the use of social workers and "institutions in the community," to assist the discharged patient in finding employment and reintegrating into the community.[16]

On the other hand, some people felt that public health departments should assume the responsibility for aftercare programs. In "Future Policy of Psychiatric Services" submitted to deputy minister B. T. McGhie in 1944, the "Committee of Psychiatrists in the Armed Forces," suggested that: "The follow-up care of patients, discharged from the Ontario Hospitals and acute psychotic wards in General Hospitals should be taken care of by the Municipal Health Unit social worker, who should be under the guidance of the Clinic Director in this phase of her work."[17] By contrast the superintendent of the provincial hospital at London argued strongly against using social workers for aftercare and in favour of public health nurses. "The importance...of keeping these people well in their homes and of returning them to employability, or at least good social adjustment, cannot be overstressed and in my opinion should be a nursing responsibility."[18] Despite suggestions that aftercare services be linked to public health departments, little was done until the mid–1950s when the mental health division decided to experiment with using public health nurses operating out of local boards of health to provide aftercare for discharged patients. Noting that "in the past" the division had been reluctant to use boards of health in aftercare, public health personnel now observed that the mental health division was interested in cooperating with public health. The plan was to notify local medical officers of health of the date of the patient's impending discharge, to provide public health with case notes and to advance suggestions for rehabilitation and aftercare. The hospital social worker would then act as a liaison agent between the institution and public health.[19] But in 1956, when the director of community mental health, Dr. B. H. McNeel was asked if he had formulated a "definite plan," he answered that he had not.[20] A few months later, when it became apparent that social workers and rehabilitation workers were in short supply (at the St. Thomas provincial mental hospital, there were five social workers serving a patient population of about 2,000), it was suggested that an experiment be tried in Hamilton using public health nurses to provide aftercare.[21] The following spring, the medical superintendent at the St. Thomas provincial mental hospital notified the mental health division that, after reading a report of aftercare services provided by the division of community services in Kentucky, he contacted the medical officer of health in

Windsor, the nearest population center 125 miles away, about using public health nurses to perform aftercare duties.[22] According to Dr. Cleland, the public health nurses would visit patients' homes when they were in the hospital, to contact their families and to visit them when they returned home. "If the husband is in the [mental] hospital, financial problems often occur, and if the wife is in the hospital, there are very often problems related to the care of children, and the help, advice and support of a trained Public Health Nurse should be valuable."[23] However, Cleland's plans ran into opposition from the public health nurses because late in the summer, Dr. B. H. McNeel, who had recently been appointed as chief of the mental health division, wrote to Cleland telling him he thought "all of them are a little alarmed at the idea that they might be expected to do social work, to look for employment of patients and to undertake other tasks which they do not think of as part of Public Health nursing."[24] That fall, a social worker noted that the head of public health nurses in one community was "a little appalled at the prospect of losing her nurses in batches," but that she seemed to be amenable to working with the program.[25] In October, the superintendent of the provincial hospital at Hamilton wrote to the chief of the mental health division: "This program has been slowed down rather materially and off the record I don't know just what results we are going to be able to get. I am very much afraid that the situation regarding Public Health Nurses in the city is so acute that the nurses themselves feel that they can give only a minimum of time to this program."[26] Later that month, the assistant director of public health nursing wrote to the chief of the mental health division that: "The situation from the point of view of nursing staff is not good."[27] Unquestionably, the problems encountered in trying to use public health nurses to perform aftercare functions was another reason why in 1957 the mental health division decided to abandon the idea of establishing community mental health centres attached to local public health units, and to concentrate instead on utilizing the psychiatric units to perform community mental health functions.

By the early 1960s, therefore, there was no policy on aftercare for the mentally ill in the Department of Health. In the January 1959 "Proposed Revision of Mental Health Program in Ontario," the Department of Health stated that since rehabilitation began in the community, then "rehabilitation committees with leadership from public health" should be established.[28] So vague was this idea that at a meeting of the superintendents in the fall of 1959, the chief of the mental health division frankly stated: "when the Department is asked what is its policy [on aftercare]...there is none."[29] The following year, the Minister of Health attempted to rectify this by establishing a division of rehabilitation whose main responsibility was to provide vocational counselling and to help discharged patients to find employment. Dr. Dymond also expressed good intentions in the area of community mental health in a speech to the legislature.

> In looking at the ideal, to meet the needs of the mentally ill and mentally defective within its boundaries, every large community should have a comprehensive service... From this, it will be seen that the modern concept is that

> organization of mental health services should start at the community level. Now it is not possible for us to start all over again. If that were so, we would start at the community level. We must work with what we have at the present time, and again, I repeat, that that has been working backwards, trying to bring the mental hospitals closer to the community.[30]

However, for the Department of Health, community mental care meant that psychiatric hospitals and psychiatric units would provide inpatient and outpatient care, short-term night care, identification, diagnostic and educational services. Community mental health care did not mean establishing mental health services independent of psychiatric hospitals or psychiatric units. In his 1963 report on Ontario's mental health services, C. A. Roberts observed that the "present arrangements for the rehabilitation of patients in the mental hospitals are in a state of development" and he noted the "inadequacy of local [aftercare] services."[31] In 1964, Dr. J. S. Pratten, medical superintendent of Kingston, noted that the discharge rate in provincial hospitals was about 75 percent of new admissions. "Hospital outpatient, community psychiatric, medical, social work and rehabilitation services are not sufficiently developed or sufficiently integrated with psychiatric hospitals to provide adequate aftercare which the patients need."[32] Dr. Pratten pointed out that readmission rates were reaching 35 to 50 percent within a few months of leaving hospital, and he suggested that what were needed were closer contacts with public health units and with other community agencies. The following year, Stephen Lewis of the NDP noted that there were only 33 workers employed in the medical rehabilitation branch of the Department of Health, and that only three of these were qualified social workers.[33] In fact, because of the autonomy of the local public health departments there was, as one regional consultant on public health nursing put it, "no overall provincial program." The result was that public health units and the various provincial mental hospitals worked out their own service plans and this meant that there was "considerable variation throughout in the program and services for these [discharged mental] patients."[34]

Despite the attempt to redefine community mental health in terms of psychiatric units and general hospital psychiatric outpatient units, there were continuing complaints about the shortcomings of the province's aftercare policies. In the late 1960s, the opposition parties, especially the New Democratic Party, pressed the government to use the public health services as a base for an aftercare program and to employ public health nurses to follow up discharged patients. In April 1966, Stephen Lewis of the New Democratic Party complained that after 1964 the mental health branch of the Department of Health severed contact between public health workers and both the large mental hospital and the psychiatric units in the general hospitals. According to Lewis:

> The assertions of an effective mental health aftercare programme in the province of Ontario are fraudulent. They cannot possibly be handled by the hospitals themselves; everyone in this Legislature knows the problems of staffing in the Ontario hospitals and the follow-up of patients into the community. They ignore

> the one major department of government which is available, which has the personnel and which could do the job... Public health wants to help; public health is rejected. Public health nurses could be stationed permanently in Ontario hospitals. Mental health clinics could be attached to public health units.[35]

However, this was clearly contrary to the policy decision taken by the director of mental health service, Dr. H. W. Henderson. In a speech to the Ontario Public Health Association in October 1965, Dr. Henderson emphasized the central role to be played by the psychiatric units in the general hospitals and by psychiatrists and general practitioners in community mental health policy. For Henderson, the term community mental health referred to services delivered by the psychiatric units and by the outpatient services of the large institutions. He criticized the idea that public health workers should be involved in "routine reporting of all discharges from a mental hospital," and suggested instead that the public health worker deal only with patients who had been specifically referred by a psychiatrist or family doctor, and that the worker would be under their supervision.[36] Henderson also criticized the idea that mental health clinics could play a preventive role. Rather, he argued, this "usually boils down to the referral of problems the agency doesn't know what to do with." Instead, the "comprehensive community psychiatric centers," by which Henderson meant the psychiatric units, were better equipped to diagnose and treat mentally ill people. Henderson also criticized school boards for establishing "child adjustment services" and hiring psychologists, social workers and psychiatrists. "I do not believe," he said, "the local public health authority should attempt to carry this responsibility or add psychologists to their team for this purpose. Within the school health program, the public health nurse does have the opportunity of giving support and guidance to the child and family..." And he emphasized the dominant role of the psychiatrist: "The two most important influences on the nature of the mental health program to be developed in a given community will be those exerted by the psychiatrist in charge of the clinical service and the community itself."[37] One official with the Department of Health at this time noted that the problem of confidentiality gave rise to problems between the aftercare workers employed by the hospitals and the public health service. Public health workers would ask the hospital for the names of discharged patients, but the hospitals were reluctant to turn over the lists to public health.[38]

Problems in the Community

By the 1970s, the operational meaning of community care had become a subject of debate. Whereas in the 1960s, the term "community care" was used by the mental health division to refer to psychiatric units, outpatient facilities in the large hospitals, and to the Homes for Special Care Program, by the 1970s, opposition critics used it to refer to vocational rehabilitation, halfway houses, recreation facilities and a whole myriad of community services beyond those encompassed in the Ministry's definition.

The conflict between the two meanings of the term can be illustrated by looking at the legislative debates during this period. In the spring of 1967, NDP MPP Stephen Lewis, said:

> Community mental health: Now there, Mr. Speaker, is the biggest joke of all. The fact is that there is a serious rupture, a serious breakdown between the public health units in the province of Ontario and most of the Ontario hospitals. Referrals for aftercare...still do not come from the Ontario hospitals to the public health units.[39]

Lewis insisted that there should be more coordination between the mental hospitals and the public health units, and that it was the proper role of the public health departments to provide aftercare services.[40] He also attacked the medical model of care, arguing that community mental health should be removed from the hospital and located in the community, and he continued to stress the central role of the public health units. At the same time, the Minister of Health staunchly defended the medical model, arguing that the United States and the United Kingdom "both believe that the community mental health facilities should be centered in the hospital, and they are bringing it back to this."[41]

Another way in which the Progressive Conservative Government responded to criticism was to argue that aftercare was a private rather than a public problem. In 1970, when Minister of Health Thomas Wells was asked in the legislature why the Ministry had granted a mere $25,000 to the White Cross, a rehabilitation division of the Canadian Mental Health Association, he replied:

> Somewhere along the line this cannot be complete government responsibility...the community has to be mobilized to play its part in helping rehabilitate them once they leave hospital... If people would go out and take people from the homes for special care and take them for a ride on Sunday, take them out for Sunday dinner sometimes, do some of these things. Now these can be mobilized by volunteers in the community."[42]

But J. R. Smith of the Progressive Conservative Party observed that "really, there is no community involvement programme for these people... There is nothing set up within the community to assist those people in becoming involved again as citizens."[43]

Sidney B. Handleman, another member of the Progressive Conservative Party observed that when the trustees of the Royal Ottawa Hospital proposed the establishment of a halfway house for discharged mental patients, they could not find a single example in the province.[44] In reply, Rene Brunelle, the Minister of Social and Family Services, admitted that "it has been brought to our attention very forcibly in the last few months that in view of the large number of these persons who are coming back into their own communities...the present provision of the existing grants may not be adequate."[45]

In 1974, the Minister for Health, F. R. Miller, replied to a question concerning the care and rehabilitation of discharged patients saying, "it is ministry policy to assist in halfway houses for psychiatric patients."[46]

However, the government was still not committed to a coherent program of community care, and indeed, had been frightened by negative publicity concerning a patient who had been released on a "loosened warrant" and then committed a murder.[47] "The problem is," the Minister of Health stated in late 1974, "where do you keep a person for his benefit, in the community or in the hospital?"[48] He noted that the Queen Street Mental Health Centre had been "running an interesting study" to determine whether a person recovered faster in a hospital or in the community. Moreover, the Minister backtracked on his statement of the previous June concerning government policy toward halfway houses, for he now explained that it was very difficult to get communities to accept homes for "emotionally disturbed people."[49] Yet, he did not suggest that the government alter the provincial Planning Act and require municipalities to allow group homes or halfway houses. Rather, he said, "most of all, we need community understanding of what it is we are trying to do."[50] In 1979, when a New Democratic Party spokesman suggested an amendment to the Planning Act, the Provincial Secretary for Social Development replied: "It is not our desire to mandate in this way. The philosophy and the intent of this government is to achieve our objectives through co-operation with municipalities."[51]

Although the various Ministers of Health continued to defend government policy in the legislature, behind the scenes there were problems.

Many of the people discharged from the large mental institutions were elderly. Some were sent to nursing and residential homes under the Homes for Special Care Program, but others were finding their way into municipal homes for the aged. However, these were the responsibility of the Ministry of Community and Social Services (MCSS), and the Ministry of Health had not coordinated its discharge policies with MCSS. According to Lawrence Crawford, the provincial director of the homes for the aged, chronic care facilities "either do not exist or are overcrowded." Elderly patients were being discharged into the homes for the aged thus making it difficult to admit people who lived in the community. In the summer of 1973, the director told the homes to refuse admission to discharged patients "since the available bed accommodation should be used, in the first instance, for people actually living in the community who lack other necessary care facilities... At least people in a psychiatric hospital are receiving the basic essentials of shelter, good nutrition and adequate supervision."[52] In a later memo, Crawford stated: "We do not believe that the discharge of a long-stay psychiatric patient from an Ontario Hospital to a Home for the Aged is a return to the community."[53] In commenting on these remarks, the director of the psychiatric hospitals branch of the Ministry of Health observed that they demonstrated "something very far wrong in communications between the two Ministries which, after all, have been placed in a common secretariat of Social Development, presumably for the reason, among others, that such mal-communication would be lessened or completely done away with."[54]

In addition to problems with the homes for the aged, the Ministry of Health was criticized by MCSS for poor coordination with municipal welfare authorities.

In a summer 1973 meeting between the director of the psychiatric hospitals branch of the Ministry of Health and the director of the municipal welfare administration branch of MCSS, the MCSS official pointed out that some hospitals were discharging patients in groups, throwing them suddenly on municipal welfare systems without any prior consultation or cooperation. He also noted that some of the "lodging homes" used by discharged patients were "quite unsuitable" and he asked whether they should not be "more rigorously inspected and brought up to certain standards." He specifically complained that a plan worked out between the St. Thomas Hospital and the City of Windsor concerning discharged patients was not working well and "cooperation might be described as unsatisfactory." Both sides in the discussion also agreed that "the whole matter of halfway houses, hostels and supervised community-based residences for psychiatric patients and ex-patients of the hospital system requires a determined review and policy setting at high levels in the Social Development Secretariat." However, he also noted that attempts to establish a "senior committee" to deal with the question had not succeeded.[55]

Clearly, there were major problems with deinstitutionalization and community mental health services. It is true that in 1976/1977 the Ministry of Health spent $36.3 million on community mental health, but the vast majority of these funds were allocated to services located either in psychiatric hospitals or in general hospitals. However, the Minister did admit that "[c]ommunity-based programs require adequate support services, such as vocational and recreational activities, aftercare and medication maintenance services, and a sufficient range of residential accommodation."[56]

In 1959, the chief of mental health services had admitted that the province had no aftercare policy. A few years later, in 1963, *More for the Mind* emphasized the need for services for mentally ill people in the community. Despite its vagueness about the specifics of such services and its emphasis on the central role of the psychiatrist in administering them, the Tyhurst Report did provide an outline of a network of hospital and community services coordinated through a series of local and regional mental health councils. But practically nothing was done about community services over the following two decades. In 1975, the assistant deputy minister for health services admitted in a letter to the Ontario Medical Association that, "of course, there has been no concrete planning on the provision of psychiatric facilities for ex-psychiatric patients. This has been done more or less on an ad hoc basis."[57]

Housing Problems

In the light of government inaction, it is not surprising that in the early 1970s, the plight of ex-patients in the community became critical. The problem was particularly acute in the Parkdale area of Toronto near the Queen Street Mental Health Centre. Here ex-patients had begun to congregate since the 1960s because of the proximity to the institution and the availability of cheap accommodation. By 1981, it was estimated that between 1,000 and 1,200 ex-psychiatric patients were living in Parkdale.[58] MPPs from that area constantly peppered the government with questions and criticisms about the lack of aftercare services and the poor housing situation. Yet, the government was reluctant to act. In March 1978, an interministerial working group (from the Ministries of Community and Social Services, Correctional Services, Education, Health, Housing, Treasury, Economics and Inter-governmental Affairs, and the Provincial Secretary for Social Development) met to gather information on, and make recommendations concerning group homes. Although the report began with the usual references to the government's concern for "community life, community service and normalization," it did little but develop a definition of what a group home was, draft a model municipal by-law liberalizing provisions for group homes, and recommend the creation of a "public awareness program" to meet neighbourhood resistance to group homes. However, the government stated quite clearly that municipalities would be asked if they wanted to adopt the model by-law—it would not be imposed by changing the Planning Act.[59] Although it was critical of the government for not doing more to get municipalities to accept group homes, the Liberal Party was equally opposed to changing the Planning Act. This left the New Democratic Party to support a formal amendment barring municipalities from discriminating against group homes.

In 1979, Provincial Secretary Margaret Birch explained the Progressive Conservative position in no uncertain terms before the legislature.

> We cannot agree with the suggestion that we introduce legislation to amend the Planning Act so that communities will be forced into accepting group homes. It is not our desire to mandate in this way. The philosophy and the intent of this government is to achieve our objectives through cooperation with municipalities.[60]

This philosophy was articulated in a slightly different fashion by Keith Norton, the Minister of Community and Social Services who in October 1979 told the legislature he was speaking for the Minister of Health. According to Norton, government's responsibility ended once a patient was discharged from the hospital. Hospital staff could assist the discharged patients to find housing, but "they are under no obligation to accept that help."[61] Dennis Timbrell, the Minister of Health, put it more succinctly: "[O]nce a person is discharged they are as free to come and go as you or I."[62] The problem was not, however, that anyone was suggesting that patients be forced to live where they did not want to live, but rather that the government refused to accept any responsibility for making available adequate housing or even to inspect and regulate existing housing for ex-patients. Ironically, at the same time as he was expounding this cold philosophy for ex-mental patients, Norton headed a Ministry which, by all accounts, provided an excellent array of community services for mentally retarded people who were then being released in large numbers from mental retardation institutions.

The controversy surrounding the closure of the Lakeshore psychiatric hospital in the fall of 1979 focused criticism on the government's unwillingness to formulate a coherent community care policy. After the closure, complaints were heard that the Ministry of Health had no plans to increase the stock of alternative housing in communities formerly in the Lakeshore catchment area.[63] The press was filled with horror stories about ex-mental patients living in poor conditions in Parkdale while the opposition parties criticized the Ministries of Health and Housing for exacerbating the housing problem through poor interministerial coordination.[64] In July 1981, a *Globe and Mail* editorial titled "Mr. Timbrell Washes His Hands" criticized the Minister of Health for not providing boarding home operators with the records of ex-psychiatric patients.[65] In August 1981, reporter Betty Jane Wylie of *The Toronto Star* assumed the guise of a discharged mental patient and took a room in a boarding home in Parkdale. Her five-part series on the degrading conditions in which ex-patients lived had a profound effect in sensitizing the public to the housing problem in Parkdale and directing further criticism toward the Ministry of Health.[66] Articles appeared in both *The Globe and Mail* and *The Toronto Star* describing the living conditions of ex-patients and criticizing the lack of community facilities. According to *The Globe and Mail*: "Housing is the single most critical problem for those newly released from hospitals like Whitby Psychiatric, Queen Street Mental Health Centre and any of the province's other 10 psychiatric hospitals."[67] The article went on to cite a study which found that housing for ex-patients did "not meet minimum standards for a healthy living environment." It also criticized the lack of coordination between Health and Community and Social Services, lack of coordination within the Ministry of Health itself and the lack of planning and regulation of commercial boarding homes where many of the ex-patients lived.[68] The article quoted Dr. Donald Anderson, a staff psychiatrist at Queen Street, who stated that welfare payments were so low that ex-patients were doubly handicapped, trying to clothe, feed and house themselves on $242 a month and at the same time trying to combat the effects of their illness.[69]

In 1978, the community mental health programs branch of the Ministry of Health commissioned Community Resources Consultants of Toronto and a team from the Clarke Institute of Psychiatry to report on the status of discharged patients in the Metropolitan Toronto area. The objective of the report was to identify "deficiencies in the provision of aftercare services" which would help in the development of new programs.

The study confirmed what many people had suspected: large numbers of ex-patients were living in deplorable conditions in the community. Twenty percent of the sample were suffering from psychosocial distress, 67 percent were unable to remain out of hospital for six months, one-third of the subjects in the sample were readmitted to a psychiatric inpatient unit during the six month period after discharge, and 38 percent were unemployed.

The psychiatric aftercare study also confirmed the findings of a consultant's study of the Lakeshore psychiatric hospital and the arguments of opposition critics: the psychiatric units in the general hospitals dealt with a quite different population from the provincial psychiatric hospital. The patients drawn from the Clarke Institute, which is mainly a psychiatric research centre, and from the general hospital psychiatric units scored higher on all measures of socio-economic and educational status than those drawn from the downtown Queen Street provincial psychiatric hospital. Twenty-eight percent of the patients from the Clarke Institute, and 35 percent and 21 percent respectively from two psychiatric units had some university education, as compared to only 6 percent of the subjects from the Queen Street Mental Health Centre. Forty-two percent of the subjects from Queen Street had less than a grade nine education as compared to 11 percent from Clarke, and 17 and 19 percent from the two psychiatric units. Seventy-eight percent of the subjects from Queen Street were employed in skilled, semi-skilled or unskilled jobs, or unemployed, compared to 60 percent from the Clarke Institute, and 39 percent and 41 percent from the psychiatric units. And whereas 42 percent of the subjects at Queen Street and 39 percent at the Clarke were women, 74 percent and 77 percent at the psychiatric units were women. The report also confirmed the New Democratic Party contention that the psychiatric units catered mainly for people with neuroses rather than patients with schizophrenia: 18 percent and 11 percent of the subjects at the two psychiatric units suffered from schizophrenia, compared to 44 percent at the Clarke and 45 percent at Queen Street.[70] Finally, critics had suggested that the psychiatric units were extremely reluctant to take violent or disruptive cases of mental illness. The study showed that in the psychiatric units, 9 percent and 20 percent of the admissions were involuntary, while 30 percent were involuntary at Queen Street and 28 percent at the Clarke Institute.[71]

One of the most interesting findings was that, once released from hospital, almost all the ex-patients were treated with some form of chemotherapy. "Thus," the authors concluded, "we are seeing the impact of an illness model upon the aftercare system. Subjects are not seen as disabled or handicapped. Rather they are seen as sick and in need of ongoing treatment."[72] A subsequent 1983 study noted that "the most common form of aftercare available to the discharged psychiatric patient was chemotherapy."[73] As a result patients had to constantly return to the hospital for treatment and in this way they became dependent on the hospital. Discharged patients continued to "see themselves as sick and to function in accordance with the rules of illness behaviour." In order to prevent this "institutional transference" the authors suggested that aftercare services should be more balanced, oriented toward rehabilitation and education and separated from the medical hospital and medical care services.

Another major problem for ex-patients was the lack of government-subsidized or nonprofit residential alternatives to the commercial boarding homes which housed many discharged patients. The study suggested that boarding home standards be developed and that a "community-based aftercare agency" monitor the commercial homes. There was also a lack of recreational facilities and vocational rehabilitation services caused by a "shortage of funds," with twenty times more being spent on psychiatric hospitals than on community-based programs.[74] In the face of these findings, the government stuck to its guns: it refused to contemplate passing legislation preventing municipalities from enacting by-laws which either severely restricted or banned group homes, it tried to fob off the problems of housing and aftercare onto municipal governments, and it still refused to improve community services for discharged patients.

None of this was surprising. The Progressive Conservative government argued that legislation could not change social attitudes; rather, encouragement and education were the necessary preliminaries to social change. When Tony Ruprecht of the Liberal Party criticized the Provincial Secretary for Social Development for doing nothing about the housing problems of discharged patients, Margaret Birch replied that the unlicensed boarding homes in Parkdale were "the responsibility of the Metropolitan Toronto government... That is not a provincial responsibility. It is a responsibility of the municipality."[75]

The problem was that the Progressive Conservatives wished to leave to the community the responsibility for providing community services, and to the individual discharged patient the responsibility for availing him/herself of them. According to Margaret Birch: "I think this all begins with a much better discharge policy. Only those who are able to cope in the community should be discharged."[76] For Birch the source of the difficulties lay in poor discharge planning policies, not in a lack of community or residential services. "I firmly believe, and I think I have the support of my colleagues in this, that the discharge policy is a medical judgment and that no one should be discharged from any institution into the community unless there is a guarantee that either that person is able to cope in the community or the services to help that person are there."[77]

In social policy terms, Birch was arguing for what Richard Titmuss the English social policy theorist once called the "residual model" of welfare. In the residual model people are expected to meet their needs and deal with their problems by relying first on their own resources, then on the private market, and only lastly resorting to public services.[78] As the critics pointed out, however, the trouble was that ex-mental patients were barely able to cope with their own needs, there were no or inadequate services in the community and, the community was sometimes actively hostile to ex-patients. Moreover, there was evidence that the government undermined attempts at providing such services. According to Liberal MPP Tony Ruprecht, in 1980 the Ministry of Health eliminated a 1975 program whereby staff at the Queen Street Mental Health Centre had informally inspected and rated boarding homes for discharged patients and established a list of recommended homes.[79]

Compounding the problem was the fact that as housing prices rose, boarding homes were sold or renovated, thus diminishing the number of boarding home beds available to ex-patients. According to John Trainor, a social worker at Queen Street, 2,200 beds in suitable homes were available in Toronto to ex-patients in 1980, but a year later, 200 beds had been lost. He reported that a study which had ranked the quality of available beds on a scale of 0 to 12, with 12 signifying the best quality, had found that 95 percent of the beds ranked four or less.[80] The lack of facilities was so great, and the problems of discharged patients so pressing that in November 1981, the Ministry of Health decided to put thirty to forty patients from Metropolitan Toronto into a private retirement home in Ajax, a small town outside Toronto, and about sixty into "cottages" at the Whitby provincial psychiatric hospital, located a few miles out of the town of Whitby.[81] However, it did so after rejecting the advice of the Supportive Housing Coalition, a non-profit group which had found housing for ex-patients, but at a rate five dollars per day higher than the Ministry of Health was willing to pay.[82]

According to Ron Ballantyne, the executive director of Community Resources Consultants and a member of the Supportive Housing Coalition: "There's no indication they're [the Ministry of Health] making any effort to find housing inside Metro Toronto. It makes no sense for patients to be moved from a community they are familiar with to unfamiliar surroundings. You can raise the political question too—why aren't they using vacant buildings at Lakeshore psychiatric hospital? Because a rest home is a business, I think it's fair to assume that the owner is doing this for profit."[83]

The problem was, as New Democratic Party MPP Ross McClellan put it to Minister of Health Timbrell in the fall of 1981, that the government acted only when there was a crisis. Lacking any specific plans or policies in the mental health field, it was constantly caught short by events and forced to scramble for ad hoc solutions. Typically, it then established a task force or study commission to formulate long-term policies which were eventually ignored. According to McClellan: "It would be a little more reassuring if we saw some evidence that planning is taking place in advance of the crisis rather than in the midst of the crisis."[84]

Problems with aftercare services and particularly with housing for ex-psychiatric patients continued to plague the government in the 1980s. In May 1982, the Supportive Housing Coalition and the City of Toronto Department of Public Health published *The Housing Gap*. The study confirmed previous findings that there were insufficient services in the community for discharged patients. Ironically, further gaps in service were identified thanks to an assessment and referral unit established by the government at the Queen Street Mental Health Centre in response to criticisms in the psychiatric aftercare report. It found that 50 percent of 62 cases processed during the first three months of its operation by the assessment and referral unit needed 24-hour supervision, while eleven of these patients remained in Queen Street for lack of accommodation or were subsequently returned to the Centre. Five community programs reported that from 28 to 60 percent of their clients had difficulty in finding suitable accommodation. It was also found that more than half of the patients discharged from the Queen Street Mental Health Centre and from the Clarke Institute during the research study were on welfare.[85] This accorded well with the psychiatric aftercare study which found that only 38 percent of their subjects were employed. But the crucial problem remained the lack of affordable accommodation. Houselink, an alternative community housing operation reported that whereas in 1981 applicants for accommodation had to wait five to six weeks before being housed, by the spring of 1982 they had to wait between two to three months. Houselink concluded that "[v]irtually every dimension of the housing situation examined affirmed the need for increased supportive housing."[86] The report also recommended that the Ministry of Health become the lead ministry in coordinating support services for discharged patients in the community, that the Ministry of Community and Social Services increase allowance rates for discharged patients, and that Health establish a 24-hour mental health crisis team to respond to emergencies in boarding homes and hostels.

Another problem was the poor liaison between institutions and boarding homes. Hostel staff complained to the investigators that hospitals did not provide sufficient information about ex-patients, that "referring staff were frequently evasive about the person's current problems and that, in some cases, the person was referred before they [*sic*] were ready."[87]

In this case, however, the lack of liaison led to bad publicity for ex-patients. Articles began to appear suggesting that some ex-patients were a danger to the community.[88] In July 1981, *The Globe and Mail* ran a feature article on patients discharged from Queen Street who had a history of attempted arson. The article discussed one patient who had been referred by the institution to two separate boarding homes where, in the first case he threatened arson, and in the second actually incinerated the owner's automobile.[89] The difficulty was, the article pointed out, that Queen Street had no centralized discharge procedure. Moreover, an unnamed staff member at the institution claimed: "It becomes a fine line between quick treatment and dumping people and I think we've definitely crossed the line to dumping in the past year." Almost exactly a year later, *The Toronto Star* ran an article headed "Ex-mental patient neighbors scare us, residents say."[90] The article concerned neighbourhood opposition to an application for a rooming house in the Parkdale area, and it mentioned that the rooming house had already been visited on several occasions by the police and by ambulances. Two weeks later *The Toronto Star* reported on opposition to the establishment of a halfway house for ex-psychiatric patients in the High Park area of Toronto. Among those opposing the home was Liberal MPP Tony Ruprecht who had in the past criticized the government for not providing enough community care facilities for mentally ill people. In this case, Ruprecht claimed that he was not opposed to the principle of group homes but rather was contesting the disproportionate number of group homes that had been established in his High Park area.[91]

By the early 1980s, therefore, mental health policy had emerged as a major social policy issue. Growing numbers of ex-mental patients had been discharged from the large mental institutions and had congregated in specific areas of downtown Toronto. Their plight aroused residents who looked for help to local and provincial politicians. In 1981 *The Toronto Star* and *The Globe and Mail* ran an unusually large number of articles on mental health policy and in a series of editorials called on the government to look into the situation. Since the government was in the midst of an austerity program, the underfunding of the provincial institutions and the sheer lack of funds for community services exacerbated the situation and put further pressure on the government. In line with Progressive Conservative ideology, however, the government was reluctant to force compliance from municipalities on the group home program. For years the Ministry of Health had defined community care in terms of the psychiatric units in the general hospitals and the Homes for Special Care Program. It had now become glaringly apparent that neither the psychiatric units nor the homes for special care could in any way be described as providing community services for mentally ill people. The government was finally shown to have no coherent aftercare program at all.

Notes

1 See S. M. Rose, "Deciphering Deinstitutionalization: Complexities in Policy and Program Analysis," *Milbank Memorial Fund Quarterly/Health and Society* 57 (1979): 429–460; Gary J. Clarke, "In Defense of Deinstitutionalization," *Ibid.*, 461–479, and Alex Richman and Pamela Harris, "Mental Hospital Deinstitutionalization in Canada," *International Journal of Mental Health* 11 (1983): 64–83. This was a special issue devoted to deinstitutionalization.

2 Andrew Scull, *Decarceration (*Englewood Cliffs, N.J: Polity Press, 1973) 134.

3 Clarke 461–478.

4 Department of Health, Mental Health Division, *Annual Report*, 1971, p. 16. See also Department of Health, 41st *Annual Report,* "Patients in Residence in Ontario Hospitals and Ontario Hospital Schools (1937–1960), 1964."

5 K. M. McGregor, says that the decline began in 1958. See "Trends in Mental Hospitals," *Canadian Psychiatric Association Journal* 9 (1964): 331–335.

6 AO, RG 10, 10–20-A–5, November 4, 1971, Keith Kerns, Head, Mental Hospital Statistics Unit to H. W. Henderson, re: Annual Report for Psychiatric Units and Community Psychiatric Hospitals.

7 Interview, Dr. Henry Durost.

8 Douglas Bennett, "Deinstitutionalization in Two Cultures," *Milbank Memorial Fund Quarterly/ Health and Society* 57 (1979): 516–532.

9 Alexander Leighton refers to this as "communityism," that is, an overly optimistic notion of the community response to mentally ill people. Alexander Leighton, *Caring for Mentally Ill People* (Cambridge: Cambridge, University Press, 1982) 207.

10 Interview, Dr. S. Freeman.

11 Interview, Anonymous.

12 Interview, Dr. John Deadman.

13 *Debates*, June 6, 1975, p. 2687.

[14] AO, RG 10, Series 107, February 1, 1939, Dr. R. C. Montgomery, Director Hospitals Division to Dr. Sellars, quotes Dr. B. T. McGhie saying that the clinics attempt to "assist materially in the re-establishment of mental hospital patients and…[w]herever possible the clinics carry on this work indirectly, by means of consultation with the family physician."

[15] AO, RG 10, Series 107, November 7, 1949, J. E. Gamble, Director, the After Care Department, Ontario Hospital, London, "Bridging the Gap between the Hospital and the Community," 4 pages.

[16] See WHO Technical Report Series, No. 73, *The Community Mental Hospital*, Third Report of the Expert Committee on Mental Health, September, 1953, p. 22.

[17] AO, RG 10, Series 107, May 8, 1944, "Future Policy of Psychiatric Services in Ontario," p. 7. See also the Superintendents' Conference of April 25, 1945, where Dr. G. Stevenson suggested that aftercare provision be "much more comprehensive than in the past" and that "it might fairly well dovetail with the proposed County Health Units, each of which would consist of a fairly large staff, including psychologists, psychiatrists, etc."

[18] AO, RG 10, B. 55, HS 5–1, March 31, 1945, Superintendent, Ontario Hospital, London, to Director, Hospitals Division.

[19] The question of using public health workers in an aftercare program was raised at a meeting between representatives of public health and the mental health division in 1956. See "Minutes of a meeting held between representatives of the Public Health Administration, the Public Health Nursing Branch and the Division of Mental Health—October 5, 1956." AO, RG 10, B.115, Gen P–2–8–2.

[20] "Minutes of a Meeting…"

[21] AO, RG 10, HS S–6, October, 19, 1956, Minutes, Superintendents' Conference.

[22] AO, RG 10, B. 115, Gen. P–2–8–2, March 14, 1957, Dr. C. A. Cleland, Medical Superintendent, St. Thomas, to Dr. Marian I. Templin, Assistant Medical Officer of Health, Board of Health, Windsor.

[23] AO, RG 10, B. 115, Gen. P–2–8–2, June 1957, C. A. Cleland, M.D., Medical Superintendent, St. Thomas to Secretaries Medical Societies, Sarnia, Chatham and Windsor, "Sample Letter."

[24] AO, RG 10, B. 115, Gen. P–2–8–2, August 21, 1957, B. H. McNeel, Chief, Mental Health Division to Dr. C. A. Cleland, Superintendent, St. Thomas.

[25] AO, RG 10, B. 115, Gen. P–2–8–2, September 16, 1957, J. Taylor, Social Worker, to Miss Isabel Black, Assistant Director, Division of Public Health Nursing.

[26] AO, RG 10, B. 115, Gen. P–2–8–2, J. N. Senn, Superintendent, OH Hamilton, to Dr. B. H. McNeel, Chief, Mental Health Division.

[27] AO, RG 10, B. 115, P–2–8–2, October 30, 1957, Miss Isabel Black, Assistant Director, Division of Public Health Nursing, to B. H. McNeel.

[28] AO, RG 10, Series 5, January 1959, "Proposed Revision of Mental Health Program in Ontario."

[29] AO, RG 10, B. 165, HS S–6, March 6, 1959, Dr. B. H. McNeel at Superintendents' Conference.

[30] *Debates*, February 11, 1958, p. 289.

[31] C. A. Roberts "Report," p. CR–40–41.

[32] Dr. J. S. Pratten, *Canada's Mental Health*, January–February, 1964, cited in *Debates*, February 25, 1964.

[33] *Debates*, June 14, 1965, p. 4127.

[34] AO, RG 10, P–2–8–2, September 2, 1965, Leora Wright, Regional Consultant, Public Health Nursing Branch to Dr. Colin Smith, University of Saskatchewan.

[35] *Debates*, April 28, 1966, p. 2753.

[36] H. W. Henderson, "Community Mental Health—Administrative Implications," *Canadian Journal of Public Health* 57 (1966): 145–152.

[37] Henderson 151.

[38] Interview, Ray Berry.

[39] *Debates*, April 13, 1967, p. 2139.

[40] *Debates*, April 24, 1967, pp. 2548 ff.

[41] *Debates*, May 6, 1968, p. 2547.

[42] *Debates*, Committee on Social Development Policy, October 19, 1970, pp. S–1574–1576.

[43] *Debates*, Social Development Committee, October 19, 1970, S–1481.

[44] *Debates*, Committee on Social Development, June 6, 1972, p. S–957.

[45] *Debates*, Social Development Committee, June 6, 1972, p. S–957.

[46] *Debates*, April 22, 1974, p. 1207.

[47] *Debates*, December 19, 1974, p. 6761.

[48] *Debates*, December 19, 1974, p. 6761.

[49] *Debates*, December 19, 1974, p. 6732.

[50] *Debates*, June 6, 1975, p. 2689.

[51] *Debates*, October 18, 1979, p. 3610.

[52] AO, RG 10–108, B7, June 5, 1973, "Remarks of Mr. Lawrence Crawford, Director, Homes for the Aged—Office on Aging Branch, 6th Conference on Co-operation in the Provision of Health Services," MCSS.

[53] AO, RG 10, B7, June 18, 1973, Lawrence Crawford, Director, Homes for the Aged—Office on Aging Branch to Administrators and Home Physicians, Charitable and Municipal Homes for the Aged, Re: Admissions from Psychiatric Facilities.

[54] AO, RG 10, B. 108, B7, June 8, 1973, Dr. G. A. Ives, Director Psychiatric Hospitals Branch to Mr. G. J. Chatfield, General Manager, Direct Services Branch, Re: Statement by Mr. L. Crawford.

[55] AO, RG 10–108, B. 7, July 9, 1973, Dr. G. A. Ives, Director Psychiatric Hospitals Branch to Mr. G. J. Chatfield, General Manager, Direct Services Division.

[56] *Debates*, December 14, 1976, p. 5704.

[57] AO, RG 10, (12.4), March 14, 1975, Letter from W. Alan Backley, Assistant Deputy Minister, Health Services to Dr. Thomas Porter, General Secretary, Ontario Medical Association.

[58] *The Globe and Mail* 31 March 1981.

[59] Secretariat for Social Development, "Group Homes: Report of the Interministerial Working Group," June 16, 1978.

[60] *Debates*, October 18, 1979, p. 3610.

[61] *Debates*, October 18, 1979, p. 3615.

[62] *Debates*, October 18, 1979, p. 3618.

[63] *Debates*, October 18, 1979, p. 3613.

[64] Liberal MPP Tony Ruprecht criticized Provincial Secretary for Social Development, Margaret Birch: "In my view, this is a classic case of the need for coordination, if ever there was one: and of course coordination is your primary mandate and function, as you yourself have acknowledged." *Debates*, June 3, 1981.

[65] *The Globe and Mail* 29 July 1981.

[66] Former Assistant Deputy Minister Dr. Boyd Suttie says the series had a profound effect on people in the Ministry. Interview, Dr. Boyd Suttie.

[67] *The Globe and Mail* 13 March 1981. The study was conducted by John Trainor, a social worker at Queen Street, Ron Ballantyne from Community Resources Consultants and Dr. Henry Durost, medical director at the Queen Street Mental Health Centre.

[68] Some years later, the Metropolitan Toronto District Health Council found after interviews at psychiatric units that "planning mental health care often takes place in isolation. A recent illustration...may be seen in the failed attempt of teaching hospitals to set up a common bed registry. Apparently this failure was due to a lack of trust and to the long established custom of independent hospital operation. The problem of emergency care for patients in psychiatric crisis was often viewed in terms of a bed problem." *The Final Report of the Mayor's Action Task Force on Discharged Psychiatric Patients* (Toronto: City of Toronto, 1983) 83.

[69] In 1986, social workers John Trainor and Katherine Boydell found that, in Metro Toronto, income maintenance, housing and recreational services were biased against the chronically mentally ill. John Trainor and Katherine Boydell, "The Politics of Normalization," *Canada's Mental Health* 34 (1986): 19–23.

[70] Health Planning Policy Committee, "Health not Illness—A Green Paper for Health of Ontario," New Democratic Party of Ontario, p. 59.

[71] Community Resources Consultants of Toronto and Social and Community Psychiatry Section, Clarke Institute of Psychiatry, "Psychiatric Aftercare in Metropolitan Toronto," April 1981, 31 pages. Dr. Reva Gerstein noted in 1983 that: "Both police and Nellies [a women's shelter]...identify considerable difficulty in arranging admission to the psychiatric wards of general hospitals for those who (in their view) require medical attention." *The Final Report of the Mayor's Action Task Force* 83.

[72] "Psychiatric Aftercare in Metropolitan Toronto," p. 28.

[73] *Final Report of the Mayor's Action Task Force* 120.

[74] *Ibid.*, p. 30.

[75] *Debates*, Supply Committee, June 3, 1981, p. S–110.

[76] *Debates*, Supply Committee, June 3, 1981, p. S–110.

[77] *Debates*, Supply Committee, June 3, 1981, S–109. In addition to refusing to make additional expenditures in mental health programs, the Progressive Conservatives were also frantically looking for some way to cut mental retardation costs. A confidential Ministry of Community and Social Services submission to cabinet recommended the closure of six intermediate size mental retardation facilities and emphasis on independent living. According to the document one major advantage of the proposal was that it "[m]aximizes cost sharing...", while one major disadvantage was that it "[r]elies heavily on low cost option." Ministry of Community and Social Services, "Services for the Developmentally Handicapped: A Five Year Plan," June 30, 1982. Confidential document in possession of author.

[78] Richard Titmuss, *Social Policy* (London: George Allen & Unwin, 1979) 30.

[79] *Debates*, Supply, June 3, 1981, p. S–96. See also report in *The Globe and Mail* 13 March 1981.

[80] *The Globe and Mail* 13 March 1981.

[81] *Debates*, November 23, 1981, S–757.

[82] According to John Trainor, the Supportive Housing Coalition was part of a social movement which brought together four community groups working in the area of mental health aftercare. John Trainor, Steve Lurie, Ronald Ballantyne and Dennis Long, "The Supportive Housing Coalition: A Model for Advocacy and Program Development," *Canadian Journal of Community Mental Health* 6 (1987): 93–106.

[83] *The Globe and Mail* 1 December 1981.

[84] *Debates*, Supply, November 30, 1981, p. S–831.

[85] Joint Study for the City of Toronto, Department of Public Health and The Supportive Housing Coalition, *The Housing Gap: Deficiencies in Appropriate Housing for Ex-psychiatric Patients*, May 1982.

[86] *The Housing Gap* 27.

[87] *The Housing Gap* 19.

[88] The number of articles on mental health issues in *The Toronto Star* and *The Globe and Mail* jumped from 22 in 1979 and 28 in 1980 to 61 in 1981.

[89] *The Globe and Mail* 28 July 1981.

[90] *The Toronto Star* 8 July 1982.

[91] *The Toronto Star* 27 July 1982.

10

Policy Under Attack

> I'm not at all sure [as a result of Lakeshore closing] we're not going to see Queen Street become in 10 years a lot more similar to the way it was 10 years ago. We're going to be overcrowded...nosediving as a result of a rather short-range saving which in the long run could be disastrous.
>
> Dr. Donald Anderson in 1979, quoted in *Madness* by John Marshall

> During our visit to three hospitals (Queen Street Mental Health Centre, the Whitby and North Bay Psychiatric Hospitals) we reviewed the adequacy of the individual wards. All of the self-contained wards visited were overcrowded.
>
> (Annual Report of the Provincial Auditor, 1987)

Agenda for Action

During the latter part of his tenure as Minister of Health, Dennis Timbrell was under fire over mental health policy. Voluntary organizations, trade unions and government-sponsored bodies were all highly critical of Ontario's mental health policy while reports, analyses, hearings and newspaper articles issued forth from all sides.

This flurry of activity was due not only to the impact on the community of deinstitutionalization, but to three additional important factors. First, there was a lack of information about almost every aspect of the mental health system, from statistics on the provincial psychiatric hospital system and the psychiatric units to information on the fate of discharged patients. In the charged environment of the late 1970s, when mental health policy had emerged as a leading preoccupation of pressure groups, the press and the public, the government was being pressed to provide information which it did not have. Second, although it was clear that there was a critical shortage of community facilities for discharged patients, the government was reluctant to undermine its expenditure restraint program by increasing funds for community services. Moreover, the unsuccessful attempts by Minister of Health Frank Miller to close general hospitals in the middle 1970s, and the closing of the Lakeshore Psychiatric Hospital in 1979 had alerted trade unions and other organized groups to the danger of lost jobs in the event of hospital shutdowns. Resistance to hospital closings meant the province could not

Table 10.1
Mental Health Expenditures

Year	*as percentage of total MOH expenditures*	*as percentage of total government expenditures*
74/75	12.5%	3.6%
75/76	12.6%	3.6%
76/77	11.8%	3.5%
77/78	11.0%	3.1%
78/79	10.8%	3.0%
79/80	11.1%	3.0%
80/81	10.5%	3.1%
81/82	10.5%	3.1%
82/83	10.4%	3.1%
83/84	10.3%	3.1%
84/85	10.1%	3.2%
85/86	9.8%	3.1%
86/87	9.6%	2.9%

[Source: Figures for mental health expenditures based on *Regional Allocation of Estimated Expenditures on Mental Health Services by Ministry of Health*, Ministry of Health, Information and Resources Branch, various years. Regional Allocation figures include expenditures on all mental health related programs, including OHIP payments, grants to community mental health programs, alcohol and drug programs, psychiatric hospitals and psychiatric units in general hospitals, homes for special care, grants to local health agencies, grants to associations, and research expenditures. Figures for total MOH expenditures and provincial expenditures from various *Public Accounts*.]

fund community care from savings in the hospital sector. Third, government had embarked upon a course of radical change in mental health law. With the passage of the 1967 Mental Health Act, the rights of patients in provincial facilities had been extended and psychiatric authority narrowed. Amidst all this, at the end of the 1970s, the Committee on Mental Health Services published *Agenda for Action*, one of the most critical reports on provincial mental health policy since the Hanly report of 1970.

The Committee on Mental Health Services was established by the Ontario Council of Health, a body funded by the Ministry of Health. The Committee was chaired by a member of the philosophy department from the University of Toronto, and was composed of nine members drawn from the health care field and/or the university system.

Of the 22 recommendations in the study, only a few were directly critical of government policy, with most calling for improving or extending existing services or creating new services to fill gaps. Yet in many ways the report was a damning indictment of the state of Ontario's mental health system at the end of the 1970s. *Agenda for Action* noted:

> a major difficulty has been the lack of a commonly-accepted Provincial definition of mental health services... The Government's present division of mental health services cannot be regarded as other than contradefinitional, unless mental illness in children is the equivalent of "social services needs" and mental illness in adults is really "health." Without elaborating further, until there *is* [their italics] a definition of "psychiatric services" or "social services"...no planning is (or could have been possible).[1]

The report went on to deny government claims that the Ministry of Health had made mental health a priority. "This is not confirmed," the report reads, "as policy, formally or informally in our observation." Given the fact that the Ministry of Health had no "working definition" of mental health, it followed that there could have been no clear policy regarding mental health. "Clearly, lacking is a formulation of government policy and priority, publicly stated, regarding mental health and mental illness services relative to other provincial projects, plans and programs...without policy, planning is impossible." Moreover, to the extent that government priorities are indicated by expenditure statistics, the figures from the 1970s indicate that as the decade drew to a close, the Ministry of Health was spending less rather than more each year on mental health services.

Planning requires accurate information, but the Committee on Mental Health Services discovered serious lacunae in the information collection capacities of the Ministry of Health. For some time prior to 1975 the Ministry of Health had collected outpatient data from the provincial psychiatric hospitals, but it discontinued that practice in 1975. The Committee approved of

> the Ministry of Health attempt to enumerate adult out-patient resources. In our view, this attempt is long overdue: its lack, from the time of discontinuation of this information collection until the present is inexplicable in terms of planning, particularly at a time of deinstitutionalization when out-patient services were a critical factor.

Moreover, when the Committee attempted to obtain fiscal data it was "only after three months of constant refinement of Ministry data, with the direction of one of our Committee's Task Forces" that the data was obtained "*for the first time* [their italics]...in properly adjusted form." This was not a new problem for we have seen how in 1960, the mental health sub-committee on mental health care costs complained about its inability to obtain necessary statistical information about the mental hospitals. But the Committee broadened its critique to encompass the lack of any systematic overview of the mental health system. This should be provided, it argued, through public participation and the establishment by the Ministry of "a group of knowledgeable and concerned persons to be responsible for maintaining an overview of mental services in Ontario, initiating special studies as required, and assisting in the further development of the spectrum of mental health services."

The Committee also discovered a lamentable lack of coordination between different ministries, most notably between the Ministry of Health and the MCSS. It criticized the absence of any inter-ministerial groups and recommended their establishment, "particularly in terms of service-delivery planning." It also noted that in 1978 Health decided to "delegate planning and delivery" of health services (with the exception of children's services and services for mentally retarded people) to the district health councils. The DHCs were supposed to "identify local needs, evaluate alternative programs, establish priorities, prepare comprehensive plans for the district and facilitate coordination with it." In addition, the Ministry had decided in 1978 that there would be no "master blueprint for psychiatric services in the province nor a designated amount of tax money set aside for psychiatric services" and that community mental health policy would emerge from the various DHCs. But the DHCs found it extremely difficult to work in an area that required previous coordination between Health and Community and Social Services, and where there "appears to be an internal lack of coordination and a lack of coordination between Ministries." Moreover, the Committee noted that several DHCs claimed that Health "is insensitive to District Health Council requests, advice, and need for consultation."

With regard to the actual delivery of mental health services, the Committee focussed most of its attention on the provincial psychiatric hospitals, although it did discuss the psychiatric units and community mental health services. Here again it confirmed previous criticisms. During the middle 1970s, the New Democratic Party had been particularly vociferous in arguing that a two class system of mental health care had come about, with the psychiatric units catering mainly for the middle classes and the psychiatric hospitals left to deal with the lower classes. These views had been put quite forcefully by Dr. Jan Dukszta, New Democratic Party member from Parkdale from 1971 to 1980. Not only did Dukszta represent the area with the highest concentration of discharged patients, but he was by profession a psychiatrist. On May 26, 1972 he stated:

> If you look sociologically at the type of individual who is admitted to Queen Street Mental Health Centre, it invariably has been a lower-class individual on welfare, an indigent "socially or otherwise" which I think suggests that the psychiatric units in general hospitals, in spite of the enormous money poured into them by the department...have not been pulling their weight...when you look at the type of in-patient population of these psychiatric units...they are largely middle-class.[2]

However, when questioned by the leader of the New Democratic Party about whether any studies had been done on the "income background" of people seeking mental health care in the province, the Minister, Richard Potter replied that no such studies had been done.[3] Despite this, the Committee noted that "the perception suggests that we have operating in Ontario...a two class system which over-services the upper and middle classes...while under-servicing a large number of working class persons with severe or incapacitating problems by way of the provincial psychiatric hospital."[4]

The Committee on Mental Health Services also joined a long list of individuals and organizations which had, since 1963, recommended that the Department of Health divest itself of responsibility for the provincial psychiatric hospitals. In 1971, Minister of Health Thomas Wells stated that regional boards would operate the provincial psychiatric hospitals along the same lines as boards of governors in the public hospitals.[5] In 1974, Minister of Health F. R. Miller said in the legislature: "I think the whole future of the Ontario Hospitals as such is really under review in our ministry right now, whether in fact district units should operate under our ministry. I think if you check back to two years ago...it was stated that the ministry should get out of direct services such as the Ontario Hospitals, if, and when it could."[6] In 1974/75 the annual report of the Ministry of Health stated that the psychiatric hospitals branch "began to examine the possibility of placing some or all of the...psychiatric hospitals under local community boards."[7] The same intention was expressed in the 1975 annual report. However, in 1978, the Ministry of Health told the London Psychiatric Hospital advisory board that "no divestment of the board would occur in the foreseeable future."[8] Despite the unwillingness of the Ministry of Health to divest itself of responsibility for the provincial psychiatric hospitals, the Committee on Mental Health Services stated in 1979: "We believe that the 1964 promise, made with such frequency over such a time span, should be kept."[9]

The Committee then launched into a series of criticisms of the provincial hospital system noting inadequate attention to patient welfare, inability to attract and retain qualified staff, inadequate staff-patient ratios (although the Committee complained that data supplied by the Ministry in this area was "not helpful"), and vague information on the criteria or meaning of the accreditation standards applied to the hospitals. It concluded by recommending that the Ministry of Health "divest itself of direct operation of the Provincial Psychiatric Hospitals by appointing Management Boards representative of the community served (which initially may serve as Advisory Boards or through merger with an existing public hospital.)"[10]

In discussing community services, or what it called "rehabilitation and maintenance" the Committee noted that "little has been accomplished in terms of improving the availability and accessibility of these services." With regard to life skills programs, education, vocational rehabilitation and accommodation, leisure activities, family support and other activities and programs, the Committee found an extremely uneven distribution of inadequate services. Moreover, in commenting on the Homes for Special Care Program, often touted by the province as part of its community care program, the Committee noted: "We received a number of statements expressing concern about the quality of care provided mentally ill patients in the community... Some persons commented to us that home operators in particular cases have received no special training in residential or long term care, that supervision of these Homes is not as stringent as it should be... Others commented on the lack of organized programs of social, physical and recreational activities for residents."[11] The Committee noted that public health nurses already played an important role in providing community service to mentally ill people and suggested that "public health units and their nurses could well provide the basis for extended and organized community mental health services," particularly in underserviced or geographically isolated areas. And it formally recommended that the Ministry of Health "recognize mental health care as a priority function for public health nurses."

Clearly the Committee on Mental Health Services in Ontario was repeating the criticisms of previous committees, commissions, groups and individuals: the Ministry of Health had no clearcut mental health policy, planning was non-existent, information collection was sporadic and superficial, and coordination between ministries barely existed. In light of these conclusions the Committee recommended re-establishing a mental health division "under the executive leadership of a coordinator with sufficient authority to ensure inter-intra Ministerial coordination and to act as the recognized Ministry of Health Officer responsible in matters of mental health/mental illness for the Ministry."[12]

Ironically, just at the point when the Committee was on the verge of publishing its report, a dramatic illustration of all the accumulated criticisms of the mental health system was given when the Ministry of Health decided to close the Lakeshore Psychiatric Hospital.

Closing Lakeshore

The decision to close Lakeshore had been preceded by a series of hospital closings which had been undertaken with little or no consultation with the concerned parties and the community and which, for many people, demonstrated the insensitivity of the Ministry of Health to community concerns.

According to John Maynard, who was director of the psychiatric hospitals branch in the early 1970s, there was pressure to reduce the budgets of the hospitals. However, when the decision was taken in 1975 to close the Northeastern Regional Mental Health Centre in South Porcupine (it had only been open seven years), the government did not consult with the community or with the 223 full-time employees, but merely announced the decision over the local radio station.[13] However, Maynard admits he was "disturbed" when Northeastern was closed—but staff was difficult to find.[14] The patients previously housed in Northeastern were transferred to the North Bay Psychiatric Hospital, 220 miles away, while outpatient clinics associated with the hospital were terminated. Three years after the event, the Timmins Mental Health Association noted that the 110 beds lost through the closure had been replaced by 20 beds, a number that was insufficient to cope with demands. Many people had to travel to North Bay for treatment and subsequently found it difficult to return to their local communities. The average outpatient caseload for social workers was 160, and there was no accommodation for discharged patients except for one home for special care.[15] That year the Goderich Psychiatric Hospital was closed in the same climate of community outrage and government indifference. Mackinnon Phillips Hospital was transferred to Owen Sound "on the principle that the community should take care of its own." When questioned about the way in which the Goderich closing was handled, Health Minister Frank Miller admitted: "It is very difficult to deal with some of these things with the community in advance of the decision being made, and I admit there are better ways to do it than I did. I have learned a lot about doing it in this particular case."[16] Although Miller claimed to have learned his lesson, the government was in the process of closing down the Lakeshore Hospital in Toronto with almost the same lack of consultation or regard for the concerns of staff and patients that had been shown in the previous closings.

In 1977, senior officials in the Ministry of Health decided that facilities at Lakeshore and Whitby Psychiatric Hospitals were so bad that they should either be renovated or completely rebuilt. In view of the large costs involved, about $50 million, the Ministry decided to commission a private consulting firm, McKinsey and Company, to report on the three provincial psychiatric hospitals in the Toronto region. Together, these hospitals served more than one-third of Ontario's population and provided about one-fourth of its bed capacity. The McKinsey study provides a fascinating insight into the state of the provincial psychiatric system at a time when deinstitutionalization was well under way and when mental health policy had become a focus of controversy and concern. It also demonstrates some of the contradictions of the mental health system, for on the one hand it is a damning indictment of the living conditions at the Lakeshore and Whitby hospitals, while on the other hand it praises the provincial hospitals as among the best in the western world in active treatment. Unlike Hanly who, in his 1970 report on mental health services in Ontario, suggested that the provincial hospitals might "wither away," McKinsey came down firmly on the side of renovating, improving, but above all, maintaining the provincial hospitals.

According to McKinsey, living conditions in two of the three hospitals were extremely poor. Open wards housed up to twenty-five patients at a time, without any place for their possessions and shared toilet and bathing facilities. At Lakeshore there were "virtually no recreational facilities," while at Whitby, although such facilities existed, they were "relatively inaccessible in winter because most residential cottages are not connected with the recreational buildings."[17] Neither hospital had adequate facilities for psychotherapy, occupational therapy, day hospital or outpatient programs. "Clearly," McKinsey stated,

> the conditions at both Lakeshore and Whitby would be unacceptable for any of the general hospitals in greater Toronto and Ontario overall. The seriously mentally ill served by these two hospitals are given a much lower quality of physical accommodation than are Ontarians who are hospitalized for other sickness, or who are patients in the psychiatric units of general hospitals.[18]

Rebuilt in 1970, Queen Street was excepted from these criticisms.

McKinsey also confirmed suspicions that the provincial psychiatric hospitals and the psychiatric units in the general hospitals were catering for different psychiatric populations. The "vast majority" of patients under treatment for more than a year went to the provincial hospitals while the psychiatric units treated "almost exclusively short-term patients."[19] The provincial institutions also took most of the difficult short-term patients, "those who suffer from more intractable disorders, who are more difficult to handle physically, who are more likely to harm themselves or others, and who have relatively little support in the community."[20] McKinsey found in 1975 that 51 percent of those admitted to the three provincial hospitals were diagnosed as psychotic as compared to 40 percent of those admitted to psychiatric units in teaching hospitals, and 25 percent in the non-teaching hospitals. In 1974, 39 percent of patients treated in the provincial hospitals were women as compared to 56 percent in the psychiatric units. One dramatic illustration of the difference between the large institutions and the psychiatric units was the fact that 20 percent of all admissions to Queen Street were referred by the police as opposed to 2 percent in the case of the psychiatric units.[21] Instead of providing alternatives to the psychiatric hospitals, the psychiatric units were meeting new and different categories of psychiatric need.

These findings led McKinsey to ask whether the psychiatric population in the provincial hospitals might be better treated either in psychiatric units or in some other kind of treatment facility. The conclusion was that "no other form of care capability could substantially improve upon the services now provided by the PPH system."[22] According to McKinsey the provincial psychiatric hospital system provided a level of active treatment that was unmatched in "any western country, including Sweden and the Netherlands," both considered to provide the most advanced health care in the west. Exactly how McKinsey reached this conclusion is unclear, for their report provided evidence that some provincial programs were very poorly staffed. In a submission to McKinsey, the Volunteer Association of Whitby Psychiatric Hospital pointed out that a coordinator for the psychogeriatric program was only present two half-days a week.[23] However, McKinsey recommended preserving the large institutions mainly because it appeared the psychiatric units would not or could not provide the same services as the large hospitals. McKinsey argued that there had to be *"some"* [their italics] institutions in the Toronto area to deal with the long-term, difficult patients. Since the provincial hospitals were already in place, and had both the personnel and the physical facilities to care for long-term patients, then they should be retained. Moreover, McKinsey argued that it was "not practical" for the psychiatric units to deal with the same type of patient as the large provincial facilities mainly because they lacked the physical capacity (e.g., secure facilities), and because physicians were opposed to the idea. One of the major obstacles to getting the psychiatric units to care for difficult patients derived from the fact that psychiatrists in the psychiatric units were paid on a fee-for-service basis, and used beds in the units "extensively…to treat their private patients."[24] Because "the majority of psychiatric unit patients are women with non-psychotic disorders whose stay in hospital is relatively short," there was little incentive for the psychiatrists to treat the longer-term, more difficult, generally male patients who frequented the large provincial institutions. Finally, McKinsey noted the difficulty of assigning catchment areas to the psychiatric units since the general hospitals were legally free to determine their own programs, determine the areas they wished to serve, and even to send the more difficult psychiatric patients to different facilities if they wished.

Looked at in this fashion it is not surprising that McKinsey strongly recommended retention and upgrading of the existing provincial hospital system. After all, if the psychiatric units and the provincial hospitals were catering for essentially different populations, if the psychiatric units, the private psychiatrists who used them and the boards of governors of the general hospitals which housed them could be expected to resist accepting longer-term, more difficult patients, then,

> it is essential that some institution be unequivocally assigned and held accountable for the most difficult, least therapeutically rewarding of the mentally ill because they are the type of patient most likely to be unwanted by private physicians or by hospitals and therefore "lost in the system."[25]

In the executive summary presented to the Ministry of Health on March 14, 1978, McKinsey and Company listed three options: the first two were for a system of improved community services, expansion of outpatient services, and an expansion of psychiatric units providing a broader range of services. These would lead to the eventual replacement of Lakeshore and Whitby. The third alternative was to keep Lakeshore and Whitby open, but to upgrade them with an injection of operating and capital funds. McKinsey recommended the third alternative. The first two options were rejected mainly because of the peculiar characteristics of the patients at Lakeshore and Whitby. According to McKinsey, "PPH inpatients are too ill or dangerous to be treated in non-institutional settings;" on the basis of international comparisons there were already barely enough inpatient beds in Toronto to cope with the population, and the movement toward community care had "demonstrably gone far enough—perhaps too far—in greater Toronto."[26] McKinsey also pointed out that an expansion of the psychiatric units would merely provide additional services to a quite different population than the one which frequented the provincial hospitals. In addition, McKinsey argued that the psychiatric units were not suitable for treating the kinds of patients served by the provincial hospitals. Thus, the third option would "confirm the current patient service role of Lakeshore and Whitby, providing the operating funds necessary for them to carry out that role effectively."

After receiving the McKinsey study, the Minister of Health entered into discussions with his ministerial colleagues about the future shape of mental health services. Shortly afterward, the decision was taken to ignore McKinsey's recommendations on Lakeshore, to close the hospital and transfer the inpatients to Queen Street, Whitby and Hamilton, and to rebuild the Whitby Hospital. On January 22, 1979, Minister of Health Dennis Timbrell announced that Lakeshore would be closed as of September 1, 1979. Inevitably, the decision provoked an enormous controversy, leading to wrangling in the legislature and to an unusual amount of media coverage.

One of the government's major problems was its inability to produce any internal policy documents justifying the closure. According to the Minister of Health, the province did not have the funds to rebuild both the Lakeshore and Whitby provincial hospitals, and so the decision was taken to sacrifice one and rebuild the other. But even this explanation was in contradiction to the McKinsey study, for it had taken for granted that rebuilding was not an option. Rather, McKinsey had recommended maintaining the admittedly inadequate facilities at both institutions, but increasing operating expenses. Moreover, McKinsey had noted that with some reorganization, between 125 and 150 beds might be made available for additional inpatients at Queen Street. Yet, the Minister of Health planned to transfer approximately 230 patients from Lakeshore to Queen Street. As McKinsey had observed, however, to increase the bed capacity to this limit and beyond would require cutting down on existing programs at Queen Street.

The exact process by which the decision to close Lakeshore was reached is unclear. When Ross McLellan, the NDP health critic, accused the Minister of basing it on "chit-chat" the Minister replied, "chit-chat is hardly the right expression." But when McLellan asked for evidence that senior policy staff had recommended closure of Lakeshore, the Minister of Health replied: "Essentially very little was committed to writing. It consisted of direct discussion of an evaluation of McKinsey and then a determination to make a recommendation to cabinet."[27] When pressed on the matter of documents the Minister of Health could produce only the McKinsey report, an assessment by the fire marshal's office, and a report by the Ministry of Government Services on the physical state of Lakeshore. Both the Liberals and the New Democratic Party claimed that since the decision ran directly contrary to the McKinsey recommendations, and since no policy papers could be produced justifying the closure, it had been motivated purely by economic reasons.

Moreover, the opposition parties were particularly critical of the decision to transfer patients from Lakeshore to the Hamilton Psychiatric Hospital, some 40 miles east of Toronto, and to the Whitby institution, which was about 25 miles to the east. NDP MPP Dr. Jan Dukszta argued that before closure, the Queen Street Mental Health Centre and the Lakeshore facility each had a catchment area of about one million people, while after closure, Queen Street alone would be asked to provide services to about two million people.[28] Moreover, some people who came from the Toronto area and who were treated at the Lakeshore facility would, if they were inpatients, be transferred either to Hamilton to the west or Whitby to the east, or would have to depend on new services at the Queen Street hospital. According to Dukszta, with the withdrawal of the outpatient services at Lakeshore, many of the people they serviced would "sink without a trace, without treatment often, they become invisible…they simply go into the community and produce problems for the community and themselves."[29] However, the Minister replied that $1.3 million saved from the Lakeshore closing would be devoted to improving community services to meet the eventuality that Dukszta mentioned.[30] The debate over Lakeshore dragged on during the spring and early summer of 1979, but as the Ministry had promised, it closed in the fall.

The McKinsey study had gone to great lengths to formulate ten-year master programs from 1977 to 1987 for the three hospitals in the study. Each hospital set out both mission and role statements with specific goals attached to each. According to McKinsey: "[t]hese master programs provide a challenging future for each" of the three hospitals. These programs were published in December 1977. Just three and a half years later, in June 1981, the Ministry of Health engaged yet another consulting firm, Peat, Marwick and Partners, to look at the Queen Street Mental Health Centre. Apparently, not much had changed in the interim.

Problems at Queen Street

According to Peat, Marwick, the seriously ill and chronic patients continued to be treated mainly in the provincial hospitals rather than in the psychiatric units.[31] The relationship between the psychiatric units and the provincial hospitals, frequently unclear, sometimes even hostile, remained confused. Moreover, in a surprising statement—but perhaps consultants do not read each other's reports—Peat, Marwick wrote: "The role of the Ontario psychiatric hospitals, and particularly the Queen Street Mental Health Centre, in this mental health service system, has not previously been clearly defined."[32] One of the problems apparently was that Queen Street had indiscriminately applied Maxwell Jones's therapeutic community model to patients who were not suitable for such treatment. Moreover, despite the master plan developed by McKinsey and Company only two years before, Queen Street still had not decided whether it was to be a specialized care facility or whether it would provide "a total mental health care service" to all persons in its catchment area.[33] Peat, Marwick was critical of the level of care offered by Queen Street, observing that "[a]t the present time, the Centre is not looked upon as centre of excellence providing a wide range of specialized treatment and therapy programs for the mentally ill." In its master plan for Queen Street, McKinsey had listed a number of "required" activities including coordination of discharge planning between the Centre and the community, encouraging "the maximum possible level of teaching activity" within the hospital, and encouraging the involvement of "volunteers in patient care."[34] Yet, "[n]either the staff within the Centre nor the referring agencies have a clear understanding of the role of the Centre in terms of its service, education or research commitments."[35] Moreover, the relationship between Queen Street and the general and teaching hospitals, the Clarke and "other mental health agencies is not well understood." However, what is most interesting about the report is that it assigned responsibility for some problems directly to the centralized decision-making pattern of the Ministry of Health.

Whereas the McKinsey report had merely referred to the "currently fragmented responsibilities for the mental health system" within the Ministry of Health, Peat, Marwick noted that financial management decisions were separated from personnel decisions, thus creating coordination problems.[36] Since the provincial psychiatric hospitals operated under the general direction of the psychiatric hospitals branch, many issues had to be referred to Queen's Park thus delaying the process of decision making. This in turn led to changing and inconsistent policies within the institution. For example, during the McKinsey study the volunteer association of the Whitby institution complained that: "Policy tends to come down from the Ministry reflecting the particular priorities of whichever civil servants are in power at a given moment (and that changes constantly) and is received by the hospital staff through the administrator who by his emphasis or lack of it places another set of priorities on a policy." The result was that staff were uncertain about which programs would last and which would disappear, while in some cases programs were started and volunteers recruited only to find that priorities had changed, and that money and programs had disappeared. "We feel," the volunteer association concluded, "that if policy is set locally, more consistency of operation would be possible."[37] However, Peat, Marwick noted that "[b]oth internationally and in Canada" the state assumed responsibility for operating large institutions. In Sweden an attempt to decentralize responsibility for, and to divest the state of the hospitals had resulted in a "return to more direct accountability" where the government appointed the board of governors of the institutions. Thus, Peat, Marwick was an exception in not recommending divestment, for nearly every previous study, and every study that was to follow would recommend that the government divest itself of direct responsibility for the operation of provincial psychiatric institutions.[38]

Many of the suggestions and recommendations of the Committee on Mental Health Services and of the two consulting firms were ignored. The government did not divest itself of the psychiatric hospitals, it did not appoint a committee to review mental health services in Ontario, it did not "develop, on a priority basis, comprehensive community support systems for the maintenance and rehabilitation of mentally impaired persons," it did not decentralize its planning activities for mental health and other related services to bodies such as District Health Councils, Social Planning Councils, Children's Services Committees," nor did it "appoint a senior coordinator of mental health services with authority and responsibility for developing and maintaining inter- and intra-ministerial liaison so as to ensure coordination and cooperation in the planning, development and provision of mental health services."[39] On the other hand, the government did improve its information gathering and analysis capability, it reestablished the mental health division in 1982 and, ultimately, it established community advisory boards for all provincial psychiatric hospitals.

As if to confirm the consultant's criticisms of problems at Queen Street, the last years of Timbrell's tenure as Minister of Health, were marked by controversy and dramatic incidents. On June 23, 1980, Aldo Alviani, 19, died after being given massive and eventually fatal doses of tranquilizers. In August 1981, Patricia Ellerton, 37, died at Queen Street and on December 6, 1981, Norman Davis died after receiving large doses of a series of tranquilizing drugs including paraldehyde, a tranquilizing drug which had been used since the 1920s. All three deaths occurred on weekends when Queen Street was badly understaffed—on the weekend that Davis died there were just two psychiatrists on duty attending 500 patients.[40] Within one day of Davis's death *The Globe and Mail* published a letter that had been hand delivered to Timbrell on November 13, 1981. Signed by nine current and past members of the executive of the hospital's medical staff the letter painted a dismal picture of conditions at the Queen Street Mental Health Centre. "The increased caseload has led to a deterioration in the quality of care. The medical staff no longer feel able to maintain the standards set up in our bylaws and rules and regulations." Furthermore, Dr. Frances Frank, the president of the medical staff, said that Queen Street was "being run as a plant recycling emotionally disturbed people; staff as well as patients are being depersonalized because of lack of involvement in decision-making." The authors warned that conditions at the hospital had deteriorated "so rapidly and to such an extent as to endanger its patients."[41] Although Timbrell immediately replied that he didn't believe that the conditions at Queen Street were a threat to the patients or the staff,[42] behind the scenes he had already asked a senior civil servant to "do something about mental health."[43]

In July 1981, and in the fall of 1981, *The Toronto Star* called for "probes" of mental health care.[44] Although *The Globe and Mail* had not directly called for an investigation, during the summer and fall of 1981 it too was highly critical of provincial mental health policies. However, Timbrell resisted launching a full scale investigation. Then, in November 1981 the Ontario Public Service Employee's Union (OPSEU) decided to conduct its own inquiry into "the state of mental health care in Ontario."[45] The report was released on May 20, 1982, and it was later published in book form under the title of *Madness*. Although OPSEU had already published a critical report on the mental health care system in August 1980, the 1981 inquiry was more wide-ranging, holding hearings across the province and taking submissions from a variety of groups and individuals in the mental health field. The OPSEU hearings did not reveal any dramatically new information about mental health care, although it confirmed and tied together the disparate criticisms directed against the Ministry of Health during the previous few years. The OPSEU commission endorsed the principle of deinstitutionalization, although it stipulated that community support programs should be put into place before patients were released, and it added its voice to those who had been calling for a public inquiry into the mental health care system.

At about this time, in the fall of 1981, Minister of Health Timbrell said that "something had to be done about mental health."[46] At the end of December 1981, following internal and external consultations, Dr. Boyd Suttie, assistant deputy minister of community health services, produced an eighteen-point mental health plan which he presented to Timbrell in the early part of 1982.

The proposal included putting one ministry official in charge of the ministry's mental health activities, involving the district health councils in planning for the psychiatric hospitals, beginning discussions on establishing community advisory boards for the psychiatric hospitals, creating hospital ombudsmen, (this was to become the basis of the patient advocate program) and making some tentative plans about future bed needs and policies for the psychiatric units that would protect them from cuts under the general budgetary restraint program.[47]

Although Timbrell approved of the plan, he did not have time to implement it because on February 13, 1982, after having served as Minister of Health for five years, second only in tenure to Dr. Dymond's record of eleven years, he was replaced as Minister of Health by Larry Grossman. In turn, Grossman was to serve as Minister of Health for only seventeen months before being made Treasurer in July, 1983. The radical changes that were to ensue occurred only after Timbrell left office.

Notes

1 Committee on Mental Health Services in Ontario, *Agenda for Action* (Toronto: Ontario Council of Health, 1979) 136. The criticism was provoked by the fact that children's mental health services had been transferred to the Ministry of Community and Social Services, (MCSS), while services for the adult mentally ill remained with the Ministry of Health. According to Tom Campbell, deputy minister under Dennis Timbrell from 1979 to 1981, Dr. Abbyann Lynch, Chairperson of the Committee on Mental Health Services, expressed vociferous criticisms of government mental health policy.

2 *Debates*, May 23, 1972, p. 2713.

3 *Debates*, May 23, 1972, p. 2743.

4 *Agenda for Action* 41. According to an NDP Green Paper, "patients admitted to provincial psychiatric hospitals are 'lower' in education, class and employment, than those receiving psychiatric care in general hospitals." No citation is given from this information, but it probably came from Dr. Jan Dukszta who helped write the section on psychiatry. New Democratic Party of Ontario, "Health, Not Illness: A Green Paper for Health of Ontario," 1978, p. 59.

5 Quoted in *Agenda for Action* 192.

6 *Debates*, April 16, 1974, p. 1427.

7 Cited in *Agenda for Action* 197.

8 *Agenda for Action* 194.

9 *Agenda for Action* 195.

10 *Agenda for Action* 211.

11 *Agenda for Action* 60.

12 *Agenda for Action* 151.

13 *Agenda for Action* 220.

14 Interview, John Maynard.

[15] Ontario Public Service Employee's Union, *Ontario's Mental Health Care Breakdown* (Toronto: Ontario Public Service Employee's Union, 1980) 48–49, 52.

[16] *Debates*, January 15, 1976, p. 48.

[17] McKinsey and Company, *Role Study of Lakeshore, Queen Street and Whitby Psychiatric Hospitals*, January, 1978, three volumes. I-ii.

[18] McKinsey I-iv.

[19] McKinsey I–3–2.

[20] McKinsey I–3–3.

[21] McKinsey I–3–4.

[22] McKinsey I–4–1.

[23] McKinsey V, no page.

[24] McKinsey 4–9.

[25] McKinsey 4–6.

[26] McKinsey 1–3.

[27] *Debates*, April 23, 1979, S–143.

[28] *Debates*, April 23, 1979.

[29] *Debates*, April 23, 1979, S–137.

[30] A City of Toronto report on discharged patients states that only 10 percent of the funds were put into community services. *Final Report of the Mayor's Action Task Force on Discharged Psychiatric Patients*, 1983, p. 40.

[31] Peat, Marwick and Partners, *Queen Street Mental Health Centre, Report, An Organizational Review* (1982) 3.

[32] Peat, Marwick 4.

[33] Peat, Marwick 8.

[34] McKinsey I-Q.11.

[35] Peat, Marwick 11.

[36] McKinsey I–3–6.

[37] "Submission from the Volunteer Association of Whitby Psychiatric Hospital," McKinsey V, no page.

[38] Peat, Marwick 16.

[39] *Agenda for Action* xi, xviii.

[40] *The Globe and Mail* 3 April 1982.

[41] *The Globe and Mail* 17 December 1981.

[42] *The Toronto Star* 8 December 1981.

[43] Interview, Anonymous.

[44] *The Toronto Star* 26 July 1981; 28 October 1981; 29 November 1981.

[45] The members of the commission were Cliff Pilkey, president of the Ontario Federation of Labour, Dr. Jerry Cooper, chief of psychiatry at York-Finch General Hospital, Dr. Janusz Dukszta, a psychiatrist and ex-NDP MPP, Dr. Alan Long, a psychologist on the staff of York-Finch General Hospital, Dr. Cope Schwenger, professor of public health at the University of Toronto and Betty Jane Wylie, the journalist who had in the summer of 1981 written the dramatic series of articles on conditions in Parkdale boarding homes and the treatment of ex-psychiatric patients. The report was written by John Marshall, and published under the title, *Madness*, by the Ontario Public Service Employee's Union in 1982.

[46] Interview, Dr. Boyd Suttie.

[47] Interview, Dr. Boyd Suttie.

11

End of an Era

> The state of insanity and the conditions of the asylums, at all times of interest, have attracted a great deal of attention of the Board during the last year. In their opinion, there is no class of the community whose claims upon the consideration of a civilized people are so urgent, or so deserving of regard; and they ought to be felt as being all the stronger because the sufferers themselves, unconscious of their own wants, are unable even to state much less to enforce them.
>
> Report of Board of Inspectors of Asylums, Prisons, and Public Charities, 1863

Mental Health Policy Becomes a Priority

Immediately upon becoming Minister of Health in February 1982, Larry Grossman decided to give top priority to mental health policy because "there was a crying need in the field," particularly in the area of community care.[1] He got his personal advisers and the mental health bureaucrats together and asked them what should be done. As policies were proposed, someone suggested there weren't sufficient funds available, but Grossman recalls: "I told them that Cabinet and funds were my jobs, their job was to come up with policies." Although he felt that, unlike mental retardation policy, there was a small constituency for mental health policy both inside and outside of government, Grossman decided to ask the "front-line" people like Pat Capponi, an ex-patient associated with various self-help groups in the Parkdale area of Toronto what she thought about the situation. It was not only the activists' intimate knowledge of what was happening in the community that Grossman wanted to tap, but to show them that the Progressive Conservative Party could be responsive to their needs. For a long time, he argues, front-line groups working for mentally ill people seemed to feel that the New Democratic Party was their natural ally. Grossman wanted to wean them away from the NDP and show them that they could get direct access to the government without having to "go to the NDP and give them ammunition to launch hand grenades across the floor of the House against the government."[2] Thus, Grossman began to encourage the Ontario Mental Health Association and self-help groups to apply to the Ministry for funds for specific services, such as hiring additional staff for training programs. Dr. Boyd Suttie, assistant deputy minister of public and mental health at the time recalls that Grossman's plan was to strengthen external representative bodies even if the result was that, as Suttie put it, "sometimes they would savage the hand that fed them."[3] Whereas Dennis Timbrell's method of operation was, according to one civil servant, that of a typical pressure group politician who reacts only when pushed, Grossman decided to initiate policies rather than wait for a crisis to force his hand. This civil servant regards Grossman as unusual in the depth of his feeling for the plight of mentally ill people and contends that Grossman was one of those rare ministers who had a personal interest in solving mental health problems.[4] Steve Lurie of the Metro Branch of the Mental Health Association agrees that Grossman quickly became committed to activism in mental health and that, along with his close adviser Ted Ball, he took the initiative in a wide variety of program areas.[5]

Although one psychiatrist at the Clarke Institute said Grossman had the reputation of being a "firefighter, not a long-term planner," Grossman quickly made it clear that he was going to strike out in a different direction from his predecessor.[6] He asked his civil servants to expand aftercare facilities and programs even though the Ministry would have to use funds that were already committed to other areas in Health. In early May 1982, he announced that the Ministry of Health would be the lead ministry in mental health matters ("My ministry will accept the direct responsibility for mental health head-on,") and that he was setting aside $1 million for housing and community programs for discharged patients.[7] In the legislature, Grossman stated that the Ministry of Health had funded the Supportive Housing Coalition so it could hire an executive director to implement the establishment of between 250 and 260 beds for mentally ill people in Toronto.[8] By the winter of 1982, Grossman announced the establishment of a new $430,000 advice and referral program employing fourteen people to be operated by the Queen Street Mental Health Centre out of Archway, in Parkdale.[9] One ex-civil servant estimates that during his seventeen months as Minister of Health, Grossman doubled or even tripled the number aftercare programs.[10] As well, Grossman established a patient advocate program for each of the ten provincial psychiatric hospitals. Acting as a hospital ombudsman, the patient advocate's job was to provide a "'patient friend' who informs the patient of his or her rights, acts as a mediator with the hospital staff and serves to overcome irritants before they develop into major complaints."[11] After some months, Grossman was complimented by some of his Cabinet colleagues for his activities in mental health.[12]

Grossman succeeded where Timbrell had failed in finding sufficient money to radically expand the aftercare program by, as he puts it, "stealing from other budgets." Grossman states he transferred funds within Health from communications and from research and then used them for mental health purposes. He points out that the deputy ministers in most large ministries have some discretionary funds at their disposal, and he was able direct them toward mental health policy. But he admits he did not go to Management Board for authorization because it might have given him a hard time or simply forced him to waste time going through red tape in order to obtain formal approval. With regard to the patient advocate program, Grossman acted on his own initiative without going through the formal procedure of discussion with the other social development ministers or with the Policy and Priorities Board. Grossman claims that bringing his mental health policies to the social development field for discussion would have been a waste of time. Since the Social Development Committee did not make expenditure decisions but rather discussed policy, "with four strong Ministers as we had at the time, none of them would have made any concession to the other, so the main purpose is to keep everyone informed of what is happening." As for bringing the patient advocate program before Cabinet,

> they would have said it would just cause trouble, that the patient advocates would manufacture stories and that it would get into the paper and, anyway, they needed the money for something else. The Cabinet still doesn't know that it [the patient advocate program] exists... Government is so big now that people don't have enough time for details, they have a hard time knowing what is happening outside their own ministries.[13]

Although Grossman's tenure as Minister of Health was notable for its innovative programs, the Ministry was still under fire from outside critics. The problems were the same: the large institutions were underfunded, community care facilities were inadequate, most municipalities continued to discriminate against boarding homes, while in areas like Parkdale, where municipal zoning restrictions did not apply, residents were mobilizing to prevent any further expansion of housing for ex-psychiatric patients.[14] A City of Toronto study of discharged psychiatric patients found that there was little coordination between psychiatric units, that they did not provide sufficient emergency services, and that "the general hospitals' psychiatric departments have not assumed the responsibility for the chronic population envisioned in the deinstitutionalization program."[15] (The term "program" is used here in the loosest possible sense, since the Task Force itself mentions that deinstitutionalization took place without putting in place any community support mechanisms for discharged patients).[16]

The Heseltine Report

In the spring of 1981, while the mental health system was under attack from the opposition parties and the press, Minister of Health Dennis Timbrell was questioned about mental health policy by his Cabinet colleagues.[17] In order to defuse the criticism and to get an overall idea of future directions, on June 1, 1981, he appointed Dr. Gilbert Heseltine, Chairman of the Department of Psychiatry at the University of Western Ontario, as a special consultant on mental health to the Ministry of Health.

In December 1982, Heseltine presented an interim report, and in December 1983, the Ministry released Heseltine's *Towards a Blueprint for Change: A Mental Health Policy and Program Perspective.*

Despite decades of investigations, consultants' reports, and media criticism, Heseltine described a mental health system that was underfunded, unplanned, poorly coordinated, geographically uneven and heavily weighted toward the provincial hospitals and psychiatric units as opposed to community services. At the beginning of his investigation Heseltine accepted the government's stricture that no additional funds would be made available for mental health. In an interview in *The Globe and Mail* on February 2, 1982, Heseltine said: "The realistic situation is that there is only a limited number of dollars. The day of supermarket shopping with open-ended credit is gone, and we're going to have to start being a little more discriminatory in what we purchase." Ironically, between this interview and his first report Heseltine seemed to have realized that some desirable goals could not be achieved without the injection of more funds. On five separate occasions he referred to the need for more dollars: in discussing the treatment of severely disturbed patients in the psychiatric hospitals, the need for "transitional" funds to develop community services while maintaining the same level of institutional care, the necessity for injecting funds into the "pivotal" general hospitals which would assume a key role in the system, "the provision of funds for French-language courses for anglophone mental health specialists," and the "provision of adequate income support to the psychiatrically impaired."[18] Moreover, it is hard to see how many of Heseltine's other objectives, such as improving services in the north, improving data gathering and program evaluation services, or expanding public education programs could have been achieved without the infusion of additional funds.

This apparent contradiction caused some trouble in the legislature when the report was discussed in the standing committee on social development early in 1983. When Ross McLellan of the NDP asked the Minister of Health whether he thought "you are going to get the resources from your cabinet to do the kind of massive expansion of beds in general hospitals and in the pivotal hospitals that...would be required in order to make this system operative," Larry Grossman replied that Heseltine's recommendations could be met through "reorganization of our programs and reorganization of funds." But a few minutes later when McLellan asked whether additional funding would not be necessary for the "transitional period" during which community care facilities would be established and extra beds added, Grossman replied "there has to be a front-end investment. There can't first be a front-end saving which is then reinvested. I believe that we will succeed in getting the necessary funding to make that front-end investment."[19]

The main recommendation of the interim report was that there had to be a "shift of emphasis away from the large provincial hospital to a balanced mental health delivery system."[20] After all, Ontario put a "disproportionate amount of its mental health care money into hospitals" instead of into community care.[21] Among the specific recommendations was a proposal for a major reorientation in the roles of the provincial psychiatric hospitals and the psychiatric units in the general hospitals. Certain general hospitals would be designated "pivotal hospitals" and they would become the centrepiece of mental health services in a particular area, providing additional "intramural" services for designated categories of patients as well as being the centre for community care. The provincial psychiatric hospitals would be limited to providing secure facilities, respite beds, and beds for "some patients with low prevalence disorders," and long stay patients other than those with problems associated with aging. The provincial hospitals would also provide consultation services to the pivotal hospitals.[22]

In addition to the discussion of the specifics of mental health policy, the interim report was unusually critical of government. Heseltine referred to "inconsistent leadership, [and] fragmentation of responsibilities."[23] With regard to planning, or rather the lack thereof, Heseltine repeated the same complaints about poor or scanty data that had appeared in Agenda for Action in 1979.[24] Heseltine pointed out that mental health planning was based on what he called an "add-on philosophy" whereby "facilities, services or staff" were added to the existing network without any examination of whether they were effective or appropriate.

> A major problem has been that individual practitioners, professional groups, or community representatives have been able to promote successfully their particular interests. Without an overall "masterplan" the Ministry is vulnerable to such lobbying. As a result the needs of the mental health system as a whole have been sacrificed and particular components or locations have received disproportionate resources."[25]

Farther than this, Heseltine did not go, but it is worth drawing out the implications of his remark.

The assumption was that it would have been possible to elaborate a masterplan for mental health policy. At first glance, this looks highly unlikely. After all, except for the inception of mental health policy in 1836, when Dr. Charles Duncombe laid his report on lunacy policy before the House of Assembly of Upper Canada, it would be hard to point to any time when the government followed a masterplan. Even when government did try to plan—as in the 1830s and 1840s—events soon overtook the plan and rendered it useless. During its long history, almost every observer of mental health policy in Ontario has remarked on its essentially ad hoc nature.

Yet, it is not impossible to establish an overall plan. In the 1970s, after tremendous pressure was brought to bear on the government by the Ontario Association for the Mentally Retarded, the media and the opposition parties, Robert Welch, Provincial Secretary for Social Development, did produce "Community Living for the Mentally Retarded: A New Policy Focus," or as it became known, the Welch Green Paper.[26] The Green Paper lay the groundwork for what became a radical change and improvement in mental retardation policy. Thus, masterplans can be produced—but only rarely and under unusual circumstances. The reason for the lack of a masterplan in mental health policy was not, as Heseltine believed, because there were too many mental health pressure groups, but rather because no one group or coalition of groups emerged as sufficiently strong, militant and independent enough to force the government to plan. Of course, this begs the question of why mental health pressure groups were so weak when compared, for example, with mental retardation pressure groups, but the fact was that the government had been able to ignore the recommendations of every single report done on mental health policy since 1930.

Moreover, the problem was not that the Ministry was, as Heseltine put it, "vulnerable" to lobbying—if it was there would be a much larger aftercare network than currently exists, provincial hospitals and psychiatric units would be awash with funds, and complaints would be heard about an over-extended, over-funded and pampered mental health system. Rather, policy has been incoherent and ad hoc because the pressure group network is weak, and because there is no strong constituency for a coherent mental health policy in government. Under these circumstances, policy has resulted from a shifting coalition of bureaucratic and political forces within the Ministry of Health and in the government. Moreover, the task of bureaucrats and politicians is not made any easier by the fact that there is disagreement over what constitutes mental illness and over appropriate therapeutic modalities. For example, Heseltine referred to the "disharmony amongst...professional groups over who should do what and what are the best means for achieving 'mental health'."

The *Discussion Paper* released in December 1983 was a more detailed analysis of the mental health system than was contained in the interim report. Whereas in the interim report Heseltine referred to the "marked discontent...and general dissatisfaction with the inadequacies and inequities in the delivery of mental health services," the discussion paper was much less critical of government policy, although Heseltine continued to highlight specific deficiencies in the system.[27] The reason for the difference between the two reports is that, after the interim report appeared in late 1982, there was a sharp reaction from the psychiatric units and the provincial hospitals against the concept of the pivotal hospital and the proposed role changes it implied. Individual psychiatric units did not want to play second-fiddle to the pivotal general hospital, nor did the psychiatric hospitals want to be reduced to chronic care facilities. The final report, therefore, dropped the concept of the pivotal hospital system.

Once again, the same themes reappeared: the lack of planning and coordination, the backward state of aftercare services, the lack of a clearly defined role for the provincial hospitals and deficiencies in manpower, distribution of resources, statistics and research. In 1979, *Agenda for Action* had identified five areas which "required action on a priority basis: coordination and decentralization, statistics and information, management of psychiatric hospitals, French-language services and services for northern Ontario."[28] With only minor modifications and additions, these were exactly the same areas to which Heseltine called attention.

With regard to aftercare, Heseltine noted that in 1979, *Agenda for Action* called the aftercare services "totally inadequate."[29] Yet, despite improvements, Heseltine stated that they were still "far from adequate, particularly for specific target populations such as young assaultive schizophrenics and psychogeriatrics." The major problems remained inadequate income maintenance and lack of accommodation for ex-psychiatric patients. Of course, low income or maintenance payments and lack of access to appropriate housing go together, but even in the case where government provided housing, as in the Homes for Special Care Program which, in 1983 housed approximately 4,300 ex-psychiatric patients, serious problems remained. According to Heseltine, these ranged from "resident selection, through policy, planning and evaluation... Policies and procedures are out of date, there is no defined consistency between the HSC Program policy and practices and the MOH's thrust in mental health services."[30] With regard to the provincial psychiatric hospitals and the psychiatric units, Heseltine still found "vestiges of a two-tier psychiatric service in which the poor and less advantaged tend to use the PPHs, while the more affluent and more socially adept tend to use the GHPUs [General Hospital Psychiatric Units]..."[31] There were serious variations amongst the provincial hospitals with regard to treatment levels, with three hospitals doing "very little group or individual therapy" and only minimal programs in areas such as discharge planning, or placement." The provincial hospitals had also suffered from the expenditure restraint program as the percentage increase in grants was lower than the rate of inflation from 1978/79 to 1981/82. Heseltine agreed that "[t]here might be some justification for the frequently-heard complaint from the PPHs that they are being 'starved'."[32] Yet, Heseltine was "reluctant" to recommend more funding since, he argued, better planning and a better use of resources in the hospital's catchment area were necessary. Problems with hiring sufficient numbers of qualified psychiatrists was an apparently insoluble problem given the income differential between private and public psychiatry. This problem was also compounded by the extreme difficulty in recruiting qualified psychiatrists to work at provincial institutions remote from urban areas and unattached to a university health sciences centre.

There were also problems with the psychiatric units: many lacked the emergency and outpatient services required under their mandate, and there was so much conflict over the disposition of resources within the hospital that, in October 1982, the Minister of Health found that "some general hospital boards were not passing on to their psychiatric units their full share of the hospitals' global budget increases."[33]

Finally, Heseltine was very critical of the state of children's mental health services. Children's mental health services had a strange history of bouncing back and forth between the Ministries of Health and of Community and Social Services—with no consensus as to which Ministry should house them, or even whether they should even be within a Ministry rather than functioning as an autonomous service outside the ministerial structure.

Children's Mental Health Services

Prior to 1967, there was a paucity of services for children with emotional disorders in Ontario. Except for the Thistletown Hospital in Toronto, the Sunnyside Children's Centre in Kingston, and the Browndale homes established in 1954, there were few specific treatment facilities for children with emotional disorders.[34] As a result many children wound up in the adult wards of the provincial mental hospitals or in mental retardation facilities.[35] After Dr. Dymond's 1967 White Paper, the Department of Health quickly moved to improve the state of children's mental health services. In 1968 there were 12 residential treatment centres, two children's mental hospitals and six units in provincial mental hospitals for emotionally disturbed children.[36] In 1969, the Department of Health established a children services branch within the mental health division, then headed by Dr. H. W. Henderson. When the task force on psychiatric and retardation services was established at the beginning of 1972, a subcommittee on children's and adolescent services was appointed, headed by Dr. Naomi Rae-Grant, director of the children's services branch of the mental health division. Although, the previous year the Children's Mental Health Centres Act had been passed giving to the Department of Health responsibility for services for emotionally disturbed children, thereby ensuring that such services could be provided free of charge, the subcommittee agreed that "the current system for delivery of service needs to be amended or completely overhauled."[37] Four years later, Dr. Rae-Grant wrote that "it is certainly fair to view our present uncoordinated fragmented mosaic of services on behalf of children a 'mess'...our present system...is inadequate, and where it exists, is fragmented, lacks cohesiveness and is not consistent."[38] One of the major problems was that the children's mental health centres were being used not only to provide treatment but also as a "placement bureau" for residential services. At the same time, the medical model of care for mentally retarded and mentally ill people was being subjected to severe criticism. Thus, as the normalization concept took hold, the locus of treatment was shifting from hospital to residential settings.[39] As a result of these criticisms, in 1977, responsibility for children's mental health centres was shifted from the Ministry of Health to the children's services division of the Ministry of Community and Social Services. Despite the reforms and administrative shifts, however, Heseltine claimed that "[m]ental health services for children and adolescents is one area which continues to experience discontinuity due to a lack of clarity between the two ministries, Community and Social Services and Health... In addition there is a difference in philosophy over the role of treatment in service delivery."[40] Heseltine then suggested four possible administrative changes. These included again shifting children's mental health centres back to Health, shifting only some centres to Health, an arrangement whereby the Ministry of Community and Social Services would purchase psychiatric services from Health, and finally, his own preferred option, establishing children's mental health centres as "autonomous community agencies with their own boards" funded jointly by Health and Community and Social Services. It is interesting to note the parallels with suggestions that Health divest itself of responsibility for the operation of the provincial psychiatric hospitals which could be transferred to community boards.

Proposals for Reform

In 1979, *Agenda for Action* had commented on the poor planning of mental health services, and set forth a scheme for correcting the problem. In 1983, Heseltine repeated the essentials of this scheme—mental health services should be delivered by appropriate bodies at the provincial, regional, district, local and individual levels. These services would be planned and coordinated through a series of administrative bodies from individual case managers at the individual level, through district health councils, regional area committees and the various divisions within the Ministry of Health. However regional area committees would have to be created because none yet existed. It should be emphasized that the idea of creating regional administrative bodies was not new—B. T. McGhie had made a similar proposal as far back as 1944. And, on December 15, 1971, Dr. E. W. R. Best, the director of the local health services branch of the Department of Health, had proposed the establishment of regional management committees of the Department composed of officials from hospital, medical, mental health, public health services, and health insurance services.[41] A year later, a subcommittee of the task force on psychiatric and retardation services put forward a comprehensive proposal for social development councils, including health and mental health services organized on a district, regional and provincial basis. However, any scheme for reorganization of administrative structures could not function efficiently unless the problem of divided responsibility for the provincial institutions and the psychiatric units within the Minister of Health was solved. As Heseltine pointed out, expenditures for the psychiatric units came through the institutional division which had responsibility for public and private general hospitals. There was no direct control over the psychiatric units by the mental health bureaucracy. Thus, two major components to this scheme had to be put into place if it were to work: regional area committees had to be established and linked to the individual, district and Ministry levels, and some solution had to be found to the problem of ensuring that the psychiatric units were responsible to and integrated in the Ministry's mental health bureaucracy. Since regional committees were not established and the budget for the psychiatric units continued to come through the general hospital budget, Heseltine's ideas on improving planning and coordination were never tested.

A second area in which Heseltine proposed important structural changes concerned the psychiatric hospitals. Following suggestions and recommendations that went back to the 1960s, he proposed that the Ministry of Health "should divest itself of the provincial psychiatric hospitals."[42] Heseltine admitted that central government control ensured the provision of basic, minimum psychiatric hospital services throughout the province, but there were "considerable grounds for dissatisfaction with their performance to date." Moreover, "some reasons for this dissatisfaction" derived from the fact that the Ministry exercised central control over the hospitals.[43] Heseltine set forth detailed criteria which hospitals would have to meet in order to qualify for divestment, including the development of clear objectives for the individual hospital, improvement in training programs of hospital personnel, attracting more qualified psychiatrists by allowing psychiatrists to bill on a sessional basis like private psychiatrists rather than paying them salaries, and, finally, giving the community advisory boards an increased role in influencing government policy toward the hospitals.

Heseltine was appointed under Minister of Health Dennis Timbrell, produced his first report under a second, Larry Grossman, and published his final report under a third, Keith Norton. After Grossman was appointed Treasurer, Norton took over Health on July 6, 1983, and served until February 1985, with time out for illness for two months in the fall of 1983. Allan Pope then served as Minister of Health from February 1985 until the government dissolved the legislature in May 1985. Given the rapid turnover in ministerial portfolios, it is unlikely the government could have implemented Heseltine's administrative proposals—assuming it wished to do so. In any case, the government did not divest itself of the psychiatric hospitals, the pivotal hospital concept was abandoned by Heseltine himself between the interim and final reports, and regional mental health committees were not established. *Blueprint for Change* joined *Agenda for Action, Mental Health in Ontario*, the Roberts report and countless others, forgotten and ignored on the shelves of the Ministry library.

Finally, in the summer of 1985, the Progressive Conservative Party lost its majority in the legislature and, after forty-two years of Progressive Conservative government a member of the Liberal Party took over as Minister of Health in 1985.

Notes

1 Interview, Larry Grossman.

2 Interview, Larry Grossman.

3 Interview, Dr. Boyd Suttie.

4 Interview, Anonymous.

5 Interview, Steve Lurie.

6 Dr. Donald Wasylenki, later to become clinical director and chief of psychiatry at the Whitby Psychiatric Hospital, in *The Toronto Star* 14 July 1982.

7 *The Globe and Mail* 21 May 1982.

8 *Debates*, May 20, 1982, p. 1877.

9 *Debates*, December 17, 1982, p. 6293.

10 Interview, Anonymous. In his *Blueprint* Heseltine remarks on the "substantial growth" in the number of community support programs from 1982/83 to 1983/84. Dr. Gilbert Heseltine, *Towards a Blueprint for Change: Mental Health Policy and Program Perspective* (Toronto: Ministry of Health, December 1983) 124.

[11] *Debates*, December 17, 1982, p. 6295.

[12] Interview, Anonymous.

[13] Interview, Larry Grossman.

[14] *The Toronto Star* recalled that in June 1981, the outgoing president of the Ontario Medical Association said that the provincial psychiatric hospitals were "grossly underfunded and undermanned." *The Toronto Star* 26 October 1982.

[15] *The Final Report of the Mayor's Action Task Force on Discharged Psychiatric Patients* 97.

[16] *Task Force* 40.

[17] Interview, Anonymous.

[18] Gilbert Heseltine, *Blueprint for Change: The Next Ten Years, Interim Report*, (Toronto: Ministry of Health, 1982) II–26, V–4, VII–1, VIII–7, VIII–20, IX–12 and X–29.

[19] *Debates*, Standing Committee on Social Development, January 25, 1983, S–787–789.

[20] *Interim Report* I–1.

[21] *Interim Report* II–28.

[22] *Interim Report* VIII–13.

[23] *Interim Report* I–1.

[24] *Interim Report* II–1.

[25] *Interim Report* III–11.

[26] Simmons 203 ff.

[27] *Interim Report* III–1.

[28] *Agenda for Action* 257.

[29] *Blueprint for Change* 124.

[30] *Blueprint for Change* 132.

[31] *Blueprint for Change* 84.

[32] *Blueprint for Change* 88.

[33] *Blueprint for Change* 100.

[34] Ontario, Ministry of Community and Social Services, "Three Decades of Change," November, 1983, pp. 54 ff.

[35] See Bryan McConville, "Present State," in Jalal Shamsie, *Experience and Experiment* (Toronto: Crainford, 1977) 129.

[36] "Three Decades of Change," p. 56.

[37] AO, RG 10–108, B. 3, January 25, 1972, Ministry of Health, Sub-Committee on Children's and Adolescent's Services.

[38] Dr. Naomi Rae-Grant, "Roadblocks and Stopgaps," *Canadian Psychiatric Association Journal* 21 (1976): 434.

[39] In 1976, the Ontario Association of Children's Mental Health Centres "adopted the principle of 'normalization,'as the basis for its standards." Shamsie 60.

[40] *Blueprint for Change* 226.

[41] AO, RG 10–108, B.12, December 15, 1971, Dr. E. W. R. Best, Director, Local Health Services Branch to Dr. G. K. Martin, Executive Director, Public Health Division.

[42] *Blueprint for Change* 246.

[43] Problems in organizational responsibility were cited by Heseltine to illustrate the difficulties inherent in central government control. "The PPHs are owned and operated directly by MOH, and this too has created some difficulties. There are diverse reporting relationships between the PPHs and the provincial government." *Blueprint for Change* 89.

12

Lobotomy and the Decline of Psychiatric Authority

> Lobotomies? They promised great things. They were doing them by the dozens. They just drilled a burr hole, and inserted a special type of curette, but you couldn't see what you were cutting. At Whitby their criteria were fairly relaxed, so instead of confining themselves to obsessive compulsives they were doing a lot of schizophrenics and everybody else. McKenzie didn't put the bone chips back in and depressions were noticeable. We had a lot of people at Whitby who looked like they had their horns plucked out. He was doing so many that he was going to run into all the possible problems you can run into. We had a few people die on the operating table.
>
> Former psychiatrist at Whitby psychiatric hospital

The Inception of Lobotomy

The 1970s ushered in a period of radical change in psychiatry and mental health policy. Changing ideas on the nature and meaning of insanity, the social consequences of deinstitutionalization, changes in mental health law and unprecedented criticism of government all left their mark on mental health policy. Equally important, the profession of psychiatry was now subjected to a concerted attack from antipsychiatrists such as R. D. Laing, Thomas Szasz and Erving Goffman, and from a public which had grown increasingly suspicious of and skeptical about psychiatric authority. This wave of negative sentiment did not come out of the blue—it had been building for years. After all, what explains the fact that a profession which, until the 1960s, could excise portions of an individual's brain, send a patient into a dangerous coma, repeatedly pass electricity through his or her brain, or commit an individual to a public institution for years without benefit of counsel or a hearing, was, by the 1980s, viewed with suspicion and even hostility by large numbers of people?

We have already seen how psychiatrists skirted the edges of legality and exploited their positions to the full in the administration of the radical therapies of the 1930s. However, among these therapies there was one above all which eventually caught the public's imagination and, in the end, contributed in a major way to the undermining of psychiatric authority. That procedure was lobotomy.

"Lobotomy" or "psychosurgery" has been defined as a procedure which "removes, destroys or interrupts the continuity of histologically normal brain tissue…for the purpose of altering behaviour or treating psychiatric illness."[1] The terms do not refer to such procedures when used to treat organic brain conditions, intractable physical pain, or epilepsy. Although the terms lobotomy and leucotomy are slightly different in meaning they are often used interchangeably.

Dr. Walter Freeman popularized the use of lobotomy in the United States, brushing aside the objections of those psychiatrists who argued that such a serious and irreversible procedure should be given rarely and then only if surrounded with the strongest safeguards.[2] Although Freeman's impact on the history of lobotomy was immense, (as was the disillusionment that set in afterward), the practice became widespread—and widely abused—only because mental hospitals adopted it.

From the mid–1940s to the 1960s, lobotomy operations were performed on tens of thousands of mental patients in Canada, Great Britain, and the United States. By the mid–1950s the rate at which the operation was performed began to decline. By the late 1970s it had almost disappeared in Canada and was only rarely performed in the United States. It is still performed in Great Britain.[3]

After visiting Walter Freeman and his colleague James Watt in Washington, D.C. in 1939, and viewing some of their cases, Dr. K. McKenzie, a Toronto neurosurgeon, and Dr. Lorne Procter commenced a series of 27 psychosurgical operations in 1941.[4] There was a four-year hiatus after 1944, but Dr. McKenzie resumed the operations in 1948. The reason for the pause is unclear. It may have been due to a desire to assess the results of the operation, or because McKenzie requested that nurses be assigned to a special rehabilitative ward for patients, a request that the Department of Health found impossible to meet.[5] From 1948 to 1952, 150 patients were given lobotomies at the Toronto General Hospital. Of these, 109 were women and 38 were men, the sex of the remaining three was not given. The only study of sex bias in psychosurgical operations has been conducted by Valenstein who analyzed articles on psychosurgery published in the United States between 1971 and 1976. He found that 56 percent of psychosurgical patients during that period were women and he suggests that women were overrepresented because they comprised a disproportionately large fraction of those suffering from manic-depression, a condition thought to benefit from psychosurgery.[6] However, some critics have pointed out that applying the manic-depressive label to women conceals the tendency of many psychiatrists to stereotype and denigrate women who refuse to conform to male-imposed role definitions.[7]

After 1948, McKenzie seems to have done the operation *in situ* at the Whitby and Hamilton institutions. Between 1944 and 1967, approximately 1,000 lobotomies were done at the various provincial mental hospitals.[8] An unknown number of operations were performed in general hospitals on patients admitted from the community and at the federally run Westminster Veteran's Hospital in London, Ontario. The vast majority of operations were performed by McKenzie. Beginning in 1944, L. S. Penrose began to do statistical analyses of the lobotomy operations. Occasional studies followed including one ten-year follow-up study published in 1967.[9]

The theoretical basis behind lobotomy operations was rarely discussed in the internal communications of the Department of Health; rather, the superintendents and the mental health bureaucracy were mainly concerned with establishing criteria for selecting candidates for lobotomy and with assessing the effectiveness of the operation. However, the press endeavoured to explain in layman's terms how the operation worked. On September 4, 1947, both the Toronto *Globe* and the Toronto *Telegram* quoted a local psychiatrist who explained that the brain's frontal lobes contained the "conscience of the person under treatment." According to these newspapers, the operation "deadened the conscience." However, the reporter for *The Toronto Star* wrote that "the 'conscience' is not deadened but the emotional reaction to the irritant [that produced the disease] is removed." Eleven months later, on August 20, 1948, the three major Toronto newspapers reported that the operation helped to "relieve tension and enable the person to co-operate with other persons." All the clippings in the mental health file of the public archives of Ontario give a favourable view of lobotomy. This accords with Valenstein's view that "nothing played a larger role in stimulating interest in lobotomy than the many popular articles that appeared in newspapers and magazines."[10]

From the mid–1940s to the late 1960s decisions about lobotomies, about who was to have them, how they were to be done, whether or not there were to be statistical studies of the patients, and whether the policy was to continue were made by a narrow circle of medical doctors and bureaucrats. The possibility of the relatives or dependents of the patients, of the media, the public or of politicians having any influence on policy was hardly contemplated. However, whenever there was any threat of outside influence impinging on policy, the wagons were drawn round in a circle and the attackers fended off. For example, in late 1946, the press began to publish exaggerated claims about the success of lobotomies. The Toronto *Globe* published an Associated Press dispatch from Detroit headlined: "Brain surgery may save woman from life of crime." According to the AP:

> A delicate brain operation which may transform a cigar smoking morally degenerate 28-year-old woman into a useful member of society was revealed today by staff doctors at Wayne County General Hospital...Following the operation about a month ago, the woman said her "outlook on life" had changed. Dr. Lipschutz said psychological tests prove that the woman, hitherto a confirmed liar, is now telling the truth.[11]

Articles like this, and those reporting that there was "hope for 50 percent recovery in lobotomy operations," led to enormous public pressure on the authorities and the superintendents to increase the number of operations being performed. By May 1948, the superintendent of the Ontario Hospital in New Toronto was writing to the director of the hospitals division of the provincial government: "I am getting letters from relatives regarding leucotomy operations.

The relatives are aware of the fact that this is being done over in the United States and also by the Military Hospital in Ontario and there has been considerable publicity about it. They are rather critical of the fact that no provision is made for it in Ontario Hospitals."[12] A subsequent letter from another superintendent referred to "insistent demands for drastic treatment." In August 1948, the director of the hospitals division sent a circular letter to all the superintendents warning them that: "Unless the tendency to an indiscriminate application for supposed benefit is resisted both the project and method are likely to fall into disrepute... Without the full application of medical authority at this stage judicious selection will be impeded; the idea of maximum benefit in a special treatment will be lost in expedient practice."[13] What the director of the hospitals division is saying here is clear. The superintendents must make it clear to the public that it is they, on the basis of their medical expertise, who choose the candidates for lobotomy, not the public. The alternative would be to diminish the authority of the superintendents. However, while the superintendents and the provincial authorities were resisting public pressure to increase the number of operations, and expressing concern about the possible deleterious consequences of doing them on a wholesale basis, it is apparent that the actual criteria for selecting patients for the operation were very ambiguous indeed.

The Criteria for Lobotomy

A directive to the superintendents from the director of the hospitals division on August 19, 1948 stated:

> Operative priority should be given to those cases who may be expected to return to a satisfactory home environment following the operation. Priority consideration should be given also to those patients presenting long-term hospital behaviour difficulties who, following operation [sic], may be expected to be more receptive to other forms of therapy.

This second objective is ambiguous because the purpose of the further therapy is not made explicit. If these patients were expected to leave the hospital after therapy, would they not have fallen under the first group? Apparently, some patients were to get lobotomies not because there was any expectation that they could leave the hospital, but rather because they would be easier for the staff to control. In other words, lobotomy was used as a means for calming or controlling disruptive patients. At one provincial hospital this was stated quite explicitly: "The leucotomy program at this hospital has till recently been aimed at alleviating the ward management problem with chronic disturbed patients. Hence the great majority of our operated series is comprised of such cases."[14] The superintendent of the Hamilton hospital made the same point in 1958:

> Our first thought was to give lobotomies to the chronically assaultive, destructive and soiling group of patients that more or less regularly had to be secluded. Our thought was that we probably might not be able to get too many of these patients out of hospital, but we would create an easier nursing situation in the hospital.[15]

In addition to easing the management problems for ward staff, research objectives played a role in the policy. Dr. Senn of the Hamilton hospital stated in 1958 that: "[W]e...did a group of deteriorated patients, more or less in a research project, but the results were just about what we expected and generally not too favourable."[16] Finally, patients were chosen for lobotomies simply because more appropriate candidates were not available. At the federally run Westminster Veteran's Hospital in London, Ontario, Dr. H. B. Carscallen noted, in 1948:

> [T]he formal clinical diagnosis has not played a major role, as far as the choosing of the candidates for lobotomy is concerned. Under this form of therapy it is realized that the predominantly affective states, such as manic depressive psychosis and involuntary melancholia, afford better prospects for recovery than certain other psychotic conditions. It so happens, that the incidence of the purely affective disorders at present resident in Westminster Hospital is extremely low... This does not depress us in the least, though it may suggest a less favourable group prognosis with lobotomy. We are therefore left, to all intents and purposes, with a schizophrenic group of a very chronic or malignant type. We have been fully cognizant of the gravity of the illnesses we have been treating. We have also realized that we would be unwise to set our sights too high as far as the ultimate statistics are concerned. Nevertheless it was the feeling of the medical staff that any patient from this group who showed at least some potentialities for improvement, warranted the benefits of the operation.[17]

Thus, the criteria regarding who should or should not be selected for a lobotomy were very broad indeed, and in the end, the main criterion seemed to have been that the candidate was a chronic patient who had been unresponsive to previous methods of treatment. There were, however, some restrictions. In his 1948 memorandum, the director of hospitals had stated that: "As a general rule, patients of the following diagnostic groups should not be considered for the operation: (a) psychopaths, (b) alcoholic and drug addicts, (c) homosexual and other sexual deviates and (d) psychosis with organic cerebral pathology."[18] Of course, there is no way of knowing how closely these guidelines were followed, and given the possibility that some individuals might have presented other symptoms in addition to those listed above, some of those on the exclusionary list may have undergone psychosurgery.

The paternalism of the asylum authorities also extended into the realm of consent. As we have seen, in the 1940s superintendents routinely ordered the administration of insulin, metrazol or electroshock therapy without seeking consent. The situation was different with regard to lobotomy, however, since a lobotomy was considered a surgical procedure which had to be performed in a hospital. The law required the written consent either of the patient or of his legally constituted representative. However, according to the provincial solicitor, the law permitted the superintendent to act as the "committee of the patient" and, as such, "could direct the course of treatment of the patient."[19]

During the 1950s there was correspondence between various superintendents and the Department of Health regarding the question of consent in lobotomy operations. In 1953, the provincial solicitor wrote to the assistant director of the hospitals division: "In the case of lobotomy operations where consent cannot be secured I think the superintendent should satisfy himself beyond any doubt that the patient concerned will benefit materially from the surgical interference... I think an independent opinion should be secured on the point as well."[20] There is no evidence that much account was taken of this latter point, and given the superintendents' belief that lack of consent should not prevent them from giving treatment, it is probable that legal niceties did not constitute a major obstacle to the lobotomy program.

The Decline of Lobotomy

By the mid–1950s lobotomy operations were being gradually abandoned in Ontario and the rest of North America. According to Valenstein, "the rate had started to decline before 1955 and...it dropped very significantly after 1955."[21] Whereas prior to that date an estimated 1,000 operations were performed each year, John Donnelly showed that 330 procedures were carried out in the U.S. and Canada in 1971, and 370 in 1973.[22]

These figures exclude procedures that might have been carried out by neurosurgeons not contacted by Donnelly. Although statistics for Ontario for the 1950s are not available, the Hanly report noted in 1966: "Prefrontal lobotomy is no longer used by the vast majority of psychiatrists except in the most unusual circumstances and when all other treatment methods have failed."[23] Statistics do show that between 1968 and 1972, a total of 17 lobotomy operations were performed, six of these in 1972. Three operations were performed in Toronto in 1981.[24] Very few operations were performed in Canada or the United States after the mid–1970s. However, during the late 1960s German scientists operated on the "mating center" of male pedophiliacs, homosexuals and men with symptoms of "hypersexuality."[25] In the 1970s, psychosurgical operations were performed in order to treat obesity, alcoholism and drug addiction, anorexia nervosa, and, of course, violence.[26] From 1977 to 1982, 13 patients were referred to the Clarke Institute of Psychiatry in Toronto for psychosurgery. Eight of these patients were diagnosed as "obsessive-compulsive," one as paranoid schizophrenic and four as suffering from "primary affective disorder."[27] Of these 13, six were men and seven were women. In 1981, psychosurgical procedures were performed on three women with primary affective disorder with agitated depression by Dr. Kenneth Livingston, a Toronto neurosurgeon. One patient died before the three-year follow-up could be completed, as a result of "unrelated causes," one failed to respond to surgery and one patient showed "dramatic initial improvement but rapidly reverted to her preoperative state."[28] Dr. Livingston's death shortly after the procedures were performed seems to have ended any further attempts at psychosurgery in Ontario. According to Valenstein, between 200 and 250 operations were performed in the United Kingdom each year between 1973 and 1975. Statistics from England and Wales show that from 1979 to 1982, psychosurgical procedures were performed on 207 informal (voluntary) and 4 detained patients.[29]

Lobotomy almost disappeared in North America because the psychoactive drugs proved a more effective method for easing the nursing and management problems within the mental hospitals and for discharging large numbers of patients. Insofar as the administration of psychosurgery was intended to pacify disruptive patients and to calm violent ones, then the procedure was not ineffective. Nor did psychosurgery decline because it had become controversial; psychosurgery did not become a political issue until the 1970s, long after the decline had begun.[30] Thus, the antipsychiatry writings of Foucault, Goffman, Laing and Szasz had little impact on the rate of administering psychosurgery, since their major works all appeared within a few years of each other after 1960. According to Valenstein: "Although psychosurgery did continue at a relatively low level throughout the 1960s, the topic received virtually no public attention at all."[31]

The Politicization of Lobotomy

The psychosurgery question became politicized at almost the same moment when the psychiatric community was abandoning the procedure. In this sense, the public controversy surrounding lobotomy was a case of driving nails into an already sealed coffin. For example, in July 1974, the Church of Scientology in Toronto and various human rights commissions affiliated to the Church in Denmark and Sweden protested to Canadian authorities about the use of psychosurgery in Ontario. After a brief flurry of messages between the Canadian embassies in Sweden and Denmark, and some preliminary newspaper articles in Toronto, it turned out that no lobotomies had been performed in provincial psychiatric hospitals since 1972.[32] In the United States, the issue of psychosurgery was kept alive by the popular press and by films such as *One Flew Over the Cuckoo's Nest*. Moreover, amidst the urban riots of the 1960s, suggestions by two well-known neurosurgeons that research was needed to determine whether brain damage might lead some people to participate in riots aroused enormous controversy and was seen as further cause for suspicion that the psychiatric profession was politically biased.[33]

By the 1970s, there were a series of attempts to restrict and regulate psychosurgery. In the 1973 U.S. landmark case of Kaimowitz vs. Department of Health, a Michigan court ruled that an involuntary patient could never give informed consent to a psychosurgical procedure. At the same time, in the early 1970s, the states of Oregon and California passed laws establishing psychosurgery review committees to vet applications from both voluntary and involuntary patients.[34]

In 1977, the United States National Commission for the Protection of Human Subjects of Biomedical and Behavioral Research recommended the establishment of a national psychosurgery advisory board to vet applications for psychosurgery from voluntary patients, and it recommended that the operation be performed only if individual institutional review boards had established the competence of the surgeon, the appropriateness of the surgery, pre-and postoperative assessments and that the patient was fully informed of the operation and had given consent. The Commission did not advise against psychosurgery for consenting, involuntary patients, although it did suggest that the procedure not be performed "over a patient's objection."[35] In contrast to the political controversy that occurred in the 1970s in the United States, and except for the continuing pressure from the Scientologists there was little discussion of psychosurgery in Ontario. In view of the debate in the United States, however, the Canadian Psychiatric Association examined the issue and in 1978 recommended that psychosurgery be made available to consenting voluntary patients "in much the same way as other surgical procedures."[36] It also recommended that psychosurgery review boards be established to vet applications from involuntary patients, mentally handicapped people, prisoners and minors.

The Ban on Lobotomy

In 1978, the Ontario Council of Health's Legal Task Force submitted an interim report to the government at the same time as new amendments to the Mental Health Act were placed before the legislature. While committee hearings on the proposed changes to the Act were taking place the Legal Task Force recommended that although "a case exists for precluding performance of the procedure (psychosurgery) upon surrogate consent on behalf of an involuntary patient," it recommended that psychosurgery still be available to voluntary patients and to "fully, informed, competent," involuntary patients giving personal consent.[37] For the latter, the Legal Task Force suggested that a psychosurgery review board be established, composed of not less than two members of the medical staff of the mental hospital, a lawyer, and "up to perhaps two other persons, such as [a] chaplain or layperson."[38] However, the recommendations of the Canadian Psychiatric Association and the Ontario Council of Health were ignored as the government pressed ahead and banned psychosurgery for involuntary patients. The circumstances leading up to this ban were as follows.

In February 1977, the new Minister of Health, Dennis R. Timbrell supported the recommendation of his legal adviser Gilbert Sharpe that psychosurgery be banned. Testimony before the legislative social development policy committee in 1978 on amendments to the Mental Health Act disclosed widespread abuses of compulsory treatment powers. During the hearings amendments were adopted prohibiting the administration of psychosurgery in Ontario mental hospitals even in the case where involuntary patients or their "nearest relative" gave their consent. The political situation in Ontario also militated in favour of the expansion of patients' rights. The 1977 provincial election had produced a minority government headed by the Progressive Conservatives but dependent on the support of the opposition New Democratic and Liberal parties. In committee hearings on the Mental Health Act, both opposition parties supported the government amendments.[39]

What is highly unusual about these legislative attempts to regulate psychosurgery is the establishment of psychosurgery review boards to vet applications for the operation from consenting patients. Even more unusual is the provision in Oregon and Great Britain, and the initial suggestion in Ontario that the psychosurgery review boards include non-medical personnel. Quite clearly, if it were merely a case of ensuring that the candidate for psychosurgery, or those responsible for him/her, had understood the nature and possible consequences of the operation, and had willingly consented, then a review board composed entirely of medical doctors or of doctors and some lawyers would have sufficed. But, as two authors of an article on psychosurgery have asked, what were the reasons "for this largely unprecedented intrusion into medical practice?"[40]

The answer is that the presence of laypeople on the boards was supposed to ensure that candidates for psychosurgery had not been chosen for political reasons or for reasons that had little to do with psychiatry or medicine. According to D. S. Rushmer, chairman of the Oregon psychosurgery board, behind the bill establishing the board was "the unspoken allegation that those who performed organic therapies...would use their skills in the service of political or social ambitions or as a final weapon in the closed closets of the penal system or the back wards of the state hospitals."[41] A 1977 position paper on psychosurgery commissioned by the Canadian Psychiatric Association alluded to the political controversy surrounding psychosurgery by stating that the objections to psychosurgery were "frequently based on ill-considered presumptions of abuse and deprivation of human rights with politico-social overtones..."[42] Recognizing the unusual nature of a procedure which required the authorization of review boards in the case of voluntary, consenting patients, the California legislature stated: "Because those who are emotionally disturbed are vulnerable to being unduly influenced, the Legislature believes the protection of their rights requires a careful process of informing and consenting in order to assure the protection and vindication of their rights."[43] A California appellate court explained the necessity for a review committee for consenting, voluntary patients by noting that the "physician's assessment of his patient's competency and voluntariness may not always be objective."[44] Moreover, the court noted that because the procedure was serious and irreversible and because "tort damages are totally inadequate," there had to be some regulation.[45] Neither Oregon nor California forbade psychosurgery on consenting involuntary patients, but so many conditions were attached to the administration of psychosurgery that it became virtually impossible to perform.

In Ontario, further restrictions on psychiatric authority and an extension of patients' rights were embodied in a 1986 bill which granted to competent patients in psychiatric hospitals the right to refuse all treatment including drug therapy and electroshock. While under previous legislation a doctor could apply to a review board in order to administer these treatments, in the 1986 act there was no appeal from the patient's decision. Curiously, while Ontario law now prevents involuntary but consenting mental patients from access to psychosurgery, there is no legislation establishing review boards for voluntary patients. Exactly the reverse obtains in Oregon and California, where review boards process applications from both voluntary and involuntary patients.

What explains the patchy legislation regarding psychosurgery? In the case of Michigan it was a court challenge which led to restrictions on psychosurgery. In other cases, such as Oregon and California, sympathetic legislatures passed laws regulating psychosurgery. In Great Britain, the medical profession decided that one way to meet the controversy over psychosurgery was to establish one or two central locations where psychosurgery would be performed under highly controlled conditions. One such centre is run by Dr. Geoffrey Knight at the Maudsley Hospital in London.

As is often the case, public policy in Ontario was affected by events in the United States. It was the powerful Ontario bureaucracy (specifically the mental health bureaucrats in the Ministry of Health) who decided to follow the example of some of the American states and impose restrictions on psychosurgery. In order to understand the difference in the positions of civil servants in Ontario and most American states it is important to remember that government at the federal and provincial level in Canada is organized along parliamentary lines, and that a disciplined party system prevails. Moreover, as the passage of the 1968 Federal Medicare Act and subsequent amendments have demonstrated, Canadian doctors and psychiatrists have nowhere near the same political power as their colleagues in the United States. Thus, once the Minister of Health agreed to the policy changes, it was an almost forgone conclusion that the amendments to the Mental Health Act would pass and that psychosurgery would effectively be banned in all public mental institutions.

Unquestionably, one reason for the recent restrictions imposed on psychosurgical operations and for the continuing attempts to circumscribe the authority of psychiatrists is the public's belief that psychiatrists have abused their authority. Archival material indicates that psychosurgery in Ontario was administered in an indiscriminate and probably illegal fashion. The highly centralized bureaucratic health system in Ontario protected the psychiatric hospitals from outside forces which might have raised questions about psychosurgery. Ironically, in the 1980s, this same bureaucracy helped bring about major reforms in mental health policy.

The Decline of Psychiatric Authority

Psychosurgical procedures were carried out during a time when what happened in the mental hospitals and in the psychiatric profession in general was determined almost exclusively by a small circle of decision-makers: psychiatrists, the superintendents of the asylums, and those few government officials concerned with mental health policy. It is true that an occasional scandal would reach the press and governments would be forced to investigate or make some changes in policy, but on the whole the daily life of mental patients in asylums passed in isolation from the media and certainly in isolation from the political realm.

This was the heyday of paternalism in psychiatry when psychiatrists or mental health policy-makers made decisions for mentally ill people without their consent, and justified those decisions in terms of the best interests of those mentally ill people. Whether the decisions taken were in the best interests of the patients is another question, but the fact is that from the middle of the nineteenth century governments assumed almost full responsibility for the care of mentally ill people. This responsibility included the right to forcibly administer treatments such as insulin coma therapy, metrazol therapy, electroshock and lobotomies to patients who would not voluntarily submit to them.

Elliot S. Valenstein notes: "There is a recurrent and disquieting theme throughout the older psychosurgical literature suggesting that problems of management played too large a role, both in the selection of patients and in the evaluation of results."[46] The evidence from Ontario indicates that psychosurgery was frequently administered for reasons that had little to do with treating the patient, and had more to do with alleviating management problems in the hospital, with research and experiment, or, in some cases, with idle curiosity.

Although each asylum superintendent was under the direct control of the Ontario Department of Health, within the individual asylum the superintendent was supreme. There was practically no outside influence on the operation of the mental health system. Until the 1970s, only the Canadian Mental Health Association and the press monitored the operation of the asylums. However, the CMHA was weak, and the press usually ignored the asylums until violence or a scandal drew their attention. Moreover, if local politicians played any role in asylum life it was usually to ensure that loyal constituents got jobs in the institution.

Thus, the mental health system in Ontario was almost hermetically sealed against outside influences, supervised and operated by a closed circle of medical doctors and medical bureaucrats and responsible to the legislature and to the public through the Minister of Health who was usually a medical doctor. This is not to suggest that decisions taken within the mental health system were based on exclusively medical grounds. In fact, the practice of medicine, however broadly defined, played a very small role in the day-to-day life of the asylum. Typically, the asylum superintendent occupied himself with the administrative matters consequent upon the governance of an institution housing anywhere from 300 to 2,000 patients. Mostly this involved a humdrum routine of housing, feeding and clothing enormous numbers of mentally ill people, preventing them from hurting themselves or others and, if possible, keeping the harmless patients occupied during the day. Although superintendents were expected to conduct regular rounds, such rounds were usually perfunctory. Pervading most asylums was an air of hopelessness and despair. It is true that a large number of patients were discharged as cured every year, but the majority of patients could expect to spend the rest of their lives in hospital. Moreover, those who worked in mental hospitals during this time emphasize how different conditions were before the inception of the neuroleptic drugs and how desperately authorities grasped at any treatment that could mitigate severe mental illness. Dr. E. Cunningham Dax, an Australian psychiatrist has attempted to explain the popularity of lobotomy in England during and immediately after the Second World War.

> First, patients were much more disturbed than we know them now and the nursing staff were few in numbers. Barbiturates were fairly new and sodium amylobarbitone was greeted as the new wonder drug. Sulphanol had gone out of fashion, but chloral, bromide and paraldehyde remained. Padded rooms were in frequent use, incontinence of urine and faeces was rife and many patients wore strong canvas clothing...some were extremely violent and tube feeding was frequent. Depressives on suicide caution cards were stripped of their possessions, spoon fed and marched from one room to another. There was sentinel walking, echolalia, flexibilitas cerea and frequent stupor with the constant danger from the catatonics. It was rare for members of staff to walk round disturbed wards unaccompanied. The second point was that in the wartime years in spite of considerable overcrowding and scanty staff, the energy and morale rose to amazing heights. Perhaps this had something to do with the mass production methods used in carrying out the vast amount of treatment by malaria, insulin, convulsive therapy, prolonged sleep and prefrontal leucotomy. Chronically ill patients suddenly became the centre of attention and there was a new feeling of therapeutic hope.[47]

However, there was another reason for the enthusiasm with which psychiatrists greeted the inception of new drug and physical therapies. By the 1930s the introduction of insulin coma therapy, metrazol and electroshock treatment led to profound changes in the status of psychiatrists and in public perceptions of the profession and of the mental hospital.

Whereas prior to the 1930s psychiatrists' expertise in the area of mental illness derived from skill in the diagnosis and classification of mental disease, that is, in nosology, now, with the introduction of new drugs and techniques their claims to authority could be given a scientific validation. However, as the public began to learn about the actual effects on patients of heroic treatments such as insulin, metrazol and electroshock, the image of the psychiatrist became more ambiguous, a mixture of Dr. Kildare and Dr. Moreau. It is within this context that the introduction of lobotomy must be understood.

By the 1940s, lobotomy was seen as a major and valuable addition to the physician's armamentarium. After all, psychiatrists constantly complained that they were paid less and had lower prestige than doctors practicing physical medicine. It was only natural, therefore, that the superintendents, the medical officers of the various asylums and the medical men who staffed the Ministry of Health from the Minister on down would give an enthusiastic reception to a medical, indeed a surgical procedure which helped to blur the distinction between the practice of physical and psychiatric medicine. Eventually, the neuroleptic drugs obviated the need for psychosurgery. Later, the furor over psychosurgery in the 1970s in the United States led Canadian policymakers to apply American lessons even before there was any widespread public pressure for action.

More recently, the fact that psychiatrists in Ontario and elsewhere have been powerless to reverse legal restrictions on the administration of psychosurgery and to stop the trend toward giving patients greater rights in the areas of committal and treatment illustrates the radical change in public attitudes toward psychiatry that has occurred over the past two decades. From the vantage point of the 1980s, it can be seen that restrictions on the use of psychosurgery were the thin edge of the wedge in the movement to reduce psychiatric paternalism and to grant to mental patients the right to refuse treatment unconditionally. As the Canadian Position Paper on Psychosurgery put it: "The prevalent negative attitude toward psychosurgery is almost certainly part of a wider general anti-psychiatric attitude." There is no sign of that attitude changing.

Notes

1 Ontario, *Statutes*, 1982, chapter 262, section 35, paragraph 1.

2 When in 1940 a journalist asked the New York Academy of Medicine about the operation "he was surprised to discover bitter opposition—labels such as 'crime' and 'criminals' were mentioned." Jack D. Pressman, "Sufficient Promise: John F. Fulton and the Origins of Psychosurgery," *Bulletin of the History of Medicine* 62 (1988): 17.

3 Elliot S. Valenstein, "Historical Perspectives," in *The Psychosurgery Debate,* edited by E. Valenstein (San Francisco: W. H. Freeman, 1980). See also. W. H. Freeman and P. Bean, *Mental Disorder and Legal Control* (New York: Cambridge UP, 1986).

4 I incorrectly stated in a 1987 article in the *Journal of Health Politics, Policy and Law*, that McKenzie conducted the first operations in 1944. The correct date and an interesting discussion of the inception of psychosurgery in Ontario can be found in "The Rise and Decline of Psychosurgery in Ontario," an unpublished paper by Mr. Geoffrey Reaume, Graduate Programme in History, University of Toronto. McKenzie reported on the first series of operations in a book review of Freeman and Watt's *Psychosurgery* in the *American Journal of Psychiatry* 101 (1944): 280–281; and in Kenneth G. McKenzie, M. D. and Lorne Proctor, M. D., "Bilateral Frontal Lobe Leucotomy in the Treatment of Mental Disease," *Canadian Medical Association Journal* 55 (1946): 432–441.

5 AO, RG 10–107, Gen. 1–9–8, January 3, 1947, R. C. Montgomery, to file.

6 *The Psychosurgery Debate* 101.

7 "To the psychiatric profession, a return to mental health for a woman is a return to satisfaction with her role as wife and/or mother, and contained in that assessment is the biased view that that is the entirety of women's role." Di Hudson, "The Psychocontrol of Women: Lobotomy as a Method of Social Control," *Catcall* [U.K.] 16 (1984): 22,

8 This figure is based on my own calculations. There is no single source giving the total number of lobotomies performed in Ontario's psychiatric hospitals, but one can arrive at a rough estimate based on information in the AO for the various provincial hospitals.

9 Abraham Miller, "The Lobotomy Patient—A Decade Later: A Follow-up Study of a Research Project Started in 1948," *The Canadian Medical Association Journal* 96 (1967) 1095–1103.

10 Elliot Valenstein, *Great and Desperate Cures* (New York: Basic Books, 1986): 154.

11 *Globe* 7 December 1946.

[12] AO, RG 10–107, Gen. 1–9–8, August 19, 1948, Dr. R. C. Montgomery to all Superintendents.

[13] R. C. Montgomery to all Superintendents.

[14] AO, RG 10, Series 37, Box 7, December 1957, David N. W. Doig, "Review of Leucotomy Operations: 1952–1957."

[15] AO, RG 10, B. 115, Gen. P–2–8–2, December 15, 1958, J. N. Senn, superintendent Ontario Hospital, Hamilton, to Dr. B. McNeel Chief, Mental Health Division. Participants in the lobotomy program at the Hamilton Hospital published their results in the *Canadian Psychiatric Association Journal* in 1958. Because so many patients were "a great problem to those who care for them," the authors wrote, "it was felt that there was need for a Leucotomy program which concentrated on the disturbed patients who present a difficult nursing problem, not so much to get the patients out of hospital as to relieve the overall nursing program...Primarily, we wished to find out if...arduous nursing tasks could be alleviated by bilateral Leucotomy." The program began in 1952 and a series of 200 patients were given the operation. Two patients died eight days after the operation. The authors concluded: "Our experience with the Leucotomy program for the chronically disturbed patients has been very gratifying. Assaultiveness, destructiveness and noisiness have been greatly reduced. Much less symptomatic electroshock is required. Most patients are more content and easily managed. Many are living out of the hospital who probably would otherwise have required indefinite care... The program is paying for itself financially, apart from the emotional and social profits." B. A. Boyd, W. H. Weber, and K. G. McKenzie, "Leucotomy—its Therapeutic Value on the Disturbed Wards of a Mental Hospital," *Canadian Psychiatric Association Journal*, 3 (1958): 170–179.

[16] AO, RG 10, B. 115, Gen. P–2–8–2, December 15, 1958. In the late 1960s, 60 patients from the London Hospital, and 60 from the St. Thomas Hospital were the subjects of an experiment to determine the relative effectiveness of two kinds of lobotomy operations. The results were mixed. In addition the experimenters reported "the usual findings of having the poorest results in the cases of schizophrenia was borne out..." Thus, the experimenters subjected to the operation schizophrenic patients, knowing full well that the prognosis for success was poor. See G. E. Hobbs, C. G. Drake, J. M. Wanklin and G. G. Essert, "Bilateral vs. Bimedial Lobotomy," *Canadian Psychiatric Association Journal* 5 (1960): 80–84.

[17] AO, RG 10, B.53, HS 2–1, 1948, Dr. H. B. Carscallen, "Preliminary Report on Prefrontal Lobotomy at Westminster Hospital."

[18] AO, RG 10–107, B. 7, Gen. 1–9–8, August 19, 1948, Dr. R. C. Montgomery to all Superintendents.

[19] AO, RG 10–107, B. 7, Gen. 1–9–8, April 21, 1948, C. Walker, Provincial Solicitor, to R. C. Montgomery.

[20] AO, RG 10, B. 115, Gen. P–2–8–1, December 15, 1953, C. Walker to C. H. Lewis, Assistant Director, Hospitals Division.

[21] Valenstein, *The Psychosurgery Debate* 29.

[22] John Donnelly, "The Incidence of Psychosurgery in the United States, 1971–1973," *American Journal of Psychiatry* 135 (1978): 1476–79.

[23] C. Hanly, *Mental Health in Ontario* (Toronto: Committee on the Healing Arts, 1970) 38.

[24] AO, RG 10–108, September 4, 1974, G. J. Chatfield, General Manager, Direct Services to S. W. Martin, Deputy Minister of Health. Of the 17 lobotomies performed between 1968 and 1974, 13 were performed at the Kingston psychiatric hospital which had links with the medical school at Queen's University, three at the Lakeshore psychiatric hospital and one at the Hamilton psychiatric hospital. The three patients involved in the 1981 operations were assessed by the Psychosomatic Medicine Unit at the Clarke Institute. See Peter Prendergast and Padraig Darby, "Psychosurgery—The Clarke Institute Experience," 1985. Unpublished manuscript kindly provided by Dr. Prendergast. For specific studies of lobotomy patients in the 1950s and 1960s, see A. Miller, M.D. "Lobotomy—A Clinical Study," Ontario Department of Health, 1954?, 107 pages; A. Miller, M. D. "The Lobotomy Patient—A Decade Later: A Follow-up Study of a Research Project Started in 1948," *Canadian Medical Association Journal* 96 (1967): 1095–1103 and K. G. McKenzie and G. Kaczanowski, "Prefrontal Leukotomy: A Five Year Controlled Study," in *Canadian Medical Association Journal* 91 (1964): 1193–1196.

[25] Inge Rieber and Volkmar Sigusch, "Psychosurgery on Sex Offenders and Sexual 'Deviants' in West Germany," *Archives of Sexual Behavior* 8 (1979): 523–527.

[26] Valenstein, *The Psychosurgery Debate* 89–107.

[27] P. Prendergast and P. Darby, "Psychosurgery—the Clarke Experience," 1985.

[28] Prendergast 7.

[29] P. Bean 144.

[30] Kenneth Livingston, "The Frontal Lobes Revisited," *Archives of Neurology* 20 (1969): 90–95.

[31] Valenstein *The Psychosurgery Debate* 39.

[32] AO, RG 10–108. Documents in the AO lobotomy files include communications in July 1974, between the Under-Secretary of State for External Affairs, Ottawa and the Canadian Embassies in Copenhagen and Stockholm concerning protests by the Danish and Swedish Citizen's Commission on Human Rights concerning psychosurgery in Canada. These groups were sponsored by the Church of Scientology.

[33] V. Mark, W. H. Sweet and F. R. Ervin, "The Role of Brain Disease in Riots and Urban Violence," *Journal of the American Medical Association* 226 (1967): 895.

[34] Robert J. Grimm, "Regulation of Psychosurgery," and F. C. Pizzulli, "Psychosurgery Legislation and Case Law," in Valenstein, *The Psychosurgery Debate* 421–438; 374.

[35] Grimm 432–433.

[36] Canadian Psychiatric Association, "Position paper: Psychosurgery, the Position of the Canadian Psychiatric Association," *Canadian Journal of Psychiatry* 24 (1978): 361.

[37] Committee on Mental Health Services in Ontario, Legal Task Force, *Report* (Toronto: Ontario Council of Health, 1979) v-vi.

[38] *Report* 70.

[39] See Standing Social Development Committee, Hearings on Bill 19, the Mental Health Amendment Act, June 1978.

[40] D. Carrol and M. A. J. O'Callaghan, "Regulating Psychosurgery: Ethical, Social and Scientific Considerations," *Medicine and Law* 3 (1984): 193–204.

[41] Grimm 423.

[42] J. D. Earp, "Position Statement on Psychosurgery to be Considered by the Board of Directors of the Canadian Psychiatric Association," Unpublished manuscript, 1977.

[43] F. C. Pizzuli, "Psychosurgery Legislation and Case Law," in Valenstein, *The Psychosurgery Debate* 373.

[44] Pizzuli 379.

[45] G. J. Annas, "Informed Consent and Review Committees," in Valenstein, *The Psychosurgery Debate* 497.

[46] Valenstein, *The Psychosurgery Debate* 35.

[47] Dr. E. Cunningham Dax, "The History of Prefrontal Leucotomy," in J. Sidney Smith and L. G. Kiloh, editors, *Psychosurgery and Society* (London: Pergamon, 1977) 20.

13

The Politics of Mental Health Law

> In any remodeling of provincial psychiatric services, the question of legal formalities deserves serious consideration. The legal formalities now required for the treatment of psychiatric patients in hospitals are often painful to patients and their relatives and prejudicial to patients' interests. These formalities have contributed to the separation of psychiatry from general medicine and foster the so-called stigma attached to mental illness. A psychiatric disability is the only kind of sickness which requires a separate and individual process of law to get a patient under treatment in a hospital.
>
> Canadian House of Commons Special Committee on Social Security, "Minutes of Proceedings and Evidence," May 18, 1943

A Brief History

Until recently, changes in mental health law resulted from the efforts of psychiatrists, civil servants and those few politicians interested in the question. Except for rare occasions, as in 1938, when the press took up the cause of John R. Green and Premier Hepburn himself became involved, mental health law was rarely the topic of public debate.

The result was that, until the late 1960s, the grounds for committal were so broad and the legal rights of patients so limited that mental patients were almost as constrained as prisoners in the criminal justice system. According to Dr. C. A. Roberts:

> It didn't occur to me with a certified patient, any more than with a prisoner, that there was any question of asking them whether or not they wanted treatment. They had been brought to hospital mentally ill, incapable of judgment or decision, so they were treated. That was true of mental hospitals, prisons, homes for the aged, and county homes. Formalized consents were a postwar development.[1]

A brief look at selections from earlier Ontario statutes illustrates the degree to which mentally ill people were rendered helpless by the law.

In 1937, under Section 25 (1) of the Mental Hospitals Act it was possible for anyone to lay an "information" before a justice of the peace regarding a person "suspected or believed by the person laying the information to be mentally ill or mentally defective." At that point, the justice of the peace might issue a warrant for the police to "apprehend" and forcibly bring a person before a magistrate for an examination. Then, with no recourse to a lawyer or to any other independent authority, if found to be mentally ill by two "medical practitioners" the person would be certified and committed, that is, incarcerated in a provincial psychiatric hospital. Once in hospital the patient was virtually a prisoner, with the superintendent granted "full control over and the custody and care of the person of every patient" in the institution. This meant that patients could be forcibly subjected to an array of drastic treatments such as insulin coma therapy, metrazol, electroshock, wet packs and even, as we have seen, psychosurgery. Patients could lose control of their property, they were stripped of their right to vote in provincial and federal elections, barred from practicing as funeral directors, police officers, accountants, medical doctors, or pharmacists and they could be deported from the province or from Canada. Even the language used in the 1937 Mental Health Act was analogous to that used in criminal law. People were "suspected" of being mentally ill. "Warrants" were issued to "apprehend" suspects. Patients "escaped" from the institution, people could be fined for "abetting" an escapee. Patients could also be placed on "probation" or "apprehended" and brought back if they again became mentally ill. When authorities did become concerned about mental health law it was mainly in relation to mentally ill people in trouble with the law and with the lack of mental health services for prisoners in jail or on probation or because of the lack of sufficient examination facilities in courts.

However, by the early 1960s, mental health laws came under attack from two quarters: from antipsychiatrists such as Thomas Szasz, who cast doubt on the very meaning of the term "mental illness," and from the Canadian Mental Health Association, concerned about questions of civil liberties. Thus, in 1962, the National Scientific Planning Council of the Canadian Mental Health Association, the same body which had established the Tyhurst Committee in 1958, established a committee on legislation and psychiatric disorder. Composed exclusively of doctors and lawyers, the committee produced reports on mental health and the law in 1964, 1967 and 1969. A revised and updated version of their work was published in 1973.[2]

It is interesting to note that in the early 1960s, the CMHA aimed at achieving two apparently contradictory objectives: to facilitate the apprehension, examination and committal of certain classes of mentally ill people, but also to protect their civil liberties through the establishment of hospital review boards. The first goal was prompted by complaints from psychiatrists about the cumbersome procedures regarding involuntary patients. As the Committee on Legislation and Psychiatric Disorder put it in 1964: "Many of the practices of the past laid undue stress on the protection of personal liberty because committal to a hospital was for many years, and the judicial order, or certificates of two or three physicians, were of indefinite effect."[3] Thus, the committee recommended, and the Ontario statutes ultimately included, changes whereby the number of physicians involved in the process of removal, examination and committal was reduced from two to one. Whereas in 1959, an "alleged mentally ill or mentally defective person" had to appear before a magistrate or a justice of the peace, and be examined by two physicians, the committee recommended that the "opinion" of a single physician that "a person is probably mentally ill *and* a danger to himself and others *and* in need of medical attention" [italics in original] was sufficient for the person to be forcibly removed to a hospital for examination, to be certified and then held for examination for 72 hours, for a further 30 days, and for increasingly longer intervals after that.[4] Of course, the major difference is that in 1959 the criterion of dangerousness was not a necessary prerequisite for the intervention of police and courts, whereas by the early 1960s it was felt that mentally ill people should not be compelled to undergo hospitalization and treatment unless dangerousness to self or others was present. Moreover, in 1964, the committee suggested that hospital review boards be established so that certified patients might obtain a hearing and, in the event of an unsatisfactory decision, appeal to the courts.

It was not just increasing concern about civil liberties and suspicion of psychiatrists exceeding their authority that prompted a new look at mental health laws, but developments within the mental health system itself. The continued expansion of the psychiatric unit system and the treatment there of "unwilling" patients raised the question of whether the general hospital administration or the psychiatric unit staff were responsible for obtaining consent for treatment procedures.[5] Questions of liability were also raised concerning foster homes, boarding homes, halfway houses, approved homes and residential centres.[6]

According to Barry Swadron, who helped draft the 1967 Mental Health Act, Minister of Health Matthew Dymond and "the mental health administration" began to think about reforming existing mental health law in the late 1950s.[7] In 1966, responding to criticism from the NDP's Stephen Lewis about confusion in drafting the new mental health act, Dr. Dymond stated that the 1966 Act "arose out of a statement of my own made in February 1959 when I stated that it was my intention to remove legal entanglements from mentally ill patients in every possible way that I could. One of the first things that I proposed in that programme was that every patient detained against his will should have the right—at least the rights of a criminal—and I stated: Many patients admitted to a hospital for the mentally ill are bereft of even the rights of a criminal."[8] In 1966, therefore, with the work of the CMHA committee on legislation and psychiatric disorder in the background, Swadron began to work with the CMHA and the Canadian Association for the Mentally Retarded on a draft law that was to become the 1967 Mental Health Act.[9] Many provisions of the new Act embodied the recommendations of the Committee on Legislation and Psychiatric Disorder. The role of the courts in deciding the question of mental illness was drastically reduced, the signature of only one physician was necessary to admit an involuntary patient for examination or for committal, and provisions were included for the establishment of hospital review boards—although there was no provision for appealing board decisions to the courts.[10] Unlike previous occasions when mental health law was only cursorily debated in the legislature, there were lengthy discussions in 1966 about the proposed act. Some of it reflected growing suspicion of psychiatric authority. For example, Liberal F. R. Oliver objected to the proposed inclusion of two psychiatrists on the board of review.

> I am thinking back to a case that came up in my riding, the Fawcett case. That man was examined by, I think, a dozen or more psychiatrists. Perhaps seven out of the twelve who examined him said he was properly a patient for the Penetang institution...and four or five said that he was not. I mean there is a great variance of opinion among psychiatrists themselves just as there is among members of this House... I cannot understand why this board should not be something in the form of a jury—a jury of laymen, for instance, perhaps a legal man to interpret the legal entanglements but certainly not a group of professional men because their minds are fixed.[11]

What is interesting about these remarks is that they express a sentiment which, however widespread it might have been in the general public, hitherto had not been expressed in the legislature. Thirteen years later, the legal task force established by the Committee on Mental Health Services stated: "We also consider that in general psychiatrists should no longer continue to serve as members and as expert advisors to the review board." As of 1988, however, that recommendation had not been followed and psychiatrists continued to be represented on review boards.[12]

For a few years after the passage of the 1967 Mental Health Act, mental health law again disappeared into obscurity, becoming the concern mainly of those few lawyers interested in the question and of government civil servants trying to iron out inconsistencies, close gaps or clarify obscurities.

Mental Health Law in the 1970s and 1980s

The next major wave of reform began in the late 1970s and continued until the middle of the 1980s. During this period there was a clear trend in the direction of restricting psychiatric authority and extending patients' rights. The grounds for compulsory psychiatric assessment and committal were narrowed, the right to refuse or to challenge treatment was extended and appeal procedures were broadened—although, according to Carla McKague, a lawyer active in the mental health field, there was one step backward in 1978 when, for the first time, the law made it possible to give an involuntary patient treatment without consent.[13]

The initiative for reform came first from Minister of Health Dennis Timbrell, and the issue was soon joined by a variety of consumer and patients' rights groups, and professional organizations, particularly psychiatrists and medical doctors. The Canadian Civil Liberties Association which, according to Barry Swadron, had not been interested in mental health law in 1967, also joined the fray.[14] Although mental health law would inevitably have become a focus of attention with the passage of the Charter of Rights and Freedoms, it was mere chance that mental health law became an issue in the mid–1970s.

In May 1975, lawyer Gilbert Sharpe was employed as a consultant to the Ministry of Health and was asked to visit the various psychiatric hospitals in the province to discuss with administrators and medical directors the operation of the 1967 Mental Health Act.[15] Sharpe found that most doctors assumed, "wrongly, that they had the power to forcibly treat. They rarely sought consent. When I suggested they had no authority to forcibly treat many were extremely hostile."[16] In the fall and winter of 1976 there were continuing discussions about the status of mental health law, and in 1976 the Ministry appointed a committee to propose guidelines. After becoming Minister of Health in 1977, Dennis Timbrell asked the Ontario Council of Health to review the provincial mental health system and to enquire as well into the operation of the Act. Out of this Committee on Mental Health Services emerged a research group which produced *Agenda for Action*, and a legal task force which began an examination of mental health law. Thus, while Timbrell and his staff were working on specific amendments to the 1967 Mental Health Act, the legal task force was working on an overall critique of the Act. According to its report, "[m]ost of the problems are focused on a single process: the handling of the patient who, because of his mental disorder, is unwilling to be treated or even to be examined."[17]

Gilbert Sharpe recalls that after Timbrell was appointed Minister of Health, "we went to him in the sense that every area in the Ministry briefs the new Minister. He indicated that he wanted changes in this area [mental health law]."[18] Timbrell himself argues that "amendments to the mental health act in 1978 arose out of various studies that came to my attention, the involuntary committal procedures around the world, concerns raised by civil libertarians here, the media...it did not come from caucus, it did not come from Cabinet."[19] Timbrell contends that there was no pressure on him to change the law, but that he was cautioned against raising such a sensitive issue by his deputy minister who asked: "'Do you really want to touch this?' He told me the psychiatrists, doctors and some of the public would be upset. But I said I still think we ought to look at it at least."[20]

In the fall of 1977, Timbrell and his staff developed some proposals which he then took to Premier William Davis.

> Typical Davis, chomped on his cigar or his pipe, observed all this and essentially he said if you want to do it go ahead, we'll back you. We had some private discussions where he tested my resolve to see if I was really personally committed to do it or if it was because my staff wanted it. To his credit once he realized that I really wanted it, he backed it.

However, Timbrell was vigorously opposed by two medical doctors: in Cabinet by Dr. Bette Stephenson and in caucus by Dr. Robert Elgie. "The attitude generally in cabinet was, "it's your neck if you want to do it. If you blow your brains out we'll get another Minister of Health, we did it before."[21]

Timbrell then ran into trouble in the legislature. During the debate over Bill 19, "I had the leader of the opposition, who was a psychiatrist [Dr. Stuart Smith] against me, I can remember several of his speeches in the House, he was just apoplectic by the end of some of his speeches." Even then, according to Timbrell, "we got through second reading in the legislature, then it went into hearings and all hell broke loose." According to one civil servant who worked with Timbrell on the bill,

> it was an uphill fight. Timbrell was taking on his own political caucus with people like Dr. Bette Stephenson and Dr. Elgie resisting these changes, the Liberals led by a psychiatrist, didn't want the changes and the NDP was split. Some of Timbrell's advisers said "who needs this, why are we doing this?" There was a write-in campaign from many doctors complaining about what they were doing.[22]

According to Gilbert Sharpe the doctors were very upset by what they saw as restrictions on their authority to commit and to treat contained in Bill 19.

> When I drafted the basic statement of principle in the 1978 bill, saying you cannot treat patients against their will, and included a review board procedure to compel treatment against a patient's wishes, I thought I would be perceived as having helped the doctors in giving them this mechanism that hadn't existed since 1967. In fact, they reacted with hostility. Their perception was that I had changed the law, changed their practice, tied their hands because now they suddenly had to go to a board for what they had been doing automatically in the past, probably without authority. We even had letters from orthopedic surgeons saying, "don't take away our committal powers." It was bizarre.[23]

The hearings before the social development committee were contentious mainly because of disagreement over the basis on which individuals could be involuntarily admitted to a mental hospital.[24] Bill 19 was the subject of a brief debate in the legislature on June 23, 1978. At that time the Leader of the Opposition, Dr. Stuart Smith moved an amendment intended to broaden the grounds of involuntary admission far beyond the provisions in Timbrell's draft bill. At that point Premier Davis took Timbrell aside and asked him to give way on the restrictions on doctors' committal powers saying that the government had already made substantial gains for patients' rights in the Bill. According to one witness, Timbrell then told Davis he did not want to concede the point as it would open the door to the possibility of inappropriate committals and that he was willing to become a backbencher over the issue. "Essentially that meant Timbrell was willing to give up politics over this fundamental rights issue. In light of that statement, Davis supported him. They had to take a head vote on that issue...but Smith's motion to expand doctors' committal powers was defeated."[25] The vote was 17 for the amendment and 38 against. However, the amendments were so controversial that although they passed the legislature in June 1978, they were not proclaimed until 1984.

The controversy aroused by Bill 19 marked a new era in the history of mental health law, for after 1978 mental health law moved to the centre of the political stage. It has been kept there ever since because of two new, crucial factors: the formation in the 1970s of a series of sophisticated patients' rights and consumers groups and the passage of the Charter of Rights and Freedoms.

Patients' Rights Groups and the Charter

The first patients' rights groups were born in 1970 in New York and in Vancouver. By 1987, 75 such groups had been established in North America.[26] In Ontario, a number of ex-mental patients, or, as Don Weitz prefers to call them, ex-psychiatric "inmates," organized On Our Own in the late 1970s, and established the quarterly *Phoenix Rising*.[27] Concerned Friends of Ontario Citizens in Care Facilities, the Advocacy Resource Centre for the Handicapped (ARCH), People First, the Patients' Rights Organization and other organizations in Ontario began to fight for patients' rights and to challenge the existing law. Then, in 1982, the adoption of the Charter of Rights and Freedoms whetted the interest of lawyers. According to Carla McKague of ARCH,

> we have gone from a situation in 1980 when I was articling, when David Baker also of ARCH and I were the only two doing substantial amounts of mental health law, to an incredible explosion of interest. Eventually, lawyers, patient advocates and law students, formed a Committee on Legal Issues in Psychiatry (CLIP), a small group which met together informally and did a fair amount of policy discussion.[28]

Under section 15 of the Charter, the provinces were given three years to bring their statutes into line with the Charter. Ontario then drafted Bill 7, the Equality Rights Statute Law Amendment Act, an omnibus bill intended to reconcile contradictions between existing laws and the Charter. According to Carla McKague, Bill 7 originally contained only minor amendments to the Mental Health Act. But after meeting with CLIP she drafted 22 proposed amendments to the Mental Health Act. Evelyn Gigantes of the NDP put the amendments forward and the Liberals expressed their support. The proposed changes to the Mental Health Act gave patients access to their records, restricted the ability of doctors to restrain patients and provided for a review of decisions on incompetency. One of the most important and controversial changes granted the right to refuse treatment to involuntary competent patients, or to the relative of an involuntary incompetent patient.[29] Under previous legislation a board of review could override this refusal, but now the proposal was to remove the override power from the board of review. So great was the opposition to this last provision, that although Bill 7 passed in December 1986, the government delayed implementation of this last provision pending further debate. In January 1987, the government introduced Bill 190 which included a provision restoring the override power of the boards of review (with the exception of electroconvulsive therapy). In the debate over the bill, the psychiatric and medical community supported restoration of the override powers while psychologists, social workers, advocates and patient self-help groups were opposed.[30] Finally, in June 1987 after discussions between the Liberals and the New Democrats and a reworking of the definition of competency, Bill 190 was passed—but the right of competent involuntary patients to refuse treatment remained. However, Bill 190 provided that a board of review could override the decision of a substitute decision-maker to refuse treatment for involuntary incompetent patients. In both cases, electroconvulsive therapy could not be imposed without consent.[31]

The Patient Advocate Program

Changes in mental health law were not the only sign of developing concern for patients' rights, for in 1981 Ontario established the first Canadian psychiatric patient advocate office. The patient advocate program was a response to a series of deaths that had occurred in 1980/81 at the Queen Street Mental Health Centre. Each incident was subjected to a coroner's inquest and in each case the coroner was critical of hospital policy. The first and most dramatic case concerned Aldo Alviani, a 230-pound 19-year-old male who had a previous history of mental illness. He was admitted to the Queen Street Mental Health Centre on the morning of June 22, 1980, showing symptoms of agitated, psychotic and assaultive behaviour. He was then subjected to a procedure called rapid "neuroleptization" whereby large doses of a tranquilizing drug were administered to control his behaviour. Unfortunately, the usual doses did not work and he was administered large doses of three different drugs: the psychiatric equivalent of a general anesthetic.[32] However, his vital symptoms were not adequately monitored, he was left on an open ward and was eventually found dead some time after he had actually died. It was only because someone at the Queen Street Mental Health Centre anonymously sent the information to New Democratic Party MPP Mike Breaugh that the public learned about the Alviani incident. During the inquest it turned out that the list of drugs given to Alviani on the morning of June 23 had either been lost or stolen. The Alviani inquest focussed public attention on the lack of adequate care for patients in mental hospitals, and the question of the extent to which mentally unstable people should be coerced into accepting treatment.

One result of the Alviani inquest was the establishment of a coalition of self-help and patients' rights groups including On Our Own, Houselink Community Homes, Friends and Associates, the Ontario Association for the Mentally Retarded and the Toronto and Ontario branches of the CMHA. In December 1980, these groups presented a brief to the Minister of Health Dennis Timbrell, "Psychiatric Care in Ontario: Some Serious Concerns," recommending specific improvements in the care and treatment of psychiatric patients in provincial facilities. Moreover, the brief called on the government to launch a public investigation into treatment practices in Ontario psychiatric hospitals. According to Dr. Tyrone Turner, later to become the first provincial coordinator of the psychiatric patient advocate office, the coalition "began to put a lot of pressure on government for the advancement of patients' rights, more in that area than in the area of clinic care... They called for proclamation of two unproclaimed sections of the Mental Health Act, sections 66 and 67, for the increased legalization of safeguards, including advocacy."[33] In addition, this was a period when both *The Globe and Mail* and *The Toronto Star* were devoting a lot of attention to poor housing for ex-mental patients, the lack of community services and to bad conditions in the provincial psychiatric hospitals. *The Toronto Star* called on Minister of Health Dennis Timbrell in three separate editorials on July 26, October 28 and November 29, 1981, to initiate a probe into provincial mental institutions and it specifically referred to the Alviani case in two of those editorials. Mental health law was also coming under attack in *The Globe and Mail* which published two articles by John Weingust, a lawyer who attacked the existing state of mental health law.[34] Weingust argued that mental patients were being denied due process of law and subjected to autocratic and arbitrary decision making by psychiatrists and bureaucrats. He called for a public enquiry into the provincial psychiatric hospital system. In August 1981, and then in December 1981, two more drug-related deaths occurred at the Queen Street Mental Health Centre. At an inquest held in April 1982, Coroner Margaret Milton was quoted by *The Globe and Mail* as saying that: "Political stalling is a major stumbling block in trying to improve mental health care services in Ontario."[35] The coroner accused former Minister of Health Dennis Timbrell of stalling in replying to staff complaints about the deteriorating situation at Queen Street.

By February 1982, however, Timbrell had been replaced as Minister of Health by Larry Grossman. Although Grossman was no more inclined than Timbrell to undertake a public investigation of the provincial psychiatric hospital system, he and his advisers had decided to meet the chorus of criticism in another way.

In the fall of 1981, at Minister of Health Timbrell's behest, assistant deputy minister Boyd Suttie had produced an eighteen-point plan for improving the mental health system. Among the suggestions was one concerning "hospital ombudsmen."[36] Although Timbrell approved of the plan, he had no time to implement it because he was replaced by Larry Grossman. Dr. Suttie then presented the plan to Grossman, who gave his approval. Grossman asked his political adviser, Ted Ball, to approach Dr. Tyrone Turner, a Toronto general practitioner with wide experience with mentally ill people, to offer him the job of setting up what would become known as the psychiatric patient advocate program. The fact that Turner had run as a New Democratic Party candidate in the St. David riding of Toronto was not an obstacle to his appointment by a Progressive Conservative Minister of Health.

The psychiatric patient office was established in 1981, and Dr. Turner was appointed as provincial coordinator in November 1982. By May 1983, eleven patient advocates had been appointed. The office was organized so that the patient advocates reported directly to the provincial coordinator, who, in turn, reported directly to the deputy minister. In this way the advocates were kept independent from the hospital and the reporting relationship involved the highest levels of the mental health bureaucracy. An advisory committee consisting of mental health consumers and providers was also established as a buffer between the office and the bureaucracy.

Not only was the establishment of the patient advocate program an attempt to defuse criticism from pressure groups and the press, it also was a tactical maneuver by the Minister of Health to ease the way for the implementation of sections

66 and 67 of the 1978 Mental Health Act which, because of heated opposition from psychiatrists and the medical profession, had not been proclaimed. Section 66 ensured that patients subjected to involuntary admission to a psychiatric hospital be given the opportunity to hire counsel and to appear before a review board where the certificate could be challenged, while section 67 gave the patient access to all documents produced at a hearing and allowed the patient to appeal the decision of the review board in court. Since psychiatrists were already up in arms over the narrowed criteria for commitment embodied in the 1978 Act and the provision for review boards, it was hoped that the patient advocates would help to smooth the implementation of the new provisions, provide help to patients and mediate between the psychiatrists and the patients or their friends or relatives. According to the first annual report of the psychiatric patient advocate office: "One of the major initial tasks given to the program was to work within the system to collect information about rights violations and rights protection and to assess whether or not Section 66 and 67 of the Mental Health Act should be proclaimed." After a year of operation it became clear to the patient advocates that patients in Ontario psychiatric hospitals, particularly involuntary patients who comprised a majority of their clients, were in need of further legal protection. In addition, since the Charter of Rights and Freedoms was to go into force in April 1985, the psychiatric patient advocate office recommended that sections 66 and 67 of the Mental Health Act be proclaimed. This took effect on March 1, 1984.

Inevitably, the patient advocate program ran into criticism from psychiatrists on the one side, and patients' rights groups on the other. The conflict centered on different models of the nature of mental illness and different conceptions of the way in which mental health care should be organized. In the medical model of mental illness, the psychiatrist is the appropriate authority for determining questions of competence and the nature of the treatment to be administered. Moreover, most psychiatrists felt that because of the nature of mental illness they should be the final authority regarding the amount of clinical information that should be made available to psychiatric patients. This immediately caused problems for the patient advocate program when psychiatrists resisted giving advocates access to patient records. The impasse was solved within a week when the Minister of Health appointed the advocates "inspectors" under the Mental Health Act thereby giving them full access to patient records.[37] But this only confirmed psychiatrists in their opinion that the treatment of mental illness was being removed from the purview of medical doctors and was becoming part of a legal merry-go-round where medicine was irrelevant. In 1984, the director of the forensic unit at the Oak Ridge division of the Ontario Medical Centre at Penetanguishine complained:

> The advocate is a frustration and an irritant. I felt I was my patient's best advocate, that I was acting in his best interests, and now all of a sudden this guy can come and look over my shoulder with rather sweeping powers and ask for explanations... The checks and balances are being carried to such extremes that

> we're inhibited from doing our job. It takes a hell of a lot longer to treat a patient but the treatment ends up the same—you just have to jump through a lot more hoops.[38]

From an entirely different perspective, antipsychiatrist advocates such as Don Weitz criticized the advocate program for being,

> caught in a conflict of interest. They're employed by the Ministry of Health, the Ministry funds the institutions. We've recommended all along that the advocates must be independent and should operate out of legal aid clinics. People in psychiatric institutions are prisoners, mental illness is a euphemism for people who don't conform.[39]

Whatever the criticisms, the psychiatric patient advocate program was a clear success, and by the summer of 1987 a review of advocacy recommended the formation of a provincial advocacy office and the extension of advocacy programs to a wide variety of disabled groups in the province, as well as to patients in psychiatric units in general hospitals and in the community.[40]

The Impetus for Reform

What explains the enormously increased pace of reform in mental health law and the extension of patients' rights in the late 1970s and 1980s? In the first instance, the impetus for change came from within the Ministry of Health itself, from Ministers of Health Dymond, Timbrell and Grossman. All three ministers took an interest in mental health policy, saw themselves as reformers and set their civil servants to work on various aspects of mental health law. Despite the fact that the plight of mentally ill people had rarely evoked popular support, there were political advantages to be gained from showing an interest in mental health reform. Undertaking reforms in the mental health system is, as one psychiatrist put it, "do-able." It is much easier than, for example, trying to control costs in the hospital sector or to reform the system of general medicine.[41] Of course, there are risks and penalties, as Timbrell discovered in the 1978 debates, but it is easier to confront the opposition of psychiatrists in the case of mental health reforms than the opposition of general practitioners in trying to reform the general health care system. Moreover, by the 1980s, when there was increasing criticism of government inaction in areas such as housing for ex-psychiatric patients, reforming the law could give the appearance of responding to criticism without, however, incurring the financial costs of making major changes in policy. Finally, increasing the scope of patients' rights necessarily meant a decline in psychiatric authority, and this was a subtle way for government to reduce the political influence of psychiatrists whose power, like any profession, depends partly on status and prestige.[42]

A second reason for the increasing pace of reform was pressure from patients' rights groups, consumer groups, public interest lawyers and the press. Changes in mental health law in Ontario reflected changes in the United States. There, court challenges to psychiatric authority and constitutional appeals had helped expand patients' rights, and had led to reforms in mental health statutes, particularly in the northeast and some of the western states such as California and Oregon.

A third reason was the impending implementation in April 1985 of the Charter of Rights and Freedoms. It was clear to the Ontario authorities that if they did not take the initiative in bringing mental health law into accord with the Charter, then the courts would do the job for them.

The last reason was the continuing, almost inexorable decline in psychiatric authority. Ever since the rise of the antipsychiatric movement of the 1960s, psychiatric prestige and authority had been under attack. Psychiatrists themselves contributed to this trend by testifying on opposite sides in dramatic murder or political assassination trials and suggesting that there were psychiatric solutions for urban violence. At the same time, scholarly critics like Rosenham in his famous article "On Being Sane in Insane Places" exposed psychiatry to ridicule.[43] Furthermore, the argument of the antipsychiatrists that mental illness is a myth re-enforced a conservative tendency to reject pleas of insanity in court cases and to force people take responsibility for their actions. In these circumstances psychiatrists and psychiatry were forced on the defensive.

Thus, radical changes in mental health law came about through a combination of circumstances, some structural, some contingent. There is no doubt that the existence of patients' rights organizations and the adoption of the Charter paved the way to law reform. But these changes might have occurred later or in a much more attenuated form if Ministers of Health Dymond, Timbrell and Grossman had not taken a personal interest in reform.

Notes

1 Interview, Dr. C. A. Roberts.

2 See Barry B. Swadron, *The Law and Mental Disorder* (Toronto: The Canadian Mental Health Association, 1973).

3 Committee on Legislation and Psychiatric Disorder, *The Law and Mental Disorder* (Toronto: Canadian Mental Health Association, 1964) 16. The members of the Committee were F. C. R. Chalke, J. Dewan, F. S. Lawson, Barry Swadron, F. K. Turner and J. D. Griffin. Except for Swadron and Turner who were lawyers, the remaining members of the Committee were physicians.

4 Statutes of Ontario, "An Act to Amend the Mental Hospitals Act," Chapter 57, Section 1 amending Section 26, subsection 2 of the Mental Hospitals Act.

5 *The Law and Mental Disorder* 10.

6 *The Law and Mental Disorder* 11.

7 Interview, Barry Swadron.

[8] *Debates*, April 6, 1966, p. 2329. A search of Hansard for 1959 did not turn up this statement, but Dr. Dymond may well have made the statement elsewhere.

[9] *The Mental Health Act, 1967*, was not proclaimed until June 1, 1968.

[10] Statutes of Ontario, *The Mental Health Act, 1967*.

[11] *Debates*, April 6, 1966, p. 2328.

[12] *Legal Task Force* 39.

[13] Carla McKague, "Civil Rights Endangered in Mental Health Bill," *The Globe and Mail* 20 April 1987.

[14] Interview, Barry Swadron.

[15] According to Minister of Health Frank Miller before the Standing Social Development Committee, *Debates*, June 7, 1978.

[16] Interview, Gilbert Sharpe.

[17] *Legal Task Force* vii.

[18] Interview, Gilbert Sharpe.

[19] Interview, Dennis Timbrell.

[20] *Ibid.*

[21] Interview, Dennis Timbrell.

[22] Interview, Gilbert Sharpe.

[23] Interview, Gilbert Sharpe.

[24] During the Social Development Committee hearings in June, 1978, Timbrell stated he had received 1,200 letters concerning Bill 19. Standing Social Development Committee, Bill 19, the Mental Health Amendment Act, June 7, 1978.

[25] Interview, Gilbert Sharpe.

[26] Harvey Savage and Carla McKague, *Mental Health Law in Canada* (Toronto: Butterworths, 1987) 238.

[27] Interview, Don Weitz.

[28] Interview, Carla McKague.

[29] According to Carla McKague, the amendment removing from the board of review the right to override patient refusals of treatment came about in a situation of extreme confusion. Originally defeated in committee, the amendment was revived before third reading of Bill 7 by Evelyn Gigantes of the NDP. Although the Progressive Conservatives had originally decided to oppose it, when it came to the floor of the legislature, the PCs mistakenly assumed that the amendment merely removed the right of a board of review to override a patient's refusal of ECT, and left intact the remaining override powers. "But they [the Tories] suddenly found that the board couldn't override on anything, and they tried to reopen it on the floor of the house." They failed.

[30] Groups opposing the amendment included the Ontario Medical Association, the Ontario Psychiatric Association, the Ontario Hospital Association and Ontario Friends of Schizophrenics. Supporting the amendment were the Ontario Psychological Association, Ontario Association of Professional Workers, Criminal Lawyer's Association, Ontario Association for Community Living, Concerned Friends of Ontario Citizens in Care Facilities, the Association of Advocates, Advocacy Centre for the Elderly, the Civil Liberties Association, Advocacy Centre for the Handicapped and various patient advocate and mental health self-help groups—"about 50 in all." Interview, Carla McKague.

[31] On Bill 190 see Carla McKague, "Bill 190: In Plain English," *Re-Action* Winter (1988): 8–9.

[32] Interview, Dr. Tyrone Turner.

[33] Interview, Dr. Tyrone Turner.

[34] See "The Shameful Case of the Mentally Ill," and "The Unjust Mental Health System in Ontario," 22 June 1981, and 10 December 1981 *The Globe and Mail.*

[35] *The Globe and Mail* 3 April 1982.

[36] Dr. Tyrone Turner says that he saw a discussion paper in the Ministry of Health from 1979 which talked about a "patient's friend," and a paper in 1980–81 that talked about a "patient's representative." Interview.

[37] Interview, Dr. Tyrone Turner.

[38] Quoted in "The Struggle for Mental Patient's Rights" by Judy Steed, *The Globe and Mail* 6 February 1984.

[39] Donald Weitz in *The Globe and Mail* 6 February 1984.

[40] See Ontario Ministry of the Attorney General, "You've Got a Friend," Report of the Review of Advocacy for Vulnerable Adults, 1987 published by Ontario Ministry of the Attorney General.

[41] Interview, Dr. Tyrone Turner.

[42] Psychiatrists are organized in the Ontario Psychiatric Hospitals and Hospital Schools Medical Staff Associations, and the general hospital psychiatrists in the Association of General Hospital Psychiatric Services.

[43] D. L. Rosenham, "On Being Sane in Insane Places," *Science*, 179 (1973): 250–258.

PART IV: CONCLUSIONS

14

Conclusion

> The public system of social assistance and insurance, grotesquely inadequate as it is, is the only framework which relates to the mass of the population. Almost every pressure group and campaign in the modern era which works seriously towards the goal of betterment in health and social welfare has to pose its objectives in terms of demands upon the state.
>
> Peter Sedgwick in Psycho Politics, *1982*

Incrementalism versus planning

In March 1987, the provincial auditor severely criticized almost every aspect of Ontario's mental health care program. The auditor noted a number of "significant problems in the psychiatric hospitals," including a "stressful work environment, below standard facilities," and the fact that 25 percent of patients might have been released from hospital if alternative care facilities had been available in the community. He also observed that the "psychiatric hospitals are becoming clogged with occupancy rates averaging 90 percent." Things were not much better in the community. The Homes for Special Care Program did not provide rehabilitation services to patients and "did not promote patient independence." Because of the tight housing market in Ontario's urban centers, there was a severe lack of affordable housing for discharged patients, while the existing boarding and rooming houses, "from a rehabilitative point of view...were unsuitable." Although the auditor recommended that more patients should be discharged to community care, he also noted that "even given [a] significant increase in funding, there was still a serious lack of adequate community services in the Province." Finally, he criticized the Ministry of Health because it "did not have the comprehensive information system needed to collect sufficient data either for managing existing facilities and services or for planning new ones."[1]

Thus, almost sixty years after Dr. B. T. McGhie inaugurated the approved homes program and four decades after his unsuccessful proposal for a comprehensive system of community mental health care, Ontario's mental health system was still unbalanced, with the psychiatric hospitals and the psychiatric units predominating over a weak community mental health care system.

Table 14.1 shows the proportion of mental health expenditures devoted to provincial psychiatric hospitals, community mental health programs and psychiatric units. Despite hospital closings during the 1970s, the proportion of total

Table 14.1*
Mental Health Expenditures as a Percentage of MOH Expenditure (Distribution of mental health expenditures across three major health programs in parenthesis)

Units	Psychiatric Hospitals	Grants to Community Mental Health	Psychiatric Units in General Hospitals
74/75	4.9 (39.3)	2.1 (17.0)	2.0 (16.5)
75/76	4.7 (37.8)	2.19 (17.4)	2.27 (17.6)
76/77**	4.3 (36.4)	1.90 (16.1)	2.27 (19.1)
77/78	4.1 (37.2)	.98 (8.9)	2.40 (22.1)
78/79	4.0 (36.9)	.65 (6.1)	2.64 (24.3)
79/80	3.9 (36.0)	.70 (6.4)	2.58 (23.2)
80/81**	3.8 (35.9)	.66 (6.3)	2.36 (22.3)
81/82	3.9 (37.7)	.30 (2.8)	2.54 (24.0)
82/83	4.0 (38.4)	.34 (3.3)	2.28 (21.8)
83/84	3.8 (37.8)	.39 (3.8)	2.25 (21.8)
84/85	3.7 (36.8)	.51 (5.0)	2.22 (21.9)
85/86	3.6 (36.9)	.44 (4.5)	2.16 (22.0)
86/87	3.4 (35.2)	.48 (4.9)	2.18 (22.5)

(*) Statistics from Ministry of Health, Information Resources and Services *Branch, Regional Allocation of Estimated Expenditures on Mental Health Services by Ministry of Health,* fiscal years 1974/75 to 1986/87. The Ministry breaks down mental health expenditures into 10 separate categories, three of which, psychiatric hospitals, community mental health programs and general hospital psychiatric units, are included in this table. Omitted are OHIP payments, alcohol and drug programs, homes for special care, local health agencies, grants to associations, research grants, and health resources development.

(**) In 1976/77 children's mental health was transferred to MCSS, while after 1980/81 a number of items previously included under community mental health were transferred to a different category.

mental health funds devoted to psychiatric hospitals declined only slightly from 1974/75. However, the psychiatric hospitals got slightly less of total Health dollars almost every year after 1974/75. Expenditures on psychiatric units rose until the 1978/78, held fairly steady for a few years, declined slightly and have held again on a slightly lower plateau.

Since 1930, reports on the mental health system had warned of serious problems and proposed the establishment of a community mental health system, but governments always adopted short-term measures in response to immediate problems. Not once in the half-century under consideration did the government attempt to formulate and then implement a coherent long-term plan for mental health services in Ontario. For more than half a century, incremental politics has been the order of the day in mental health policymaking.

For some scholars, the lack of a long-term plan is not only not a cause for alarm, but is a positive virtue. Braybrooke and Lindblom argue that wide-ranging, comprehensive decision-making is irrational and dangerous to democracy: irrational, because plans have to be based on current values and it is impossible to predict what values people will hold in the future; dangerous to democracy because rigidly adhered-to plans may lead eventually to wrenching dislocations of existing processes and institutions.[2]

Although Braybrooke and Lindblom are highly skeptical of the possibility or wisdom of nonincremental politics, or what they call "synoptic" or "utopian" styles of decision-making, there have been occasions in Canada when coherent, long-term and radical reforms have been successfully carried through.[3] Health and hospital insurance in Saskatchewan, Medicare at the federal level, the reform of mental health care in Quebec in the 1960s and the reform of mental retardation policy in Ontario in the 1970s are just a few examples.[4] Thus, one must be cautious about assuming that incrementalism is inherent to, or is functional for democracy and see it for what it is, a style of decision-making that reflects political and ideological values.

One way to look at the issue of incremental versus synoptic styles of decision making is to approach the question hypothetically. Since 1930, a myriad of suggestions for reforming mental health services have been put forward. If we ask whether the mental health system would be better or worse off now if those schemes had been implemented, the answer is that it would probably be better off. In only one area—recommending an expansion in psychiatric hospital bed capacity—did some of the early reports go wrong. On the other hand, without exception, every major proposal recommended the establishment of a coherent, integrated and multifunctional network of community services—something we have yet to see in Ontario. After the 1950s, every scheme recommended a reduction in the size of the large provincial hospitals and their divestment to some sort of community board. Most recommended the establishment of community mental health boards to link community care services with provincial hospitals and the psychiatric units. Thus, contrary to the proponents of incrementalism, synoptic planning does not always misjudge the values or needs of future generations, nor, when examined retrospectively, were they prescriptions for disaster. If at some time in the past the government had attempted to formulate long-term plans it is likely that exercise would have led to wider debate and to greater participation by involved parties in policymaking than has hitherto been the case. Synoptic, long-term planning is neither irrational nor contrary to democracy. Why, then, has incrementalism carried the day?

There are a number of explanations.

Politicians have notoriously short time horizons—in interview after interview, bureaucrats, psychiatrists and mental health professionals complained that the

Minister of Health and the government of the day never planned more than four years in advance, that is, until the next election. Bureaucrats said Ministers of Health were interested in mental health policy only when the opposition parties raised tough questions in the legislature, or when the *Globe and Mail* or the *Toronto Star* carried articles exposing a scandal or publicizing defects in the mental health system. In that case, the deputy minister had to immediately prepare a response for the legislature and the press. Mental health policy might suddenly emerge as a priority—but only as long as it took to resolve a crisis. Otherwise, it was generally ignored.

Moreover, there was no powerful pressure group in the community to speak up for mental health. In the general health care system medical doctors, hospitals and business pressure groups connected with medicine have a profound influence on policy and restrict the freedom of action of the Ministry of Health. By contrast, in mental health policy the absence of important interest groups, at least until the early 1980s, meant that mental health policy was peculiarly subject to the personality and views of whoever happened to be the Minister of Health. If the Minister of Health was not overly interested in mental health policy—which was the case with virtually all Ministers of Health until Dr. Dymond arrived in 1958—then mental health policy was of low priority, and mental health expenditures were used, among other things, to boost political support for the government. But even if the minister wanted to formulate a coherent policy he might run up against formidable structural obstacles.

Every component of the political-bureaucratic system at Queen's Park has an interest in perpetuating the status quo. What to the outsider looks like a lack of coherence or even chaos, to the insider looks orderly and rational. Most politicians see their main task as ensuring their own and their party's re-election. If funds become available for, say, the construction of a large provincial hospital, then a politician who has no personal interest in or commitment to mental health might see it as his/her job to get that institution built in an area where it will create jobs and win political support for the party. Policymaking may also be confused when different ministries try to achieve different objectives in the same policy field. The Ministries of Health and Public Works both participated in mental health policy. But the major objective of Public Works was to build large, inexpensive institutions which would be of political benefit to the government, while Health wanted institutions which would provide a beneficial therapeutic environment for mentally ill people. An institution which might look like a failure to Health might turn look like a resounding success for Public Works.

If, as was usually the case with mental health policy, there are no pressure groups powerful enough to force politicians to take account of the needs of mentally ill people—the fact that the projected institution is miles from the nearest town and therefore provides the worst kind of therapeutic climate for the residents, that it is too big, that it is ugly, poorly designed, even inhumane—if no person or group is powerful enough to threaten political penalties, then the original decision will stand. The lack of outside pressure groups or of an ideological commitment to mental health by the government also means that mental health will lose out in the complex negotiations that take place in the corridors of power over the allocation of funds.

The expenditure process

Some insight into how funds are allocated can be gained by looking at the expenditure process under the Tories during the 1970s, after the implementation of the COGP report.

The higher levels of government—Premier, Cabinet, the Treasurer and other bodies decided on the allocation of funds among the various ministries. Then individual ministries battled over the distribution of funds amongst intraministerial programs and services. The allocation of funds to the various ministries began with Management Board, which was created as a result of the COGP report. Management Board consisted of ministers from the various policy fields, the Minister of Finance and Intergovernmental Affairs and the Minister of Revenue and Government Services. Its job was to prepare a rough forecast of how much the government could spend assuming no increase in the provincial budget. While Treasury officials would prepare forecasts of expected future provincial revenue and costs, the ministers would prepare their budgets, submitting a statement of what they would need in order to continue operating at the same level as the previous year, the appropriate increment for the cost of living, how much they would need for past commitments that would require additional funds, and then any extras needed for the year.[5] This process could begin as early as March. The information would go to Management Board and later to the Policy and Priorities Board which, according to Hugh Segal "would take a first cut...and recommend total allocations for each of the three policy fields plus those ministries not operating within a formal policy field, and return these to the secretariats."[6] The policy secretariats would then arrange meetings with the various ministers in the policy fields and intense negotiations would take place over budgetary allocations for the individual ministries in the field. According to Segal it was at the secretariat level that trade-offs would occur in the Social Development field between Health, Education and the Ministry of Community and Social Services. Then the budget would go back to the Policy and Priorities Board which would produce a statement of the estimates for the next fiscal year. By December, Management Board would go to the various ministries and discuss specific budgetary figures.[7] But even by this late date, the budgetary process would continue. As ex-deputy minister of health Graham Scott put it:

> There is constant lobbying on a whole series of fronts. Let's say we have gone through the process and the budget is struck, you have to come back with detailed estimates in January, you then use that to signal that the world is coming to an end. Usually the minister and the deputy and some senior assistant deputy ministers go to fight. The minister fights it on a policy level and the civil servants supply facts and figures.

This process is not quite as unemotional as it might seem. According to Scott: "You ask them how many more broken windows they want in Parkdale. How much more they want the Solicitor-General to have to provide for the police to deal with the problems in Parkdale. You might suggest that blood is going to run in the streets." Since Management Board always has funds in reserve, if a particular Ministry can make a good case, funds will provided for pressing needs.

This raises the question of the basis on which trade-offs occur, that is, what determines whether money originally intended for Education, for example, goes to Health, or vice versa. Talking about the late 1970s, Graham Scott says: "In terms of deinstitutionalization, public concern helped policymakers in shifting resources at a time when there wasn't much discretionary money floating around in government. There were stacked up projects on the waiting list and a low priority like mental health on the public mind wasn't going to the top of the list. But public concern and recognition of the problem...made money available that otherwise wasn't going to be available and came out of the hides of other ministries for some projects that had been waiting for a long time."

The availability of funds was also subject to the vagaries of the provincial economy.

> When the Ministry puts in its budget, it says we need this amount to do what we did last year and this amount as the appropriate increment for the cost of living and then this amount for extra commitments coming home to roost. Normally, you get two kinds of answers: "We didn't fund any of those extras you asked for, but if revenues look up during the year then we might come up with the money." Or, if construction is down they may beef up their capital expenditures during the year and suddenly a "no" to the new wing at, for example, Brockville becomes a "yes" if there is more money and they want to stimulate the construction industry in eastern Ontario.

But even after the budget was cleared through Management Board and Policy and Priorities, this was by no means the end of the allocation process, for as Hugh Segal points out, "the personal style of Premier Davis meant that, despite the bureaucratic and political processes in place, every minister sensed that he or she had a direct line of appeal to Cabinet and to the Premier personally in the event the whole process did not produce a result that was responsive to his or her own view of political or departmental priorities." According to Segal this process of appealing to the Premier could go on until November. Finally, extra funds could sometimes be obtained from a sympathetic Treasurer. Larry Grossman maintains that while he was Treasurer from 1983 to 1985 he "threw some money mental health's way." One ex-deputy treasurer states that sometimes extra funds of hundreds of millions of dollars can be made available for programs which are politically necessitous and which were not sufficiently funded when the ministry's budget was established. At one point this senior civil servant states he begged the Ministry of Social and Community Services to establish province-wide centres to deal with child abuse, promising a nearly blank cheque for funds.

But officials said they needed more studies, and they never took advantage of the offer.[8]

Even after an individual ministry's budget is established, lobbying for additional funds continues. Now, instead of battles between the ministry and Management Board, the conflict shifts to within the ministry. Here the battle can become extremely heated, as civil servants fight to protect their own programs while at the same time trying to force cuts in programs competing for funds. In this process policy arguments can quickly degenerate into internal wrangling and back-biting, and ultimately lead to resentment or to personal feuds.

Usually, the minister makes the final decision on intraministry allocations, although he is expected to keep Management Board and the Treasury informed of changes. For example, during his seventeen months as Minister of Health, Larry Grossman was able to use a number of techniques to put several million dollars into mental health services. In some cases he used money from areas that were underspent, in other cases he took money intended for one program and redirected it toward mental health. One civil servant pointed out that Grossman was able to increase subsidies for housing for ex-psychiatric patients even though the money was not available in that year's budget since he knew that the actual financing would not have to be done until two or three years down the road.[9] Moreover, if money does not have to be spent until the following year then cash flow can be used for a project before it has to be accounted for in the following year—when additional funds might become available to cover the deficit. Dr. Boyd Suttie, a former assistant deputy minister in the Ministry of Health stated that "the assistant deputy ministers in any ministry know where the little money pots are hidden and whether as the fiscal year draws to a close, there is a surplus to cash flow requirements...the assistant deputy minister level is one of the most influential because he or she controls and knows the resourcing of past, present and future decisions, and this is particularly the case if tenure goes beyond two or three years." According to Dr. Suttie, an informal process of negotiation often takes place within the ministries between the assistant deputy minister for finance and the other assistant deputy ministers. There is frequently some money available either from current cash flow, from underspending in one or another area of a ministry, or even from a small inaccuracy in forecasting which, in a budget as large as, for example, the Ministry of Health can mean a surplus or a shortfall of millions of dollars. Since the assistant deputy minister for finance knows about these sources, it is sometimes possible to come up with money for a new project or additional funds for an on-going project which is a priority for the minister or the ministry's management team. However, in the end, outstanding accounts have to be settled. When Management Board realized what Grossman had done, it forced Health to restore the funds—although, ironically, it appears that after the Liberal government took power, it decided to return the funds to mental health.[10]

As is the case with the deputy minister, the assistant deputy minister has obligations to his own ministry and, through Management Board to the government. He must be convinced that allocating additional funds is not only in the interest of the ministry, but in the interest of sound government as well. In order to do this, assistant deputy ministers will try to convince the minister to throw his weight behind a particular project and program, and if successful in doing so, can then use this to lobby the assistant deputy minister of finance for additional funds.

It is also possible to reallocate money from one program to another within a ministry. According to Tom Campbell, during the 1970s, Management Board was quite tolerant of such moves and would often provide retroactive authorization.[11] Larry Grossman shifted funds around within the Ministry of Health without obtaining approval from any outside body. This occurred in 1982 after Grossman decided to give priority to mental health policy and to improve aftercare services. By diverting money from programs within the Ministry of Health to mental health, and by tapping the large amounts of discretionary funds available to the deputy minister he was able to increase substantially funding for diverse mental care organizations in the community. Moreover, by taking the risk of not keeping his colleagues abreast of his maneuvering, he ensured that he could keep the promises he made to voluntary organizations and pressure groups fighting for improved services. However, Grossman states that if there had been some criticism from within government, from his ministerial colleagues, for example, he is certain the Premier would have supported his initiatives. But he never had to ask the Premier to intercede for him since he achieved his objectives without any of his colleagues raising serious objections.[12] A recent assistant deputy minister in Health expressed surprise at the loose control exercised by central agencies over the various ministries. His experience in other jurisdictions was that the government and central agencies kept a tight grip on policy and expenditure, while in Ontario such control was perfunctory.[13]

All this indicates that published statistics on government expenditures cannot be taken literally. Statistics show a continued decline within the Ministry of Health of expenditures on mental health from 1974/75 to 1986/87. (See Table 14.1) Yet not only Grossman, but civil servants who worked in Health during the early 1980s confirm that under Grossman there was a major expansion in mental health aftercare programs. Obviously, some funds directed toward mental health do not appear under mental health expenditures, but under other, non-mental health categories. Thus, statistics indicate trends, not absolute expenditures. The hidden budgetary process tells us that government expenditure policies are never engraved in stone. No matter what any minister says, if a pressure group can put up enough fuss, if a particular issue catches the attention of the press, if the government senses the opposition parties are gaining ground in their criticism, or if key officials such as the deputy treasurer can be convinced of the need, then a previously unpopular or ignored policy may suddenly become the object of government largesse. There is always some room for maneuver on the budget. Of course, this begs the question of how pressure groups form around issues, why any particular issue becomes the focus of media concern and catches public attention, or why government will be more amenable to pressure on one issue as opposed to another. But there seems to be much more flexibility in the budgetary process than most people realize.

The Bureaucratic Process

Government's ability to bring about change is profoundly influenced by existing policy commitments. In the mental health field the dead hand of history weighs heavily on those who want to redirect policy. By the late 1960s and early 1970s it had become clear to policymakers that mental health policy could no longer be centered entirely around the psychiatric units and the provincial psychiatric hospitals, and that community care programs had to be added as the third pillar of the system. Yet the fact that nearly three-quarters of mental health expenditure went to the psychiatric hospitals and the psychiatric units constituted a formidable obstacle to a redirection of budgetary priorities toward community care. The psychiatric unit program could not be reduced because it was the centrepiece of the provincial community care program, while the provincial psychiatric hospitals were political hot potatoes which each Minister of Health tossed onto the lap of the next.[14] In 1968, the Minister of Health said: "We are certainly not going to put up any more buildings to make it bigger because the whole point of our exercise in mental health is to cut down the size of the institutions, but not to stupidly raze them if they are buildings which serve a useful purpose and I am quite certain the people of Ontario would never put up with that."[15] It is true that the province did close the Lakeshore Psychiatric Hospital in 1979, but that decision aroused enormous hostility and controversy and probably contributed to the fact that the government never again tried to close a large institution. Many of those interviewed mentioned that one of the principal reasons for the government's reluctance to contemplate closing the psychiatric hospitals was fear of the political backlash that would result from the damage inflicted on local economies and of resistance from the more than 7,000 staff members who belonged to the Ontario Public Service Employee's Union.[16]

Changes in the mental health system are also facilitated or impeded by the level at which demands are made. Whether or not a particular idea will become policy, or whether civil servants will even spend time thinking about policy alternatives depends on what level of the bureaucracy is assigned responsibility for specific tasks. If responsibility for mental health policy is set at the level of executive director of a branch or division, that is, below the level of deputy minister and assistant deputy minister, then it is less likely that mental health will be a priority than if mental health policy is the exclusive responsibility of, say, an assistant deputy minister. In the 1970s, negotiations over the Health budget took place in the Social Development Secretariat, the Policy and Priorities Board, or occasionally in Cabinet or with the Premier himself. Yet, from 1972 to 1982, the lack of a specific division or bureau to speak for mental health was a severe disadvantage. At the level of *nomenklatura*, therefore, the establishment of a mental health branch or division is a first step toward giving some coherence and visibility to mental health policy.

In a critique of the bureaucratic process, *Agenda for Action* noted that after the mental health division was disbanded, five major reorganizations of mental health services took place from 1972 to 1978. The result seems to have been near-chaos. Concerning the adult mental health planning team, it observed that "its self-perception is that of a voluntary group, with no authority, attempting to bring together some individuals within the Ministry concerned with mental health policy and program."[17] The report also noted that it had "extreme difficulty in determining the inter-relationships of the various groups within the Ministry relative to coordination of...planning." Plans were produced by the various branches within the ministry, but these were prepared separately and sent up the chain of command with little or no prior consultation or coordination.[18] The result was that "an ad hoc situation relying on results and activities determines priorities."[19] Of course, the presence of a specific department for mental health will to a certain extent guarantee high visibility for policy, but high levels of funding for, or improvements in mental health do not necessarily follow. One of the problems is that mental health policy encompasses disparate policy strands. The psychiatric units in general hospitals, for example, are funded by the hospitals and thus they are not taken directly into account during the mental health expenditure process. Moreover, unless there is some commitment to mental health on the part of government, the presence of a mental health branch or division will have little impact on policy. In the absence of such a division, there is little chance that mental health programs will get much attention. On balance, though, the existence of a specific mental health organization does at least provide a focus for outside pressure groups, the media and consumers.[20]

Mental Health Politics

Beginning in the late 1960s in North America there was a secular decline in the number of inpatient beds in mental hospitals. In Ontario the decline in inpatient beds began in earnest in the 1960s, and it has continued inexorably since then. Many of those discharged from the psychiatric institutions were transferred to residential units in the hospitals and then to the homes for special care. By this time, Health defined community care as referring to the psychiatric units in the general hospitals and to the Homes for Special Care Program. Few people in Health thought of aftercare in terms of providing suitable housing, recreation, vocational rehabilitation or counselling and referral services for ex-patients. Meanwhile, there was an increasing number of complaints about the presence of ex-patients in urban centres. Many of these ex-patients were poor and/or unemployed. Opposed in principle to providing public services except as a last resort, lacking any ideological commitment to community services for mentally ill people, the Progressive Conservative Government remained passive as ex-patients languished in the community, barely surviving on welfare, living in dirty or run-down boarding homes, prey to thieves and muggers or to their own disabilities and handicaps. Of course, this was not unique to Ontario since similar complaints were being heard throughout North America. Except during Grossman's tenure as Minister of Health, the Progressive Conservatives dragged their feet on the issue.

Is there something historically inevitable about the fate of mentally ill people? Could things have turned out differently? Although analogies are never identities, the inertia that characterized mental health policy during this time was in marked contrast to the developments in mental retardation policy. Since the early 1970s the government of Ontario had followed a coherent plan of deinstitutionalization and community care. Of course, the plan and its implementation were not perfect, but by the 1980s mental retardation services in Ontario were probably the best in Canada and among the best in North America.

What explains this difference? A number of reasons can be given.

No one contests the idea that in the 1970s and into the 1980s the Ontario Association for the Mentally Retarded was one of the most powerful pressure groups in Ontario and certainly the most powerful group speaking for the rights of handicapped people in Ontario. With an enormous and ramified provincial organization manned by devoted volunteers, supported by members of the business and cultural community, many with contacts at the highest levels of government, the OAMR enjoyed a degree of legitimacy and political influence clearly lacking to the CMHA or to the mental health self-help groups that had begun to spring up in the 1970s. Ironically, the OAMR seemed to gain in importance as it attacked the large mental retardation institutions, pressed the government to deinstitutionalize mentally retarded people and to establish community services.[21] In addition, unlike mental health policy where the government had successfully shelved every major report ever produced, the publication of the Williston Report in 1971 galvanized Robert Welch, Provincial Secretary for Social Development, into making major reforms in mental retardation policy in 1973.[22] By contrast, in the late 1970s and early 1980s, neither the CMHA nor the OMHA took the lead in criticizing the government for its lack of aftercare policies, but rather left the field to other pressure and self-help groups.[23] Indeed, many self-help groups criticized the Ontario Division of the CMHA for being too close to the government, especially in view of the fact that in the late 1970s and early 1980s approximately 75 percent of OMHA funds came from government. Thus, while the OAMR helped effectuate the transfer of mental retardation services from the Ministry of Health to the Ministry of Community and Social Services and helped establish a community care system, the mental health pressure groups were unable, despite all the publicity and public discussion in the 1970s, to bring about any major change in mental health policy. Until the 1970s, with the exception of the Ontario Mental Health Association, there were few pressure groups in the field, and they were generally small and politically weak. Although the CMHA claimed to speak for mentally ill people, almost all the civil servants and politicians interviewed agreed that the CMHA and its provincial and local branches were not taken seriously by government.

Ex-Minister of Health Larry Grossman stated that in the 1970s there was no constituency for mental health either within or outside government.[24] In their 1977 report on three provincial hospitals, the McKinsey and Company consulting firm noted that psychiatric hospitals were peculiarly vulnerable to budget cuts because their constituencies were "relatively small and have little political power" and because they tended to serve "society's forgotten and unwanted individuals."[25] Graham Scott, formerly deputy minister of health under Dennis Timbrell, Larry Grossman and Keith Norton says that any of the major general hospitals, Toronto General Hospital, or Etobicoke Hospital for example, have more political clout than the Ontario Division of the Canadian Mental Health Association.[26] According to Scott the public is not interested in the plight of the psychiatric hospitals and as a result it is extremely hard for even the most sympathetic Minister of Health to get the Cabinet to provide funds for mental health policy.[27] When, in 1979, Minister of Health Dennis Timbrell was asked by Liberal MPP Sean Conway if, on the hypothesis that additional funds were available, he would still have decided to close the Lakeshore Psychiatric Hospital, Timbrell replied: "Obviously, I can't escape budgetary considerations; even if we were in a time when money was supposedly plentiful or boundless, every year you would still have to make a decision as to your priorities and where to spend the money available."[28] Implicit in Timbrell's reply was the assumption that funds for mental health were not a top priority in the Ministry of Health.

The relationship between political priorities and outside pressure can be illustrated by the following story about American President Franklin Delano Roosevelt. One day he met with representatives of various pressure groups to discuss a particular issue. At the end of their meeting, Roosevelt told them he was completely converted to their views and to their policy recommendations. "But," he said, "all you have to do now is go out and make me do it." As the anecdote makes clear, whether or not something becomes a political priority depends not only on whether one has made a convincing case, but even more on the political clout a particular constituency can muster.

Of course, it is hypothetically possible for policies to be formulated even in the absence of pressure, but in the case of mental health there were a number of factors which militated in favour of incrementalism. One of the most important was the tendency of governments to use mental health policy as a means toward economic or political goals which had little to do with the needs of mentally ill people. Because the Department of Public Works (now Government Services) determined the location, size and design of psychiatric hospitals, mental health bureaucrats were unable to make crucial decisions affecting the delivery of mental health services. Because the major budgetary decisions concerning mental health were made by the Treasurer and the Cabinet, and because the Minister of Health was not necessarily committed to any coherent view of mental health policy, mental health frequently subserved objectives which had little to do with the best interests of mentally ill people. A further obstacle to coherent planning and policy formulation derived from the fact that mentally ill people do not all necessarily come within the purview of the Ministry of Health. Once they left the institution, discharged patients who ran into trouble with the law would become the responsibility of the Ministry of Correctional Services; those who had trouble finding housing or who were forced to live in inadequate rooming houses came to the attention of the Ministry of Housing; while those who were forced to go on welfare fell under the aegis of the Ministry of Community and Social Services. The obvious solution, and it was one proposed by the Committee on Mental Health Services in 1979, was the establishment of interministerial committees. But these committees are notoriously ineffective. If they are constituted at a low or middle level of the bureaucracy, then those who staff them are often unable or unwilling to commit their ministries to a course of action, while high level committees often come to grief because ministers or their deputies are reluctant to fund or take responsibility for clients who they think are the responsibility of other ministries. By the early 1980s, however, because of incidents at the Queen Street Mental Health Centre, the increasing presence of ex-patients in urban centres, and negative press coverage, mental health policy had emerged as a major social policy issue.

For years the Ministry of Health had defined community care in terms of the psychiatric units in the general hospitals and the homes for special care. But now there was immense pressure on government to do something. It was at this point that Larry Grossman entered the scene, declared that the Ministry of Health was the lead ministry in mental health matters, tried to help change public perceptions of mentally ill people (by giving funds to the Ontario Division of the Canadian Mental Health Association for a publicity campaign), actively promoted the establishment of independent pressure groups and advocacy agencies, and established the patient advocate program in the provincial psychiatric hospitals. Although Grossman made some structural changes in policy and increased the number of housing units for mentally ill people, community mental health continued to suffer from underfunding.

Nor did major changes occur in the psychiatric hospital system. One of the most puzzling aspects of mental health policy is that while there has been near-unanimous support for divestment of the provincial psychiatric hospitals, government has been reluctant to act. The benefits of divestment are clear: greater sensitivity to community needs, an improved and more flexible management structure, better possibility of recruiting qualified staff, and relieving government of having to take responsibility for every fault or scandal in the provincial system.[29] But against that the Ministry of Health has had to weigh the costs.

The Ontario Public Service Employees Union would have opposed divestment fearing loss of jobs, union benefits or even, ultimately, a move toward privatization of the provincial hospitals. There were concerns that if they were divested to local management boards, the provincial psychiatric hospitals would refuse to continue accepting a disproportionate number of chronic, severely ill, and violent or disruptive patients.[30] If divestment occurred the management boards would demand funds to improve conditions. In addition, some civil servants who worked in the psychiatric hospital sector opposed divestment for fear of losing their jobs, while some politicians saw the provincial hospitals as sources of political patronage. Moreover, according to Steve Lurie of the Metro branch of the Canadian Mental Health Association, if the psychiatric hospitals were divested to the community it would be practically impossible to drastically reduce their size or to close them as community boards would pressure publicly for increased funding and would resist closure or downsizing as happened in the case of the failed attempt to close general hospitals in the 1970s.[31] Whatever the reason, within and without government there was very little political pressure to move toward divestment. John Maynard, formerly director of the psychiatric hospitals branch in the Ministry of Health says that in the 1970s he was given a mandate to begin the process of divestment. "The word came from the deputy minister and then through the assistant deputy minister of institutional health services... The mental health people were set up to go in that direction, the thrust was in that direction... They said carry on, keep pushing the community advisory boards—but there was no great pressure on us to do it."[32] One explanation for this lethargy is that the government and the various Ministers of Health have paid lip service to divestment, but given the low level of management and the poor conditions in the psychiatric hospitals as well as the rudimentary state of the community advisory boards, it was thought best to wait until the success of the shift could be assured.[33] Whatever the reasons, there was no great outside political pressure for divestment, nor did any Minister of Health make divestment a top priority.

Ideology and Mental Health

Another obstacle to reform in the mental health system is ideology.

From 1943 to 1985, the province of Ontario was governed by the Progressive Conservative Party, and if the ideology of the PCs continues to baffle even the most sophisticated observer, it would be wrong to assume that it had no impact at all.

The ideology of any political party can be visualized as a building punctuated with windows, doors and access ramps. The windows allow those on the outside to look in and those on the inside to look out. The doors open to invited guests and the ramps make it easier for particularly favoured guests to enter. Each political party's ideological structure is designed differently from another. That is, some individuals and groups on the outside find it easier to look into, or get access to the building than other groups. In interviews with civil servants and with Progressive Conservative politicians, one theme recurred—regret over the fact that more funds could not be spend on mental health policy and blame for the public for not pressing harder for expenditures. These views were honestly expressed—those interviewed were genuinely sorry that more funds were not allocated and most of them had fought as hard as they could to increase expenditures. There is also some truth to the lament about public indifference, for the public is generally not interested in or particularly sympathetic to mentally ill people or to ex-patients. However, if one looks at the structure of Progressive Conservative ideology over the past four decades, there was little sign of windows, doors or ramps providing access to mental health groups. That is, the structure barred rather than eased the way for mental health issues to become an important part of Progressive Conservative ideology. Although a scholarly study of that remarkable party has yet to be written, one thing is clear: the PCs did not put mental health policy at the top of their political agenda. Although they were not resistant to change, they had to be pushed and unless pushed would do little else than keep pace with what was happening in other progressive jurisdictions in North America. "Progressive" jurisdictions because in that mysterious osmotic way that seems to have been the secret of their success, the PCs were extraordinarily skilled at adopting ideas from other parties if they thought they would gain rather than lose political support. Of course, one might say the same of any other political party, but with this difference—it is hard to establish what were the limits to the PC ideology.[34] In contrast to other jurisdictions, the Ontario Tories were so much the natural party of government, indeed they *were* the government, that given enough pressure or the perception of difficulties on the horizon, suitable policies would be adopted no matter what their provenance—within limits, of course, for there were limits. The Tories never did countenance changing the Planning Act so as to force municipalities to allow group homes for ex-psychiatric patients in residential neighbourhoods. Nor did they ever contemplate spending vast sums of money on mental health community care facilities. Nor were they interested in decentralizing decision-making responsibility for mental health policy to psychiatric hospital boards or community mental health centers. But who can doubt that if the PCs felt they could win support in Metropolitan Toronto by embarking on a crash program of aftercare, that they would have implemented an aftercare policy? After all, exactly that policy was followed with regard to mentally retarded people without major repercussions in society or the party.

Put another way, the PCs raised incrementalism almost to the level of ideology. As one assistant deputy minister with wide experience in other jurisdictions put it, "the Ontario bureaucracy is the most cautious in Canada." He was amazed at the step-by-step nature of decision-making, the absolute refusal, or perhaps inability, to make any long-term strategic plans or to contemplate any kind of radical change in the system. And he concludes that this style of decision-making was both characteristic, and partly the reason for the success, of the PCs.[35]

It is also argued that one reason for the stop-and-go nature of Tory decision-making in mental health can be found in public indifference to mental health policy. But public opinion is a two-way street; political parties are the objects, as well as partly the creators of public opinion—they are not merely passive receptors of public opinion and public pressure. As well as providing access to outside pressures, the doors and ramps in the party's ideological structure permit the troops to leave the building and do battle in society. However, with some exceptions, the Progressive Conservative troops did not win fame battling to improve conditions in the psychiatric hospitals, to eliminate or ameliorate the two-tier system that differentiates the psychiatric hospitals from the psychiatric units, or to expand and improve services to ex-psychiatric patients in the community. The party's windows faced on to different perspectives, and their doors and ramps were largely inaccessible to mental health issues.

Thus, the 1980s was a period of consolidation rather than of rapid change. The mental health care system was like a slanted tripod, sitting on two firm legs and one spindly one. Despite the continued increase in absolute dollar expenditures on mental health policy, the provincial psychiatric hospitals and the psychiatric units got the lion's share of funds, with aftercare and community services coming a poor third. Unlike mental retardation policy which had undergone a revolution both in the way the problem was conceptualized, (with mental retardation no longer defined as an illness but as a condition) and in administrative responses (from a medical-hospital model of care to a normalization-residential model of care), mental health policy seemed unable to break loose from the mold that had congealed in the late 1960s and 1970s. Certainly, the antipsychiatric revolution had undermined psychiatric authority. One has only to compare the legal rights of mentally ill people in the 1960s with their rights in the 1980s to see how much, in the sphere of law, things had changed.[36] But in the political arena, mental health policy still aroused little interest or passion.

In the 1980s there was a double movement. On one side the Ministry of Health began to marginally improve community services, especially housing, for mentally ill people and ex-patients. During this time there was an explosion in the number of self-help and voluntary groups working for mentally ill people. On the other side, ratepayers' associations and the municipalities resisted extending community services and housing into neighbourhoods. Whereas pressure groups fighting for mentally retarded people won their great victories in 1974, groups fighting for mentally ill people made some tactical gains, but they won no great battles. Despite the unanimous recommendations of every consultant, expert or academic that the provincial hospitals be divested to community boards, the psychiatric hospitals were still run from Queen's Park. Despite the obvious crying need, the proportion of mental health funds expended on community services continued, near the end of the 1980s, to rank fifth after the provincial psychiatric hospitals, psychiatric units, payments to physicians for psychiatric services and the Homes for Special Care Program. Despite continued complaints from outlying parts of the province, there remained major geographical inequities in the distribution of facilities and of manpower. Despite years of criticism, the Ministry of Health still seemed unable to work out a coherent plan for the future.

Ill-prepared, entered into from generous, or sometimes cynical motives, deinstitutionalization led to the release of thousands of ex-psychiatric patients from provincial institutions. Protected by laws which limited the ability of authorities to commit them involuntarily to a mental hospital, many mentally ill people wandered the streets dressed in rags, living in doorways and barely able to fend for themselves. Although one might have expected the public to react by demanding an expansion of community facilities, such has not been the case. Rather, an increasing number of psychiatrists, supported by the police and other authorities are asking for a relaxation of laws restricting involuntary commitment. Moreover, some people argue that running down the institutions was a bad idea, that the large provincial psychiatric hospitals have a crucial role to play in the mental health system, and that they should be expanded and improved.

In the midst of this, the government responded only half-heartedly to outside pressures. The major reforms of the Grossman era—the extension of community services, the establishment of the patient advocate system, the declaration that the Ministry of Health would be the lead Ministry in mental health matters, the upgrading of mental health by appointing an assistant deputy minister for mental health, marked a high tide for mental health policy in the 1980s. But the Progressive Conservative government left office with mental health policy still in a state of unplanned, uncoordinated and underfunded confusion.

A Way Out?

Is it possible to correct this situation? In principle, it is. In 1969, in his classic work on American liberalism, Theodore Lowi discussed the question: "Why liberal governments cannot plan."[37] The American system of separation of powers, an undisciplined political party system, enormously powerful interest groups, federalism, a reluctance to embody concrete standards in statute law, a preference for delegation of power and, above all, a public philosophy that is opposed to long-term planning are all obstacles in the way of any kind of coherent planning in the United States. But, in Ontario, few of these obstacles exist. We have a parliamentary system of government and coherent, disciplined political parties. Federalism is largely irrelevant because mental health policy is under the jurisdiction of the province while there is little evidence that the public would oppose long-term planning in mental health policy. But the Progressive Conservatives never used statutory instruments to set clear performance standards for the provincial psychiatric hospitals, the psychiatric units and community mental health services. We have already noted that in 1979 *Agenda for Action* complained about the lack of specific policy statements by government concerning definitions of mental health, mental health services or priorities in mental health care. One will search in vain for any statement of performance standards for mental health services in the current statutes of Ontario. The Mental Health Act is mainly concerned with establishing procedures and safeguards concerning involuntary commitment to psychiatric hospitals, while the Mental Hospitals Act is devoted to delineating the lines of authority between government and the hospitals, and within the hospital system. Yet it is not impossible for statutes to establish precise, substantive policy goals and the administrative structure to achieve these goals. For example, the Ontario Vocational Rehabilitation Services statute stipulates that:

> A rehabilitation program shall be established to provide a) goods or services to enable a disabled person to become capable of pursuing regularly a substantially

gainful occupation; b) services for the assessment of the individual medical, social and psychological needs of a disabled person and for the formulation of the vocational rehabilitation services likely to be required to meet his needs; c) rehabilitation counselling, including guidance and adjustment services, and assistance in obtaining and succeeding in, a substantially gainful occupation..."[38]

There is one very good reason why governments have been reluctant to include performance standards or service objectives in statutes—fear of legal action. As long as government mental health policy is confined to ministerial statements or the occasional Ministry of Health position paper then those dissatisfied with policy have no alternative but to seek changes through the political rather than the legal system. Of course, embodying positive entitlements in statutes is merely formal, the substantive provision of such entitlements will depend on the depth of government's commitment, on the degree of political pressure that can be brought to bear and on using the courts to enforce compliance with the statute. As Lowi puts it:

> Laws change the rules of the game. Laws make government an institution apart: a government of laws is not a simple expression of the political process. A good clear statute puts the government on one side as opposed to the other side, it redistributes advantages and disadvantages, it slants and redefines the terms of bargaining... Law sets priorities. Laws deliberately set some goals and values above others.[39]

It is not only the lack of substantive legislation that contributes to vagueness in policy; the lack of coherent, long-term planning is a major defect in policy. In a 1987 review of mental health services for Metro Toronto, the Canadian Mental Health Association observed that there was a "lack of an articulated and shared Provincial philosophy guiding the development of mental health services, resulting in fragmentation of services; no plan for Metropolitan Toronto to guide and assist service providers in planning and program development; no responsible local authority with accountability for managing the system [and] no generally accepted model of service."[40] Of course, long-term planning is not a panacea for all the problems of mental health policy. But the argument here is that many positive effects occur when government commits itself to long-term planning. First, all interested parties are forced to define their terms and clarify their objectives. This is particularly important in the field of mental health where contending ideas on mental illness, including the notion that mental illness does not exist, have serious and quite different political consequences. Second, the attempt to formulate a plan necessarily forces negotiation and compromise. Asking for the moon is easy when one does not have to make hard choices and resolve differences of opinion. Thus, participation in the planning process can bring groups and individuals into salutary contact with reality. Third, a democratic planning process means that real consultation and participation takes place. Fourth, planning increases political visibility. This can result in government paying more attention to a specific policy area and even to increased funding. Fifth, planning should aim to achieve exactly what planning means: the establishment of long-term objectives, greater coordination and integration of programs and services, continual monitoring of these programs and services, a clarification of administrative responsibility and, one would hope, participation at all levels of service consumers and interested groups.

But what if planning turns out to be impossible: if no agreement can be reached on definitions and concepts, if the division between service providers and consumers is too wide, if groups are not willing to make concessions in the process of negotiation and if government is unwilling to make any kind of commitment to implement the results of the planning process? Even an impasse in planning would be helpful, for it could lead to a reformulation of the parameters of mental health policy. It may be that the very terms "mental health" and "mental illness" are outmoded or no longer useful and that one will have to engage in a process of redefining and reconceptualizing the problem to be dealt with and the nature of the policy that is under discussion. If no compromise can be reached between interested parties then it might be that the lack of planning in the past had more to do with the problematical nature of mental health or mental health policy than with bad faith on the part of government or the indifference of the public. Finally, if the government refuses to carry through on the plan, then the question will be returned to the political arena where the struggle will continue in order to convince the public that mental health policy is a vital issue for our time.

Exactly how planning should take place in is up to the government. What is not needed is another report which tells us for the hundredth time that the mental health care system is unbalanced, that community care is underfunded, uncoordinated and in need of repair. What is badly needed is a coherent, long-term plan for change and a government that is, for the first time, seriously committed to righting the imbalance in the mental health system.

Notes

1 Office of the Provincial Auditor, *Annual Report of the Provincial Auditor of Ontario for the year ended March 31, 1987*, (Toronto: Queen's Printer, 1987) 78–89.

2 David Braybrooke and Charles Lindblom, *A Strategy of Decision* (New York: Free Press, 1963) 73ff.

3 For a critique of incrementalism as both a theory of decision-making and an ideology see Robert E. Goodin, *Political Theory and Public Policy* (Chicago: University of Chicago Press, 1982) 19–38.

4 On the politics of mental health in Quebec see Françoise Boudreau, *De l'Asile à La Santé Mentale* (Montreal: Editions Saint-Martin, 1984) 85 ff. On mental retardation policy see Harvey G. Simmons, *From Asylum to Welfare* (Downsview: National Institute on Mental Retardation, 1982) 192–215.

5 Interview, Graham Scott.

[6] Hugh Segal, "The Evolving Ontario Cabinet," in MacDonald, *The Government and Politics of Ontario* (Toronto: Nelson Canada, 1985) 73.

[7] Segal 73–74.

[8] Interview, Anonymous.

[9] Interview, Anonymous.

[10] Interview, Dr. Boyd Suttie.

[11] Interview, Tom Campbell.

[12] Interview, Larry Grossman. However, a highly placed civil servant who served in the Ministry of Health during this time thinks that Grossman did in fact eventually clear some of his initiatives with his Cabinet colleagues and with Premier Davis. Interview, Anonymous.

[13] Interview, Anonymous.

[14] In 1973, for example, there was some talk about closing the Whitby Psychiatric Hospital. At a meeting of the Psychiatric Hospitals Branch of the Ministry of Health, "Dr. Ives indicated that the preparation of in-house proposals regarding the future of Whitby Psychiatric Hospital presented problems in that experts would recommend phasing out over a period of three to five years, but the interim proposals and political ramifications would require careful review in so far as Whitby could be seen as a having major significance as a local industry." AO, RG 10–20-A–5, Psychiatric Hospitals Branch, Directors Reference Files 1968–1977, Volume 2.

[15] Dr. Matthew Dymond, in *Debates*, May 6, 1968, 2547.

[16] Figures on staff from *Agenda for Action* 118–119.

[17] *Agenda for Action* 149.

[18] According to one civil servant who entered the Ministry in 1978: "I came about the time Lakeshore was shut down and I have a vague recollection of some of the staff from the program development branch and from the program advisory branch having to go to a meeting to talk about the closure because no one else would go. I can still remember thinking this is the most asinine, ill-begotten idea and none of the honchos are around to take the heat and they send out staff that have nothing to do with the decision. I don't think there was really any central thinking about mental health and its effects on the health care system or what that system should look like until the mental health area was set up afterward." Interview, Anonymous.

[19] The McKinsey and Company Report also referred to organizational problems: "Organizationally... within the Ministry of Health currently fragmented responsibilities for the mental health system might be unified to provide both a managerial overview and a common process of funding." McKinsey and Company, "Role Study of Lakeshore, Queen Street and Whitby Psychiatric Hospitals," Volume I, 1978, p. 2–6.

[20] Assigning to a specific branch, division or ministry, responsibility for a policy can be interpreted as making a political statement. For example, if one agrees with the anti-psychiatrists that mental illness is a myth, and that those who officials call mentally ill are really people with a serious problems in living, then the task of policymakers should be to improve services provided by the Ministries of Health,

Community and Social Services, Correctional Services, and Housing, rather than establish a central mental health division.

21 By 1970 funds saved in the mental health area were being diverted to mental retardation. According to the minutes of a meeting of the mental health division "reallocation of funds from the review of the psychiatric hospitals forecasts...that approximately $249,260 would be surplus at the end of the fiscal year. It was agreed that $50,000 be set aside for unforseen expenses, $100,000 in reserve...and $100,000 to be reallocated to the Retardation Services Branch." RG 10, 20-A–5, Psychiatric Hospitals Branch, Minutes of Meeting of Mental Health Division, February 3, 1970.

22 Simmons 192–208.

23 Among the most vocal in support of mentally ill people were the Parkdale Activity and Recreation Centre, the London-based Self Esteem Through Independence, the Association for the Friends and Relatives of the Mentally Ill in Ottawa, Friends of Schizophrenics, the Supportive Housing Coalition and On Our Own.

24 Interview, L. Grossman.

25 McKinsey and Company I, 7–3

26 A familiar scenario appeared in 1988 when the Liberals tried to reduce hospital expenditures. The Ontario Hospital Association immediately mobilized public opposition, citing public opinion surveys showing the vast majority of Ontarians opposed to closing hospital beds and favoring increased government financing. The past chairman of the OHA also noted patients had to be put on waiting lists for scarce, expensive equipment. The next step was for human interest stories to appear in the press concerning patients whose lives were put at risk by cutbacks.

Whether the Liberals will be any more successful in reducing hospital expenditures than their predecessors remains to be seen. But the ability of the OHA and its allies to respond effectively and massively to government is in marked contrast to pressure groups representing the mentally ill. See "Tight Budgets Force Hospitals To Ration Services, OHA Says," *Globe and Mail* 18 October 1988.

On September 22, 1988, in a speech to hospital administrators, Ted Ball, former assistant to Larry Grossman said: "I know your traditional modus operandi. Having worked at the Ministry of Health and in the Treasury, I've had some opportunity to watch some of you up close." Ball then sketched a scenario where a "charismatic doctor" would talk a reluctant hospital board into acquiring an expensive piece of new equipment. The board would later find itself with a deficit. "The hospital would then turn around and label this deficit as a clear indication of 'government underfunding'—and a delegation would be dispatched to Queen's Park to talk turkey with the politicians. At those meetings, the government would be told that unless they covered this 'underfunding' by paying off the deficit, the hospital would have no choice but to cut back on certain services. They might even be forced to move the obstetrics ward onto the front lawn. Then the media would have a field day denouncing the government's 'heartless refusal to fund the hospital's properly.' Some people would call that blackmail. Well, that's exactly what it was." Quoted in *The Patient's Advocate* [Newsletter of the Patients' Rights Association] Fall (1988).

27 Interview, Graham Scott. Some American sources argue that because mental health care costs are diffused throughout the population, while benefits are clearly focused on specific providers such as trade unions or psychiatrists, mental health programs will be

"overly supplied" by the political system. It may be true that governments are reluctant to cut costs drastically by, for example, closing large institutions for fear of trade union or professional reaction. But it is also true that by the 1980s lay and professional opinion alike was still divided over the advisability of closing all large institutions and relying for mental health care exclusively on community care facilities and services. For a brief survey of the political economy literature on mental health, see Richard Frank and Mark S. Kamlet, "Nonmarket Resource Allocation in Mental Health Care," *American Behavioral Scientist* 30 (1986): 201–230.

[28] *Debates*, April 23, 1979, S–129.

[29] On divestment see Andrew Vaz, "The Divestment of Psychiatric Hospitals: Some Policy Considerations," MS, Health Administration, University of Toronto, December 10, 1984.

[30] See Vaz 20. The McKinsey and Company Report noted: "[A]vailable data—unfortunately less than is desirable—indicate that psychiatric hospitals treat the 'more difficult' to manage short-term inpatients." McKinsey and Company I, 3–3. Interview, Graham Scott.

[31] Interview, Steve Lurie.

[32] Interview, John Maynard.

[33] Interview, Anonymous.

[34] One of the problems in defining the philosophy of Conservatism is that Conservatives themselves have a hard time defining it, and even take pride in its amorphous quality. In many ways, the Ontario Progressive Conservative Party resembles the British Conservative Party before Margaret Thatcher. In *The Case for Conservatism* Quinton Hogg (Lord Hailsham) wrote that: "Conservatism is not so much a philosophy as an attitude," and he observed that Conservatives rejected all ideologies. Conservatism is "empirical and at times even frankly experimental." Quinton Hogg, *The Case for Conservatism* (London: Penguin Books, 1948): 13. One observer of English Conservatism wrote that one of its major characteristics was its ability to "absorb the bulk of what has become established practice." Robert Eccleshall, "English Conservatism as Ideology," *Political Studies* 25 (1977): 62–83. Conservatives of all stripes know that this political philosophy, or rather attitude, opens the Conservatives up to accusations of opportunism or mere pragmatism.

[35] Interview, Anonymous.

[36] However, there is some evidence that there has been a reaction against the extension of civil rights to mental patients. According to an American study, since the early 1980s most states had considered tightening the law on involuntary commitment while, by 1987, seven states had actually passed such laws. Frank and Kamlet 201–230.

[37] Theodore Lowi, *The End of Liberalism* (New York: W. W. Norton and Co., 1969) 101–190.

[38] Revised Statutes of Ontario, 1980, revised 1984, Chapter 525, section 5.

[39] Lowi 125–126.

[40] Canadian Mental Health Association, Metropolitan Toronto Branch, "Review of the Mental Health Service System in Metropolitan Toronto," June 1987, p. iii.

Postscript

> The development of community mental health programs is...a priority...we will meet every challenge in mental health in this province.
>
> *Murray Elston*, Minister of Health, before Ontario Legislature, November 20, 1985

Recent Developments in Mental Health Policy

I have argued that over the past half century, Ontario's mental health system has been weighted heavily toward institutions and psychiatric services in the general hospitals and against community services. In the concluding chapter I suggested that the government should move away from incremental policymaking and formulate a coherent, long-term plan for mental health policy. I further suggested that the province look into the possibility of embodying entitlements for mental health services in future legislation.

After taking office in 1985, the new Liberal Government took a fresh look at mental health policy. Two years after making the remarks quoted above, and while under attack from the NDP for the lack of community services, the Minister of Health said: "We have...a lot of work to do with respect to our community mental health services.[1] In 1988, the new Minister of Health, Elinor Caplan, confirmed the government's commitment to community mental health. "Our emphasis in the near future will be on community-based programs so that people can receive treatment in their own community. Our efforts will be directed toward providing a planned, coordinated mental health network across Ontario."[2]

Meanwhile, in the community, groups interested in community mental health services began to coalesce. In October 1985, after a meeting of program managers of community mental health programs, the Community Mental Health Programs Federation was established with representatives from 170 community mental health programs across the province. Since that time the organization has met with the Minister of Health and mental health bureaucrats, and it has pressured the Ministry to increase community mental health funding to 12 percent of total mental health funding—more than double expenditures for 1986/87. And, during the 1987 provincial election campaign, Premier David Peterson promised to increase spending on community mental health programs from $70.3 million to $130 million over the following three years.[3]

Thus, in the fall of 1987 major changes seemed impending in mental health policy. One hopeful sign was the appointment in October 1987 of a provincial community mental health committee, chaired by Robert Graham and composed of mental health professionals from government and consumer groups. The committee's job was to formulate an action plan for community mental health services in Ontario. Its report, *Building Community Support for People: A Plan for Mental Health in Ontario* appeared in July 1988.[4] There are two major ways in which the report demonstrates, for the first time, that the Ministry of Health has learned the lessons of the past and that it is seriously interested in reforming the mental health system. First, the report recommends developing long range plans for a "community-focused mental health care system."[5] Second, the report suggests that future mental health legislation specify entitlements for community mental health services, rather than embody the vague principles that typically characterize such legislation.[6]

There are many other positive aspects to the committee's report. It places priority on providing services to those with serious or prolonged mental illness, it suggests diverting funds from inpatient services to community services and it attempts to sketch an organizational framework within which planning will take place. It recommends the establishment of a provincial advisory committee on mental health to monitor planning and to serve educational and advocacy functions. And it raises the question of whether provincial hospitals should be divested to community boards.

Furthermore, the report sets forth an organizational scheme for democratic planning of mental health policy. At the local level district health councils are to consult with interested parties, assess local needs and services and then prioritize their options.[7] However, because psychiatric hospital catchment areas overlap different district health council jurisdictions, the plan proposes the establishment of six area mental health advisory boards composed of one representative from each of the constituent district health councils.[8] These area boards, it is assumed, will resolve conflicts that may arise amongst district health councils, and develop plans regarding hospitals, psychiatric units and local services. There is one additional feature of the area boards that is unstated, but is clearly implied in the report: because the area mental health boards would be devoted entirely to mental health issues, they could constitute formidable advocacy groups for mental health services. However, the government had not yet established the area boards. If the government decides to proceed with the action plan in the absence of the area boards, then the district health councils will be unable to deal with questions regarding the future of the provincial psychiatric hospitals or to properly coordinate services amongst psychiatric hospitals, general hospital psychiatric units and local community services. In addition, the absence of a specialized body dealing exclusively with mental health needs will deprive community mental health of an important voice in the Ministry of Health administrative structure.

There are other problems as well. As one moves up the organizational hierarchy sketched in the action plan, from district health council to area mental health advisory board, and from the provincial advisory committee to the Ministry of Health, the lines of responsibility become increasingly blurred. For example, the provincial advisory committee is supposed to review the annual reports of the district health councils and area mental health advisory boards to determine how much progress has been made toward implementing the plan. But it is unclear which office in the Ministry will have day-to-day responsibility for monitoring the plan and exactly how the provincial advisory committee fits the overall administrative structure of the Ministry. Although the Ministry is supposed to develop a multi-year plan for financing mental health services for community mental health, nothing is said about where in the Ministry this will occur, nor about the basis on which spending priorities will be established for the various components of the mental health system. At some point somebody is going to have to choose among competing priorities. Who that person will be and what office will be responsible is unclear.

Part of the problem is due to confusion about the outcome of the recent Ministry reorganization. In 1979, *Agenda for Action* commented unfavourably on the number of reorganizations that had taken place in the Ministry of Health and recommended the establishment of a single office with responsibility for mental health.[9] Shortly afterward a mental health division was established, headed by an assistant deputy minister. However, in 1988, deputy minister of health Dr. Martin Barkin eliminated the mental health division and the post of assistant deputy minister for mental health, and reorganized the Ministry according to a matrix model.[10]

As part of a Spenglerian cycle of policymaking where reorganizations and new organizational theories repeat each other endlessly, the 1988 reorganization recalls the 1970s when responsibility for mental health was scattered amongst a number of program areas in the Ministry.[11] Although the current deputy minister has assured his critics that matrix planning will increase efficiency by improving coordination and clarifying lines of responsibility, in the short run reorganizations cause disruption, confusion and a lowering in morale. According to Tom Campbell, former deputy minister of health under Dennis Timbrell, it takes about two years before the bureaucracy fully adjusts to a major reorganization.[12] Given the fact that reorganizations in the Ministry of Health occur on average every three or four years, the mental health bureaucracy may not have much time to reform the system before the next reorganization gets under way. Moreover, like so much in government, the Graham report breaks little new ground. Many of its proposals had been advanced in one form or another for years—in the early 1970s, for example, subcommittees of a task force on the reorganization of the Ministry of Health proposed reforms remarkably similar to those set forth in Graham. Thus, what is wanting are not proposals for reform but rather the political will to implement them.[13]

There are additional obstacles to reforming mental health policy. Much depends on funding. *Building Community Support for People* admits that total spending on mental health has declined as a proportion of government spending and that community mental health funding directed at people with serious or prolonged mental illness (exactly those people targeted by the proposed plan) declined in relation to total mental health spending. The report sketches four possible scenarios for future expenditure policies: a decline in institutional and hospital spending, a moderate increase in community mental health funding, an increase in mental health funding, and finding additional funds through cost-sharing with other ministries or levels of government. Significantly, nothing is said about turning to the private sector to provide additional services in community mental health.

As 1988 drew to a close, however, most of the news concerning the Ministry of Health reported growing concern about excessive spending on hospitals and health care. Whether this bodes ill for the prospect of increased funding for community mental health remains to be seen, but even if the government carries through on its good intentions, further obstacles will have to be overcome on the road to providing adequate community services. Neither the provincial psychiatric hospitals nor the psychiatric units will stand idly by if the government tries to improve community mental health services at their expense. Attempting to implement the proposed plan for community mental health services could bring about a confrontation between consumer and advocacy groups on the one side, and psychiatrists and trade unions on the other. This is particularly true in a climate where, as in the United States, there seems to be a rise in the number of patients treated in large facilities rather than in community mental health centres.[14] Reports from eighteen American states conclude that mental health professionals in the 1980s no longer see community care as a panacea for mental health problems and agree that state institutions will play a major role in mental health care for the foreseeable future.[15]

Mental Health Policymaking in 1989

Mental health policymaking has become more complex than at any time in the past. The small circle of decision-makers who made policy until the 1960s has disappeared and psychiatric authority has diminished. The entry of new forces into the field of political battle, the shifting nature of the pressure groups involved in policy, and the increased sophistication (or complexity) of the debate over the nature and implications of mental health and mental illness have led to heightened controversy over policy.[16] The media has become more alert to, and sophisticated in its understanding of mental health problems. Through deinstitutionalization and the establishment of group homes the public has become increasingly aware of the problems of mental illness and mental health. The implementation of the Charter of Rights and Freedoms has opened up new areas for legal interpretations and challenges of laws bearing on mental health policy.

Within the mental health system itself various forces contend for power. The Ontario Public Service Employee's Union complains about the underfunding of the provincial psychiatric hospitals and opposes any suggestion that they should be closed. Social workers and psychologists pressure government to give them increased authority and the right to bill the provincial health insurance plan for their services. Psychiatrists in the provincial hospitals complain bitterly about low pay while general hospital psychiatrists complain about lack of coordination between psychiatric units and the large hospitals, and the lack of community services. In these circumstances, the fight for improved community care will not take place in the realm of what is just or moral or fair. If that were the case, then there would be no difficulty in finding needed extra funds. Rather, the battle will take place in the political arena, and those advocating improved community care will have to marshall enough political support to force the government to do what, in 1989, it apparently wants to do. As is always the case in the long run, political clout is the *sine qua non* of success.

Finally, as we enter the 1990s, it is possible to draw some conclusions about policymaking in mental health.

First, the days of elite policymaking in mental health are past. No longer will policy emerge out of cozy deliberations amongst a small circle of politicians and mental health bureaucrats. The number of players in the mental health game has vastly increased since the 1960s and they all expect to have their say.

Second, mental health policy will no longer subserve the narrow political ends of the government in power. Although there is no guarantee that the best interests of mentally ill people, rather than winning political support, will be taken into consideration when the Cabinet or the Minister of Health decide where and how to spend mental health funds, there are too many groups looking after the interests of mentally ill people for those interests to be entirely ignored.

Third, as psychiatric authority has declined there has been a major increase in the number and variety of alternate therapies for mentally ill people.[17] Whether this will have an impact on the psychiatric unit system remains to be seen, but it does raise questions about the necessity for locating psychiatric units in general hospitals, and about the medical model of care that the psychiatric unit system implies.

Finally, in the unbalanced tripod of services, policy is moving toward increased support for community services. But, given the major obstacles that the community mental health movement must confront, its future success is by no means guaranteed.

Notes

1 *Debates*, June 15, 1987, p. 1385.

2 Interview in *Re-Action*, [published by the Metropolitan Toronto Branch of the Canadian Mental Health Association] Winter (1988): 4.

3 Exactly how Peterson arrived at the $70 million figure for 1985/86 is not clear. He may have combined the total expenditures for Community Mental Health and Grants to Associations as listed in the Ministry of Health's "Regional Allocation of Estimated Expenditures on Mental Health." In 1985/86 the government spent $41,379,177 on Community Mental Health and $27,871,190 on Grants to Associations. These two figures when combined with some other expenditures would provide the $70 million total.

4 The letter of submission describes the report as "an action plan." *Building Community Support for People: A Plan for Mental Health in Ontario* (Toronto: The Provincial Community Mental Health Committee, 1988).

5 *Building Community Support for People* 5.

6 On December 17, 1987, Bill 50, the Community Mental Health Services Act, received second reading. Proposed by New Democratic Party MPP David Reville, a former mental patient, Bill 50 sets forth substantive goals for community mental health services. "The system shall respond to the individual as a whole person, delivering the necessary type and degree of support without regard to age or degree of disability; each person shall be considered to be entitled to live and receive age-appropriate services in the least restrictive setting, consistent with the person's needs, potential and abilities; the system shall give to each person the maximum opportunity to participate in the mainstream of community life; the system shall monitor and flexibly adjust the supports and services it provides in order to remain appropriate and responsive to each person served by the system as the person's needs change..." Reville's bill differed from previous mental health legislation in providing for specific and positive entitlements to services. At the end of 1988 it was still before the legislature although it was expected to be replaced by proposed government legislation in the same area.

7 Time and again the report emphasizes the importance of consulting with consumers and family members. However, people are appointed to and serve as district health council members as representatives of organizations, not as individuals. For that reason the report suggests that consumer and family views be "sought through a variety of mechanisms, advisory groups, public hearings/meetings, individualized questionnaires and the direct participation of clients and families served by the programs." *Building Community Support for People* 61.

8 As early as 1943, B. T. McGhie had proposed establishing a regional or district structure for mental health services. And in his 1983 report, G. F. Heseltine recommended the establishment of regional mental health committees in the six health planning regions, as well as making other suggestions which found their way into the 1988 plan. On McGhie see Chapter 1, and on Heseltine see *Towards a Blueprint for Change: A Mental Health Policy and Program Perspective* 216–217.

9 *Agenda for Action* 147 ff.

10 Ministry of Health, "A Matrix Organization for the Ministry of Health," May 1988, 10 pages.

11 The phenomenon of cycles in both attention to, and program activity in, mental health policy is examined by David A. Rochefort in "Policymaking Cycles in Mental Health: Critical Examination of a Conceptual Model," *Journal of Health Politics, Policy and Law* 13 (1988): 129–152.

[12] Interview, Tom Campbell.

[13] See Chapter 8 for a discussion of the mental health reforms set forth by the various subcommittees of the reorganization task force.

[14] Robert Rich says that in New York State, officials report that "the de facto mental health policy is one of offering inpatient and outpatient care through the institution. The CMHCs only provide a small fraction of the services provided through our mental health system; the vast majority are provided through the hospitals." Robert Rich, "Change and Stability in Mental Health Policy," *American Behavioral Scientist* 30 (1986): 122.

[15] "The vast majority of respondents in seventeen...states...strongly agreed with the proposition that 'there always will be a need for public mental hospitals...'." Robert Rich, "Change and Stability in Mental Health Policy," *American Behavioral Scientist* 30 (1986): 117.

[16] For example, in early 1989, historian Ian Dowbiggin pointed out that those who argued for a genetic basis for schizophrenia might also support reinstitutionalization of the mentally ill and beefing up psychiatric hospitals. See Ian Dowbiggin, "Back Behind Closed Doors?" *The Globe and Mail* 23 January 1989.

[17] On this phenomenon and its repercussions for psychiatry, see Robert Castel, Francoise Castel and Anne Lovell, *The Psychiatric Society* (New York: Columbia University Press, 1982).

Interviews

The following people were interviewed in the course of this study. In some cases, individuals were quoted anonymously.

Jack Allen
Ron Ballantyne
Martin Barkin
G. Bartolucci
June Beeby
Ray Berry
Barbara Blake
Anna Bloom
Erhard Busse
Tom Campbell
J. Cleghorn
Jerry Cooper
David Corder
Roman Dale
Brian Davidson
John Deadman
Millie Dorsay
Jan Dukszta
Henry Durost
Matthew Dymond
Giah Eisenstein
Ronald Farmer
Stan Freeman
J. D. Griffin
Larry Grossman
Donald Gunn
R. Ian Hector
Barry Humphries
G. Anthony Ives
Jay Kaufman
Keith Kerns
Gregory Koval
Linda Kydd
Marcel Lemieux
Steve Lurie
Abbyann Lynch
Pat Lynes
Carla McKague
Tony McLean
Lawrence MacPherson
E. V. Margetts
John Maynard
Gordon Martin
Burdette McNeel
Abraham Miller
Brian Pell
John Pratten
Peter Prendergast
Naomi Rae-Grant
David Reville
Howard Richardson
C. A. Roberts
Graham Scott
Alf Sellars
Gilbert Sharpe
Boyd Suttie
Barry Swadron
George Szablowski
Dennis Timbrell
Tyrone Turner
Donald Wasylenki
Don Weitz

Ministers of Health, 1930–1988

Dr. Forbes Elliott Godfrey, April 17, 1924—September 12, 1930
Dr. John Morrow Robb, September 12, 1930—July 10, 1934
Dr. James Albert Faulkner, July 10, 1934—October 12, 1937
Harold James Kirby, October 12, 1937—August 17, 1943
Dr. Reginald Perical Vivian, August 17, 1943—January 7, 1946
Russell Temple Kelley, January 7, 1946—August 8, 1950
Dr. Mackinnon Phillips, August 8, 1950—December 22, 1958
Dr. Matthew Bulloch Dymond, December 22, 1958—August 13, 1969
Thomas Leonard Wells, August 13, 1969—March 1, 1971
Albert Benjamin Lawrence, March 1, 1971—February 2, 1972
Dr. Richard Thomas Potter, February 2, 1972—February 26, 1972
Frank Stuart Miller, February 26, 1974—February 3, 1977
Dennis Roy Timbrell, February 3, 1977—February 13, 1982
Lawrence Sheldon Grossman, February 13, 1982—July 6, 1983
Keith Calder Norton, July 6, 1983—February 8, 1985
Thomas Leonard Wells (Acting) October 11, 1983—December 5, 1983
Allan Pope, February 8, 1985—May 1985
Murray J. Elston, June 26, 1985—September 29, 1987
Elinor Caplan, September 29, 1987 -

Index

A

adult psychiatric services subcommittee, 148
advisory boards, 145, 147, 151, 185, 192, 206, 215, 254, 264-265
advisory committee on mental health, 41, 70, 87-88, 233, 264-265
Advocacy Resource Centre for the Handicapped (ARCH), 231
aftercare, x-xi, 38-39, 43, 47, 56-57, 61, 77, 93, 117, 161-166, 168-171, 173, 175, 198, 202, 248, 250-251, 255-256
Agenda for Action, 106, 181-186, 201-202, 205-206, 229, 250, 257, 265
Ajax, 173
alcoholism, psychosurgery to control, 214
Allen, Jack, 270
Alviani, Aldo, 192, 232
American Medical Association, 96
American National Committee on Mental Hygiene, 10
American Psychiatric Association, 18, 22
amnesia, 21-22
Anderson, Dr. Donald, 170, 181
anorexia nervosa, psychosurgery to control, 214
antipsychiatry, ix, xi-xii
approved home, 3, xi, 38, 49, 158, 227, 241
architecture, 127, 133
Archway, 198
attendants, 12, 27, 106

B

Baker, David, 231
Ball, Ted, 198, 233
Ballantyne, Ron, 173, 270
Barkin, Martin, 265, 270
Bartolucci, G., 270
Beeby, June, 270
Berry, Ray, 8, 270
Best, Dr. E.W.R., 205
Bill 19, 229-230
Bill 190, 231
Birch, Margaret, 169, 172
Blake, Barbara, 270
Bloom, Anna, 270
board of health, 40, 53, 162
boarding homes, 7, x, 48-49, 161, 170, 172, 174, 199, 227, 241, 250
boards of governors, 97, 106, 145, 152, 185, 189, 192
boards of health, 58
boards of review, 10
Boston Dispensary, 66
Braybrooke, David, xiii, 243
Breaugh, Mike, 232
Brillinger, Dr., 69
British Royal Commission on the Law Relating to Mental Illness and Mental Deficiency, 160
Brown, Dr. W.C., 112
Brown, Thomas E., 4
Browndale homes, 203
Brunelle, Rene, 166
Buck, Dr. C.A., 49
Building Community Support for People, 264, 266
Busse, Erhard, 270

C

Cabinet, 107, 109, 117, 141, 197-199, 229, 245-246, 249, 252, 267
California, 215, 217
Cameron, Dr. D.E., 68
Cameron, Dr. Ewen, 70
Cameron, Dr. G.D.W., 70, 87
Campbell, 270
Campbell, Tom, 152, 248, 265
Canada Assistance Plan, 116, 145
Canadian Association for the Mentally Retarded, 227
Canadian Civil Liberties Association, 228
Canadian Mental Health Association, 50, 90-91, 96-97, 166, 219, 226, 252, 254, 258
Canadian National Committee on Mental Hygiene, 10, 16, 37, 41, 47-48, 87, 90

Canadian Psychiatric Association, 75, 130, 216-217
capitalism, 157
Caplan, Elinor, 263, 271
Capponi, Pat, 197
Carscallen, Dr. H.B., 213
Censor Board, 25
certified patient, 225-227
Channing, Dr. Walter, 66
Charron, Dr. K.C., 118, 142, 144
Charter of Rights and Freedoms, 228
chemotherapy, 171
child care workers, 75, 131
Children's Aid Societies, 48
Children's Mental Health Centres Act, 204
children's mental health services, 183, 203
chronic care facilities, 167
chronic patients, 7, xii, xiv, 17-18, 21, 39, 49, 66, 70, 109, 112, 118-119, 133, 145, 158, 191, 199, 202, 212-213, 220, 253
cinema, 24
civil servants, 151-152, 192, 198, 218, 228, 235, 245, 247-249, 251, 254
Clarke Institute, 76, 106, 170-171, 173, 191, 198, 214
Cleghorn, J, 270
Cleland, Dr. C.A., 163
clinical psychologists, 131
Coates, D.B., 98
COGP
  See Committee on Government Productivity
Committee of Psychiatrists in the Armed Forces, 162
Committee on Government Productivity, 118, 141-144, 148, 151, 245
Committee on Legal Issues in Psychiatry, 231
committee on legislation and psychiatric disorder, 226
Committee on Mental Health Services
  See Tyhurst Committee
Committee on Psychiatric Services
  See Tyhurst Committee
Committee on the Healing Arts, 125
community care, 50, 60, 75, 88-89, 91, 93-95, 117, 127, 161, 165, 167, 169, 174-175, 182, 185, 189, 197, 199-200, 241, 243, 249-251, 253, 255, 259, 266-267
community health services
  assistant deputy minister, 193
Community Living for the Mentally Retarded
  See Welch Green Paper
community mental health board, 61
Community Mental Health Centers Act, 1963, 82, 89
Community Mental Health Programs Federation, 263
community mental health services, 40, 42, 50-54, 56-61, 69, 71, 73-76, 78, 89, 94, 96-97, 126, 128, 132-133, 135, 162-166, 168, 170, 184, 186, 241-243, 253, 255, 257, 263-267
community psychiatric hospitals, 65
Community Resources Consultants, 170
compression fractures of spine, 17
Concerned Friends of Ontario Citizens in Care Facilities, 231
consent, 15, 22, 24-26, 56, 213, 215-218, 225, 227-229, 232
consultative committee on mental health, 129
Cooper, Jerry, 270
Coordinating Committee for the Organization of the Department of Health, 148
Corder, David, 144, 270
courts, 226-227, 234-236, 258
Crawford, Lawrence, 167
Cumberland, Dr. T.D., 25, 105

D

Dale, Roman, 270
Davidson, Brian, 270
Davis, Norman, 192
Davis, William, 229
Dax, Dr. E. Cunningham, 219
Deadman, John, 270
decentralization, 148, 150, 153, 202
deinstitutionalization, 132, 152, 157, 160, 162-174, 181, 183, 187, 193, 199, 209, 246, 251, 256
Department of Health, 3, ix-xii, xiv, 16-20, 22, 24-25, 44, 47-48, 51-55, 57-61, 67, 69-75, 77, 87, 90, 103, 108-109, 111-112, 114-116, 118-119, 125, 127, 129-132, 135, 142-143, 146, 148, 150, 152, 163-165, 185, 204, 210-211, 213, 215, 219
  children services branch, 204
  medical rehabilitation branch, 164
  public health division, 58
Department of National Health and Welfare, 42
  mental health division, 42
Department of Public Works, 105, 109, 127, 133, 252
Department of Reform Institutions, 133
deviants, 4, 7, xi, 157
Diethelm, Dr. Oskar, 24
director of community mental health, 126
director of hospitals, 126, 213

discharged patients, 158-174, 181, 184, 186, 198-199, 219, 241, 250, 253
Discussion Paper, 1983, 202
district health councils, 151
divestment, 106, 148, 150-152, 185, 192, 205, 243, 253-254
Dorsay, Millie, 270
drug addiction, psychosurgery to control, 214
Dukszta, Dr. Jan, 184, 190
Duncombe, Dr. Charles, 201
Durost, Henry, 270
Dymond's "Magna Carta", 103-107
Dymond, Dr. Matthew B., xiv, 56-57, 75, 77, 97, 103-107, 109, 112, 116, 130, 134, 163, 194, 204, 227, 235-236, 244, 270-271

E

Easton, Dr. N.L., 16-18, 21, 24
Edlin, Dr. J.E., 17
Eisenstein, Giah, 270
elderly people, 38, 109-112, 114-115, 119-120, 133, 158, 167
electroconvulsive therapy
See electroshock
electroshock, 3, 16, 19-22, 25, 59, 213, 217, 219-220, 226, 232
Elgie, Dr. Robert, 229
Ellerton, Patricia, 192
Elston, Murray J., 263, 271
emotionally disturbed children, 78, 106, 108, 116, 131, 133-134, 145, 204
entitlements, 263
epilepsy, 210
Equality Rights Statute Law Amendment Act, 231
Established Programs Financing Act, 74
ex-patients, 61, 157, 161-162, 168-174, 197, 250, 253, 255-256

F

Farmer, Dr. R.A., 147, 150, 270
Farrar, Dr. C.B., 16, 67, 110
Faulkner, Dr. James A., 271
federal government, 36, 39, 42-44, 51-52, 67, 69-75, 77, 87-92, 96-98, 110-116, 118-120, 125, 130-131, 144-145, 218, 226, 243
fee-for-service, 188
Felix, Robert, 88
Ferrier, William, 108
Ferris, Dr. Albert W., 66
fever cabinets, 21
films, 15
Fletcher, Dr. D.R., 8, 10, 16, 110
Foucault, Michel, 65, 215
Frank, Dr. Frances, 193
Freeman, Dr. S., 8, 270
Freeman, Dr. Walter, 210
Friends and Associates, 232
Frost, Leslie, 71, 104, 108-109
Future Organization of the Psychiatric Services, 37

G

geriatrics, 110-111, 115, 202
Gigantes, Evelyn, 231
Globe and Mail, The, 170
Godfrey, Dr. Forbes E., 271
Goffman, Erving, 160, 209
Good, Dr., 66
Gorman, Mike, 88
Graham Report, xiii, xv, 264-265
Graham, Robert, 264
Great Britain, 210, 216, 218
Green, John R., 9
Greenland, Cyril, vii
Griffin, Dr. J.D., vii, 17, 25, 50, 90, 270
Grossman, Larry, 194, 197-200, 206, 233, 235-236, 246-248, 251-253, 257, 270-271
Group for the Advancement of Psychiatry, 88
group homes, 167, 169, 172, 174-175, 255
Gruenberg, Ernest, 160
Gunn, Donald, 270

H

halfway houses, 49, 161, 165-168, 174, 227
Hall Commission
See Royal Commission on Health Services
Hamilton, Samuel W., 10-14
Hamilton, Samuel W., 12
Handleman, Sidney B., 166
Hanly Report, 131-135, 146, 182, 187, 214
Hanly, Charles M.T., 125, 131-135, 146, 182, 187, 214
Health Insurance Act, July 1972, 118
Health Protection and Promotion Act, 1983, 58
Hector, R. Ian, 270
Henderson, Dr. H.W., 52-54, 58-59, 73-76, 116, 142, 144, 147, 150-151, 165, 204
Proposed Revision of Provincial Policy, 54
Hepburn, Mitchell, 9, 11, 107, 225
Heseltine Report, 199-204, 206, 210, 212
Heseltine, Dr. G.F., 134, 199-204, 206, 210, 212
Hincks, Dr. Clarence M., 10, 14, 39, 48, 68, 110, 115
Homes for Special Care Program, 40, 114, 116-117, 119, 147, 165, 167, 175, 185, 203, 241, 250, 256
homes for the aged, 167
homosexuals, 214

Hospital Insurance and Diagnostic Services Act, 72
hospitals
- 999 Queen Street, 7, 12, 145
- Albany, New York, 66
- Allan Memorial, 68, 70
- Brantford, 57
- Brockville, 48, 104, 107, 127, 246
- Cedar Springs, 104
- Cook County, 17
- English Oxford County and City, 66
- Fort William, 12
- Goderich, 104, 108, 127, 186-187
- Hamilton, 44, 57, 69, 163, 189-190, 210, 213
- Henry Ford, Detroit, Michigan, 38, 67
- Kingston, 11-13, 18, 44, 68, 126, 164
- Lakeshore, 169-170, 173, 181, 186-187, 189-191, 249, 252
- London, 8-10, 20-21, 25, 36, 39, 44, 55, 66-69, 111, 115, 161-162, 185
- Mackinnon Phillips, 186
- Maudsley, 218
- New Toronto, 12, 16, 18, 21, 25, 211
- North Bay, 44, 108, 181, 186
- Owen Sound, 104, 108
- Port Arthur, 39, 44
- Royal Ottawa, 166
- Sault-Ste. Marie, 105
- Smith's Falls, 43-44
- South Porcupine, 108
- St. Thomas, 8, 11, 39, 44, 58, 105, 107, 162, 168
- Thistletown, 203
- Timmins, 105, 108
- Toronto General, 67, 69, 152, 210, 252
- Toronto Psychiatric, 3, 12, 22, 25, 43, 48, 55, 66-67, 110
- Verdun, 16
- Westminster Veteran's, 36, 210, 213
- Whitby, 3, 8, 10, 20, 49, 110, 170, 173, 181, 187-190, 192, 209-210
- Winnipeg General, 67
- Women's College, 72

hostels, 168, 174
House of Commons Committee on Social Security, 36
Houselink Community Homes, 174, 232
housewives, 8
Human Resource Centres, 149
Humphries, Barry, 270

I

incremental politics, 77-78, 120, 241-245, 252, 255, 263
infirmaries, 111-112
insulin coma therapy, 3, 15-20, 23-24, 213, 219-220, 226
interest groups, 78, 87-88, 97, 129, 244, 257
involuntary competent patients, 216-217, 231
involuntary patients, consent by, 215
Ives, Dr. G.A., 118, 270

J

Joint Commission on Mental Health and Illness, 75, 88
Judge Baker Child Guidance Clinic, 47
justice of the peace, 225-226

K

Kaimowitz vs. Department of Health, 215
Kaufman, Jay, 270
Kelley, Russell, 42, 271
Kempf, Dr. G.A., 10-14
Kennedy, John F., 76
Kerns, Keith, 270
Kirby, Harold J., 271
Knight, Geoffrey, 218
Koval, Gregory, 270
Kydd, Linda, 270

L

Laing, R.D., 209
Landor, Dr. Henry, 66
Langmuir, John, 66
Lawrence, Albert B., 271
Lawson, Dr. F.S., 70
Leighton, Alexander, xi
Leighton, D.C., 134
Lemieux, Marcel, 270
leucotomy
- *See* lobotomy

Lewis, Stephen, 56, 105-106, 164, 166, 227
Liberal Party, 105-106, 108, 169, 172, 174, 190, 206, 216, 228, 230-231, 247, 252
Lindblom, Charles, xiii, 77, 243
Livingston, Dr. Kenneth, 214
lobotomy, 15, 20, 23, 25, 209-215, 219-220
lodging homes, 168
Luna Circle, vii
Lurie, Steve, 198, 254, 270
Lynch, Abbyann, 270
Lynes, Pat, 270

M

MacLennan, David, 94
Macpherson, Lawrence G., 144, 146, 270
Makarchuk, M., 114
management boards, 129, 148, 150, 185, 245, 253
manic-depression, 210
Margetts, E.V., 270
Martin, Dr. Gordon, 58-60, 270

Massachusetts, 12
matrix plan, 265
Maxwell Jones, 191
Maynard, John, 186, 254, 270
McClellan, Ross, 173
McGhie, Dr. B.T., 3, x-xi, xiv, 36, 39-44, 47, 49, 53, 110, 115, 162, 205, 241
McKague, Carla, 228, 231, 270
McKenzie, Dr. K., 210
McKerracher, Dr. D.G., 60, 130
McKinsey and Company, 187-191, 252
McLean, Tony, 270
McLellan, Ross, 190
McNeel, Burdette, 53, 58, 60, 74-75, 90, 103, 162-163, 270
medical doctors, 8-10, x, 23, 37, 55, 57, 78, 88, 93, 131, 134, 143-144, 211, 217, 219, 226, 228-229, 234, 244
medical model, 91, 94, 125, 131, 144, 166, 204, 234
medical officer of health, 57
medical superintendent, 8-9, 25, 42, 103, 125, 162
Medicare Act, Federal, 218
Mental Health Act, 1937, 226
Mental Health Act, 1954, 58
Mental Health Act, 1967, 58, 143, 182, 216, 218, 227-229, 231-232
Mental Health Act, 1978, 234, 257
mental health bureaucrats, xii-xiv, 36, 42, 44, 143-144, 151, 157, 197, 211, 218, 233, 243, 252, 263, 267
mental health clinics
  travelling, 38
mental health division, 142-143
mental health law, 225-236
mental health policy, 103, 107, 130, 132, 134, 143, 145, 150-151, 158, 165, 174, 181-182, 184, 186-187, 197-199, 201-202, 209, 218, 235, 243-244, 248-259
Mental Health Study Act, 1955, 88
Mental Hospital Survey Committee, 37
Mental Hospitals Act, 9, 225, 257
mental hygiene, 38, 47, 50, 59, 65, 73
mental hygiene clinics, 36, 47
Mental Hygiene Survey of British Columbia, 67
mental retardation, 49, 51, 105, 108, 112, 116, 142-144, 147, 149-150, 158, 169, 197, 201, 204, 243, 251, 256
mental retardation policy, 106
metrazol, 3, 15-19, 21, 23, 25, 213, 219-220, 226
Midtown Manhattan Study, The, 134
Miller, Abraham, 270
Miller, Frank, 161, 166, 181, 187, 271
Milton, Margaret, 233
Minister of Planning and Development, 13
Ministry of Welfare, 111
Moniz, Egas, 31
Montgomery, Dr. R.C., 19, 68, 70
More for the Mind, xiv, 56, 58, 75, 87, 90-91, 94-95, 97-98, 103, 106, 168
municipal government, 38, 40, 43, 51-53, 60, 71, 111, 114, 120, 162, 167, 169, 171-172, 175, 199, 255-256
Myers, C.R., 47

N

National Health Grants Program, 42, 70, 72
national health insurance program, 36
National Health Service, 128, 130
National Institute of Mental Health, 87-88, 96
National Mental Health Act, 1946, 88
National Scientific Planning Council, xiv, 90, 226
NDP
  See New Democratic Party
Netherlands, 188
neuroleptic drugs, 59, 157, 160, 219-220, 232
neuropsychiatry, 43, 67
New Democratic Party, 54, 105-106, 108, 111, 114, 164, 166-167, 169, 171, 173, 184, 190, 197, 200, 216, 227, 230-233
New York, 12
Newman, Bernard, 105
normalization, 204, 256
Northeastern Region Mental Health Centre, 186
Norton, Keith, 169, 206, 252, 271
nosology, 220
nursing units, 127

O

obesity, psychosurgery to control, 214
observation units, 41
observation wards, 41
Oliver, F.R., 228
On Our Own, 231-232
One Flew Over the Cuckoo's Nest, 215
Ontario Association for the Mentally Retarded, 201
Ontario Committee on Taxation, 133
Ontario Council of Health, 144, 182
  Legal Task Force, 216
Ontario Government
  Department of Health, local health services branch, 205
  Management Board, 141, 143, 198, 245-247

Minister of Finance and Intergovernmental Affairs, 141
Minister of Social Development Policy, 141
Ministry of Community and Social Services, 128, 142, 144, 150-151, 153, 167, 169-170, 174, 183-184, 203-204, 245, 251, 253
Ministry of Government Services, 190
Ministry of Health, 170
Ministry of Public and Mental Health, assistant deputy, 197
Ministry of Social and Family Services, 166
Policy and Priorities Board, 141
Social Development Policy, 142
Ontario Health Survey Committee, 42
Ontario Hospital Association, 144
Ontario Hospital Services Commission, 74
Ontario Medical Centre
Oak Ridge division, 234
Ontario Medical Services Insurance Act, 125
Ontario Mental Health Association, 144, 197, 251
Ontario Mental Health Foundation, 144
Ontario Neuropsychiatric Association, 68
Ontario Psychiatric Association, 144
Ontario Psychological Association, 144
Ontario Public Health Association, 165
Ontario Public Service Employee's Union (OPSEU), 193
Ontario Royal Commission on Public Welfare, 47
Ontario Welfare Council, 144
Oregon, 215
organization of the mental hospital system, U.S., 128
outpatient services, 41, 43, 47-48, 50-52, 54-56, 58, 66-69, 74-75, 89, 95, 117, 133, 159, 164-165, 183, 186-187, 189-190, 203
overcrowding, 39, 41, 47, 50, 66, 106-107, 112, 119, 142, 167, 181, 220

P

paraldehyde, 192
Parkdale, 168, 170, 172, 174, 184, 197-199, 246
Parkin, John, 106
Parran, Thomas, 88
participatory democracy, 148
paternalism, 213, 218, 221
patient advocate program, 194, 198-199, 231-235
patients' rights, 217
patients' rights groups, 231-236
Patients' Rights Organization, 231
patronage
See political patronage
paying patients, 66
Peat, Marwick and Partners, 191-192
pedophiliacs, 214
Pell, Brian, 270
Penrose, L.S., 19-20, 23, 210
Peterson, David, 263
Phair, Dr. J.T., 87
Phillips, Dr. Mackinnon, 42, 55, 70-72, 103, 108, 111, 271
pivotal hospital, 202, 206
Planning Act, 167
policy ministers, 141
political patronage, 13, 254
Pope, Allan, 206, 271
postwar psychiatric service, 40
Potter, Richard T., 119, 184, 271
Pratten, Dr. John, 126, 164, 270
Prendergast, Peter, 270
Pritchard, A.M., 106
probation, 226
Procter, Dr. Lorne, 210
professional recognition, 23
Progressive Conservative Party, 106-107, 116, 120, 166, 169, 172, 175, 197, 206, 216, 233, 250, 254-255, 257
Proposed Revision of Mental Health Program in Ontario
See Dymond's "Magna Carta"
provincial expenditures, xi, 36, 90, 116
Provincial Lunatic Asylum, 7
provincial psychiatric hospitals, 78
provincial statistician
See statistics
psychiatric authority, x, xiv, 25, 93, 182, 209, 217-218, 228, 235-236, 256, 266-267
Psychiatric Care in Ontario, 232
psychiatric social workers, 41, 131
psychiatric unit system, ix-xii, xiv, 41-42, 44, 50-54, 59-61, 65-70, 72-78, 89-90, 92-95, 104-105, 117, 128-130, 132-133, 135, 142, 145, 159, 163-165, 170-171, 175, 181, 184, 187-189, 194, 199-200, 202-203, 205, 227, 235, 241, 243, 249-250, 253, 256-257, 264, 266-267
psychiatric wards, 38, 42-44, 51, 67-70, 93
Psychiatry Under Health Insurance, 36
psychogeriatric program, 188
psychopathic hospitals, 47, 51, 67
psychopathic wards, 10, 66
psychosurgery, 23, 25, 59, 209-210, 213-221, 226
psychosurgery review committees, 215
psychotherapy, 126, 131, 135, 187

psychotic wards, 162
psychotropic drugs, 132
public health, 54-61, 71, 75, 88, 93, 95, 147, 162-166, 173, 185, 205
public health centres, 38
public health nurse, 56-57, 60, 163
  assistant director, 163
public health officer, 60
Public Hospitals Act, 129
Public Works
  See Department of Public Works

Q

Queen Street Mental Health Centre, 167-168

R

radical therapies, ix, 24, 26, 209
Rae-Grant, Dr. Naomi, 204, 270
regional and local service delivery, subcommittee on, 149
regional area committees, 205
regional health units, 41, 43
regional mental health committees, 168, 206
regional mental hospitals, 104, 186
regionalization, 153
rehabilitation units, 112-113, 128, 132
reorganizations, 125, 141-144, 148, 190, 200, 205, 250, 265
Report on Ontario Mental Health Services, 115
reprivatization, 117-118
residential units, 109, 113-115, 117-120, 127, 158-160, 250
residual model, 172
review boards, 10, 215-217, 226-227, 230-231, 234
Reville, David, 270
Reynolds, H.A., 107
Richardson, Howard, 270
Richman, Dr. Alex, 90
Riddell, John K., 108
Robarts, John, 141-142
Robb, Dr. John M., 271
Roberts, C.A., 51, 69-70, 90, 97, 115, 117, 125-131, 135, 146, 164, 225, 270
Rockefeller Foundation, 68
Rogow, Arnold A., 97
Rowell-Sirois report, 42
Royal Commission on Health Services, 60, 130, 132
Royal Commission on the Operation of the Mental Health Act, 8-10
Ruprecht, Tony, 172, 174
Rushmer, D.S., 217

S

Sakel, Dr. Manfred, 15
schizophrenia, x, 15-16, 20, 76, 171
Scientology, Church of, 215
Scott, Graham, 144, 245-246, 252, 270
Scottish boarding-out system, 49
Scull, Andrew, 120, 157
self-help groups, 197
Sellars, Alf, 270
Sharpe, Gilbert, 216, 228-230, 270
Shulman, Morton, 108
Silverthorne, O.J., 25
Smith, J.R., 166
Smith, Stuart, 229
social control, 4, 6, 26, 158
social development programs and councils, 149-150, 167-169, 172, 199-200, 205, 216, 230, 245, 249, 251
social policy, 174
social services, 67, 128, 142, 144, 149-151, 153, 167, 169-170, 174, 183-184, 203-204, 245, 251, 253
social workers, 161-165, 172, 186, 231
Special Committee on Social Security, 67
staff, problem of recruiting, 132
statistics, 4, 6, 8, 16, 18-19, 23, 107, 117, 132, 146, 158, 181, 183, 202, 210-211, 213, 248
Stephenson, Dr. Bette, 229
Stewart, Dr. J.S., 18
Stirling County Study, 134
Stogdill, Dr. C.G., 88
Stokes, Dr. Aldwyn, 71
subcommittee on children's and adolescent services, 204
Sunnyside Children's Centre, 203
Supportive Housing Coalition, 173
Suttie, Boyd, 247, 270
Suttie, Dr. Boyd, 193, 196-197, 233, 247
Swadron, Barry, 227-228, 270
Sweden, 188, 192, 215
syphilis, 3, 20-21
Szablowski, George, 270
Szasz, Thomas, xi, 209, 215, 226

T

task force on mental health care costs, 144
Temple, W.H., 111
therapeutic community model, 191
Thistletown centre, 106
Timbrell, Dennis, 169-170, 173, 181, 189, 193-194, 198-199, 206, 216, 228-230, 232-233, 235-236, 252, 265, 270-271
Timmins Mental Health Association, 186
Titmuss, Richard, 172
Toronto Star, The, 170

Toronto, City of, 146, 173, 199
Towards a Blueprint for Change
See Heseltine Report
trade unions, 152
Trainor, John, 172
transinstitutionalization, 109-120
Trotter, James, 105-106
tuberculosis, 17
Turner, Tyrone, 232-233, 270
Tyhurst Committee, 58, 75, 90-98, 103, 130, 168, 182, 226, 228-229, 253

U

U.S. Joint Commission on Mental Illness and Health, 59
U.S. National Commission for the Protection of Human Subjects of Biomedical and Behavioral Research, 215
U.S. Public Health Service, 88
Unemployment Assistance, 111
unit system
See psychiatric unit system
unmarried mothers, 48-49

V

Victorian Order of Nurses, 56
violence, psychosurgery to control, 214
Vivian, Dr. Reginald, 42, 271
vocational rehabilitation, 165, 168, 171, 185, 250, 257
voluntary patients, 67, 215-217
Volunteer Association of Whitby Psychiatric Hospital, 188
von Meduna, Ladislas, 16

W

warrant, 225-226
Wasylenki, Donald, 270
Watt, James, 210
Weingust, John, 233
Weitz, Don, 231, 235
Welch Green Paper, 201
Welch, Robert, 141, 201, 251
Wells, Thomas L., 117, 166, 185, 271
White Cross, 166
Willard, Dr. J., 112
Williston Report, 251
Williston, Walter, 142, 251
Wilson, James G., 146
Winslow, C.E.A., 50
women, 8, 16, 20, 68, 171, 188, 210, 214
Workman, Dr. Joseph, 7
World Health Organization, 70
Wylie, Betty Jane, 170

Y

Young Dr. Kildare's Dilemma, 24